INTER·PERSONAL COMMUNI·CATION IN NURSING

INTER·PERSONAL COMMUNI·CATION IN NURSING

BONNIE WEAVER DULDT, R.N., Ph.D.

Professor of Nursing
Director of Graduate Studies
College of Nursing
University of North Dakota
Grand Forks, North Dakota

KIM GIFFIN, Ph.D.

Professor of Communication Studies
University of Kansas
Lawrence, Kansas

BOBBY R. PATTON, Ph.D.

Professor of Communication Studies
Chairperson of the Division of Speech and Drama
University of Kansas
Lawrence, Kansas

F. A. DAVIS COMPANY Philadelphia

Library of Congress Cataloging in Publication Data

Duldt, Bonnie Weaver.
  Interpersonal communication in nursing.

  Includes bibliographical references and index.
  1. Communication in nursing. 2. Interpersonal communication. I. Duldt, Bonnie Weaver. II. Giffin, Kim, 1918–   . III. Patton, Bobby R., 1935–
IV. Title. [DNLM: 1. Communication—Nursing texts.
2. Nurse-Patient relations. 3. Interpersonal relations—
Nursing texts. WY 87 D881i]
RT23.D84   1983   610.73'06'99   83-5213
ISBN 0-8036-2936-2

PREFACE

The nursing profession, in recent years, has moved toward a more humanistic orientation. This orientation is the philosophical basis of primary nursing, a professional role for the nurse. Primary nursing has been defined as follows:

> Primary nursing is a philosophy and a modality of humanistic health care delivery in which the client becomes a contributor to as well as a recipient of his plan of care. The client is assigned a professional nurse who cares for him utilizing the nursing process and scientific inquiry. The primary nurse has authority, autonomy and is accountable and directly available to the client. This modality may be applied in a variety of settings.[1]

Recognition of the need for increased expertise in communication skills for the professional nurse in this primary nursing role as well as traditional roles has been emphasized in the professional literature in the last decade.

In addition, we are beginning to experience a change in the paradigm or map of reality in health care, that is, movement toward the holistic health paradigm with its nontraditional views.[2] Flynn states:

> The healing process ultimately moves beyond science. . . . in the sphere of human relationships healing will be brought about and health maintained in some ways that will always remain uncertain, because such healing will be accomplished by the observer's simply being there. We need to return to . . . a society that once again recognizes the healing power of human contact.[3]

v

Holistic health emphasizes the person as a total being, integrating and interacting. To reduce the individual to parts destroys the whole. Although it is necessary in health care and research to analyze parts, there is a need to continually be aware of the whole. Holistic health acknowledges the philosophical and spiritual aspects of the total person, and assumes the individual is responsible for discovering meaning and purpose in life, for the choices made in the care of one's own health, and for changing the direction of one's life. Illness is viewed as an opportunity for reassessment, re-evaluation, and readjustment of one's goals, purposes, values, meanings in life, and behaviors.

Consequently, the person as a nurse, a healer, becomes paramount; the interpersonal communication competency of the nurse as a healer, as the one being there, becomes crucial. The role of interpersonal communication is to humanize, that is, to make human. It has a significant influence on the growth and development of one's nature and character as a human being when well; we believe this significance increases for the person when ill.

This book seeks to provide a general conceptual base that can be useful to professional nurses, students, and practitioners, as well as other groups of health-care providers. It is designed as a text for formal nursing courses that include interpersonal communication. It also seeks to serve as an excellent reference for individuals or groups of nurses who wish to study interpersonal communication in nursing in a less formal manner through continuing education or self-directed study.

We propose to deal with interpersonal communication in terms that directly influence nursing professionals in all practice areas or specialties. Because one of the innate characteristics of human beings is the ability to symbolize and use language, communication is an innate part of the nursing process, that is, assessment, planning, implementation, and evaluation.[4] We propose to identify broadly applicable concepts and principles of interpersonal communication that are of immediate relevance to any context in which a nurse functions. These concepts and principles are based on communication processes occurring among normal human beings rather than, as in psychiatric nursing contexts, individuals or groups of people who have been labeled as presenting a particular mental illness. Consequently, then, the terminology we use is more congruent with society in general rather than a particular segment of health care. We believe this emphasis on normality tends to enhance a humanistic perspective of people generally.

The following assumptions are made. First, professional nursing students are capable of comprehending and developing theoretical perspectives; undergraduates are currently doing so in other disciplines. Second, holistic health approaches and primary nursing mode of staffing are significant trends in nursing practices that are very closely aligned or derived from humanistic and existentialistic philosophical perspectives. This text provides nursing students and practitioners necessary information regarding theoretical and historical derivations of these philosophies and how humanistic perspectives can be operationalized in nursing for educational, research, and clinical application. As a result of having such knowledge, students and nurses will be able to influence the future of nursing in a more deliberate and effective manner. The discussions of these philosophies in this text provide the basis for moving toward a theory of humanistic nursing communication.

There are a number of unique aspects about this text which are worthy of note. First, in today's health-care system, there is an increasing concern about the manner in which one is received, that is, humanization versus dehumanization. This text provides definitions of these terms for nursing. Dehumanization tends to occur for both client and nurse as the complexity of organizational structure increases in the health-care system. In this text we apply communication principles to interpersonal interactions not only in the nurse-client relationship, but also in the nurse-nurse, nurse-supervisor, and nurse-colleague relationships. The perspective for nursing is communicating career-wide and life-long.

Second, a positive perspective is taken in considering how to build good relationships through interpersonal communication. Some rules are presented for developing relationships derived from recent research. Considerable attention is also given to determining ways one can evaluate and maintain a relationship.

Third, communicating in groups generally involves more risk interpersonally than one-to-one relationships. This is especially true for the nurse as a member of multidisciplinary health professional groups. Some general, practical guidelines for communicating in problem-solving and decision-making groups are provided, and therapeutic groups or psychiatric teams are also considered.

Fourth, speaking in public presents even greater risk and responsibility for a professional nurse. In public speaking, one can influence the perceptions and images of the audience and have a strong impact on events and situational outcomes. The process of developing a speech is described and procedures are suggested for developing skill in speaking persuasively before large groups.

Fifth, there are some special problems in nursing communication that are analyzed in detail: distrust, defensiveness, and barriers between people. Alienation by communication denial, anger, sexual harassment, and verbal abuse are salient concerns for contemporary nurses. Recent research provides correctives and useful strategies to achieve greater control in these dehumanizing encounters.

Sixth, interviewing, the practical application of communication in nursing practice, is discussed by considering the nurse as the interviewer as well as interviewee, and a broad, career-long perspective is taken. The process of interviewing is presented, and problem clients, such as the child or the client who rambles, are considered. Employment, evaluation, and exit interviews are discussed frankly. Authoritative advice is offered for the nurse who must face interviews associated with being an expert witness in a court of law.

Finally, we move from the practical to the abstract by suggesting a theoretical framework, the beginnings of a theory of humanistic nursing communication. In order to apply knowledge, a theory is necessary to put all the facts into an organized scheme. Processes can be understood, concepts related, and perhaps even outcomes predicted. This text seeks to provide such a structure, which we believe will be helpful in getting a grip on interpersonal communication in nursing.

We would like to thank Julie Larson, Robin Holladay, and Mary Lou Penney for their assistance in preparing the manuscript. We also wish to acknowledge the contributions of Adelaide Mickel, R.N., and other nursing clinicians, faculty, and students who have contributed ideas and examples to this text.

KG
BRP

REFERENCES

1. SOUTHERN REGIONAL ASSEMBLY FOR CONSTITUENT LEAGUES FOR NURSING TASK GROUP: *Primary Nursing: One Nurse-One Client Planning Care Together.* National League for Nursing, New York, 1977, p 65.
2. PATRICIA ANNE RANDOLPH FLYNN: *Holistic Health: The Art and Science of Care* Robert J. Brady Co., Bowie, Md, 1980, p 1.
3. Ibid., p 4.
4. H. YURA AND M. B. WALSH: *The Nursing Process: Assessing, Planning, and Implementing and Evaluating,* 2nd ed. Appleton-Century-Crofts, New York, 1973.

CONTENTS

1   HUMANISM, NURSING, AND
    COMMUNICATION   1

    Humanism   2

    Nursing   5

    Interpersonal Communication   10

        Process   11
        Existentialism and Meaning   12
        Facts and Feelings   13
        Dialogue   13

    Summary and Preview   15

    References   18

2   INTERPERSONAL PERCEPTIONS AND
    ORIENTATIONS   21

    The Process of Person Perception   22

        Sensory Bases of Person Perception   24
        Accuracy of Inferences   29
        Stereotyping   31
        Forming Impressions   34

Estimated Relationship Potential   38

Reciprocal Perspectives   40

Orientations Toward People   42

    Open-Closed   42
    Cooperative-Uncooperative   43
    Moving Toward, Away, or Against   45
    Meeting One's Interpersonal Needs   46

Summary   47

References   48

3   RESPONDING TO ENVIRONMENTAL FACTORS   51

Physical Settings   51

    Rooms and Places   52
    Chairs and Tables   54
    Time   57

Social Factors   59

    When Others Are Present   59
    Being a Member of a Group   60

Influence of the Organization   66

A Difference That Makes a Difference: Culture   68

Summary   75

References   76

4   VERBAL MESSAGES   81

Characteristics of Language   82

    Words Have Different Meanings for Different People   83
    Words Vary in Degree of Abstractness   85
    Language Is, by Its Nature, Incomplete   87
    Language Reflects Personality and Culture   88
    Language Creates a "Social Reality"   90

Understanding One Another   92

    Speaking   92
    Listening   94
    Feedback   95

Summary   96

References   96

5   NONVERBAL MESSAGES   99

The Verbal/Nonverbal Interface   100

The Science of Signs: Semiology   103

    Pragmatics   103
    Syntactics   104
    Semantics   105

Nonverbal Communication Behaviors   107

    Personal Appearance   108
    Vocal Tones   109
    Face and Eyes   111
    Postures, Gestures, and Body Language   112
    Touching   115

Use of Feedback   116

Summary   117

References   117

6   BUILDING RELATIONSHIPS   121

Analyzing a Relationship   123

    Interpersonal Involvement   123
    The Emotional Tone   125
    Control: Dominance-Submission   125
    The D-A-S-H Paradigm   126

Stages of a Relationship   128

    Rules in Dominant-Submissive Relationships   128
    Significance of the Rules   135
    Punctuation of Interaction   136
    Degree of Rigidity in a Relationship   137

Bad Habits in Relationships   138

    Manipulative Relationship Styles   139
    Relationship "Games"   140

Evaluating and Improving Relationships   142

      Calculating the Cost/Reward Ratio   143
      Improving a Relationship   143

Summary   145

References   146

7   COMMUNICATING IN GROUPS   149

Group Problem Solving and Decision Making   149

Conflict Management   159

      The Need to Encourage Conflict   160
      Some Ways of Handling Conflict   161

Planning and Running Meetings   162

Therapeutic Groups and Psychiatric Teams   162

Summary   165

References   166

8   COMMUNICATING IN PUBLIC   167

Your Vision of Yourself as a Public Speaker   167

Developing Your Speech   171

Organizing Your Ideas   175

Planning Your Introduction   175

      Gaining the Attention of Your Audience   175
      Establishing Your Credentials   177
      Focusing on Your Topic   178

Planning the Body of Your Speech   179

      Helping Listeners to Understand   180
      Coherent Patterns for Helping Listeners Solve
      a Problem   183

Planning Your Conclusion   185

      Reviewing Your Main Ideas   185

Presenting Your Speech   187

Summary   189

References   190

9   EVALUATING INTERPERSONAL
     COMMUNICATION   193

     Assessing Interpersonal Needs   193

     Assessing Communication Competencies   196

     Assessing Interactions   197

     Assessing Leadership Behavior   209

     Summary   214

     References   214

10   SPECIAL COMMUNICATION PROBLEMS   217

     Distrust and Defensiveness   217

     Communication Behaviors That Generate
     Defensiveness   218

         Conditions for Reducing Defensive Behavior   220
         Effects of Reducing Defensiveness   220

     Gaps Between Groups   221

         Barriers Between Members of Different Reference
         Groups   221
         Gaps Between Different Cultures and Subcultures   223

     Alienation

         Communication Behaviors Related to Social Alienation   225
         Alienation by Communication Denial   226
         The "Double Bind"   228
         Alienation by Anger   230
         Dealing With Anger   230

     Sex Role Problems   233

         Sexual Harassment   234
         Verbal Abuse   238

     Summary   241

     References   242

11   INTERVIEWING: PULLING IT ALL
     TOGETHER   245

     Sequence of the Interview Process   247

Situations in Which the Nurse Interviews Clients   249

Situations in Which the Nurse Is Interviewed   252

Humanizing Versus Dehumanizing   257

References   257

12   THE FUTURE OF HUMANISTIC
       NURSING   259

Assumptions   260

Definitions and Concepts About Interpersonal
Communications in Humanistic Nursing   262

Interaction (or Interdependency) of Concepts of
Communication in Humanistic Nursing   271

Humanistic Nursing—Past   272

Humanistic Nursing—Future   273

References   275

INDEX   277

1
HUMANISM, NURSING, AND COMMUNICATION

Major trends in today's American health-care systems emphasize certain business and management concepts. Efficiency, accuracy, and economy have become core concepts of health-care delivery. Efficiency and accuracy are expected in use of sophisticated medical terminology and highly trained specialists who operate modern equipment. Economy is necessary because of the spiraling costs and the increased expectations of citizens regarding accessibility of health care. In addition, major issues in our political and legal systems focus on all phases of health care: who should receive it, who should decide what is received, who should have the right to start or stop treatments, and who should pay for it? With the impact of these trends, it becomes possible to overlook the purpose of the entire system, the client or consumer.

Health-care providers in general, and nursing as a discipline and profession in particular, are basically humanitarian—that is, concerned with and focused on the well-being of people. Yet an unfortunate trend reported by both health-care consumers and providers appears to be a growing lack of concern for people. Clients frequently describe unpleasant encounters that leave them confused, insulted, irritated, and indignant when they seek care. The more the care costs, the greater the consumer's dissatisfaction. Health-care providers, especially nurses, are experiencing reality shock, burnout, anger, dismay, and job dissatisfaction. They frequently choose to resign, resulting in high annual turnover and high inactivity rates among practitioners. Regretfully, there appears to be a trend for people to interact in a dehumanizing manner in the health-care system, and this trend can be expected to continue as society moves toward a national health insurance program, toward increased numbers of clients, and toward increasing complexity of care and of the system itself.

We believe that dehumanizing processes can be counteracted by effective interpersonal communication, the key to humanizing relationships between people. A concerted effort is needed by health-care educators, especially nurse educators, to guide students in a careful exploration of interpersonal communication processes that are known to promote humanistic relationships not only between the nurse and client but also among nurses themselves. The overall goal of this text is to present cohesive, basic, introductory information, drawn from the disciplines of speech communication, interpersonal communication, and nursing, that will promote a humanistic orientation for nursing.

In this introductory chapter, we intend to establish three concepts: humanism, nursing, and interpersonal communication. We intend to show how these concepts are interrelated and how these can together enhance the caring aspects so unique to nursing.

HUMANISM

Humanism, as a concept, has not been clearly defined. Existentialist philosophers such as Jean-Paul Sartre[1] and Kierkegaard[2] focused on four major concepts: existence (being), choice, meaning (value), and nothingness (inevitable death); these concepts seem to be shared with some definitions of humanistic behavior.

Psychologists who are generally identified with humanistic psychology have also struggled to define the term. Maslow[3] notes that psychologists can profit from the study of existentialism to find "it to be not so much a totally new revelation, as a stressing, confirming, sharpening and rediscovering of trends already existing in 'Third Force psychology'." For example, he notes that existentialism particularly emphasizes the concepts of identity and experiential knowledge (subjective experience serving as the basis of abstract knowledge). Geiger,[4] a physician, states, "Even now, I am more comfortable defining the task as identifying dehumanization and fighting it, rather than identifying humanization and supporting it." Howard,[5] in attempting to define humanization as a concept, notes a number of problems in conducting research on humanistic approaches. In operationalizing the concept, he asks, "How do we judge actions that are defined by recipients as real but are false by other measurements? If a practitioner feels neutral toward a given patient, but the patient feels loved by the practitioner, how do we determine whether the provider's behavior is humanizing or dehumanizing in its consequences?"[6] Ultimately, however, we agree with Lee,[7] who states, "At the heart of humanization is our image of man, how we value man and how we treat the individual."

Historically, humanism can be traced to the 14th and 15th centuries. During this Renaissance period, scholars who have been identified with the humanist movement were reacting to the prevailing view that humans could understand the world only by the revelation of God through the Bible. The humanists recognized a person's ability to think, to reason, and thereby to improve one's state in life. This view did not require one to reject religion or belief in a higher being. Rather, it focused on people's ability to achieve excellence in the arts, literature, and other areas of learning. Out of this humanistic movement grew the humanities in academia— philosophy, literature, the arts, history, political science, and the other disciplines commonly found in universities today. The essence of being human is highly valued; human capabilities and potential are shared experiences that supersede religion, culture, economics, politics, race, and so forth. In addition, the quality of life humans experience is valued. In health care and nursing, this emphasis is translated into the caring, concerned, and thoughtful relationship that the care giver establishes with the client. The care giver values one's own ability to think, reason, and understand the client's human existence; and the care giver also values and shares in the client's state of being human.

The humanistic movement emerged again during the 1920s. A succinct statement of humanistic positions on relevant issues is found in the "Humanistic Manifesto."[8] Many of these statements seem to be viewed with alarm by conservative religious groups, who label the movement "secular" humanism. The humanists believe human need is the central issue in religion. Consequently, humanists oppose those authoritarian religions that advocate placing responsibility for human moral behavior and quality of life on God. Some religious writers urge people to accept the present state of affairs and negate attempts to change or improve the human condition. Ritual and religious dogma thus are placed above human needs and values, hence the polarization of beliefs by humanists and some factions of the religious community. However, many religious groups seem to share the humanistic perspective and consider themselves members of the movement.

To humanize means to build relations and to make contact between people; to dehumanize is to break down interrelationships and lose contact between people. Leventhal[9] has provided a model of dehumanization and its consequences in illness. He defined dehumanization as "the feeling that one is isolated from others and is regarded as a thing rather than a person."[10] The model involves normal information-processing systems as one perceives, interprets, and responds to the environment. He suggests that during illness, the information processing system malfunctions because of the illness-treatment information inputs so that self-depersonalization and depersonalization by others inevitably result. He proposes that these "dehumanizing experiences can be avoided or reduced if *specific actions* are taken to redirect the ongoing interplay between individuals' processing systems and their environments."[11]

Of particular interest are the six factors of a dehumanizing experience that Leventhal developed from clinical material and the literature. He offers these as a starting point for consideration rather than a finished, complete set of elements for dehumanization:

1. Separation of the physical and psychologic self.
2. Isolation of the psychologic self.
3. Uncertainty and cyclic thought.
4. Planlessness and loss of competency.
5. Emotional distress, hopelessness, and despair.
6. Barriers to communication.[12]

An important and relevant aspect of the human information processing system is that subjective or private experiences of the real world need to be validated or shared with others. This validation need is the heart of Festinger's social comparison theory.[13] When something unusual happens, one typically turns to another and asks, "Did you see that?" In the ensuing discussion, information is exchanged about the way each experienced the event, and a consensus is usually achieved regarding the event's cause or importance. However, illness poses a threat that is magnified by the novelty of events, the strangeness of environment and people, and the ambiguity of outcomes. Attempts to obtain validation from others often fail because another's symptoms may differ and health-care providers tend to use unfamiliar language. Sometimes it is difficult for one even to communicate because of being "at a loss for words" to describe private experiences. Attributions of negative personality traits are readily made. Clients or patients can be labeled neurotic, nervous, or "cranks" by physicians and nurses, who in turn can be labeled by the clients or patients as cold, heartless, and unconcerned. Consequently, further efforts to communicate by either client or provider seem difficult and perhaps useless; the client inevitably experiences a breakdown in continuity and adequacy of health care sought and needed.

This problem of faulty communication and dehumanization can be solved, according to Leventhal,[14] but not by major institutional changes in the health-care system. Rather, Leventhal states, "To minimize self-depersonalization and dehumanization, it is necessary to alter the content and process of person-to-person interaction and not simply to change the labels applied to the participants."[15] We support Leventhal's position and believe it has particular relevance to nursing. One important aspect of the role of the professional nurse in operationalizing a humanistic perspective is being aware of oneself as a person in the nurse-client relationship, sharing all innate characteristics of being a human with the client. Through the ability to communicate interpersonally in a humanistic manner, the nurse as a person has potential for providing positive influence upon the perceptions, beliefs, and attitudes of others. Greater awareness of one's own interpersonal influence and communication skills can be *deliberately* used to intervene with *predictable* positive results rather than with lack of awareness and with random interventions without forethought, which have unpredictable and variable results.

NURSING

Let us now define what nursing is about as a discipline and a profession. Where are we now in defining our discipline—our *emerging* discipline? According to the dictionary, a discipline is a field of study of human knowledge and inquiry. Generally, each discipline is identified by the distinct perspective it uses in viewing human beings and the environment in which they exist. Donaldson and Crowley[16] state that there is a critical need to identify a structure for nursing as a discipline in educational programs. And in their review of nursing history, they identify three emerging themes that may serve as some structure. These are a concern for patterns and processes:

1. of life, well-being, and optimum functioning of human beings— sick or well;
2. of human behavior in interaction with the environment in critical life situations; and
3. by which positive changes in health status are effected.

Donaldson and Crowley propose that these themes suggest boundaries for the discipline of nursing. Newman[17] identifies criteria for nursing theories that are similar in theme. Note the key words *human beings*—the central focus of nursing.

Nursing is currently perceived as being in the process of becoming a field of study and a profession—an emerging discipline. There seems to be consensus among scholars that a theoretical body of knowledge is an essential element for both a discipline and a profession. Johnson[18] notes the sparsity of theoretical and scientific giants in nursing's heritage upon whose work present-day nursing scholars might build. Consequently, theories and models have been borrowed from other disciplines and professions to be applied with varying degrees of appropriateness to the nursing context. Efforts toward achieving a theoretical basis in nursing have occurred only in the past 15 years. We believe that nursing as an emerging discipline is at the preconceptual level of development in its theory building. Concepts must be defined before relationship statements can be developed. And relationships among concepts are the heart of a theory.[19]

Prior to these newer efforts, nursing has *borrowed* from other disciplines. Nursing has borrowed definitions of the major concept of nursing—human being. The profession has employed definitions of humans provided by biology, psychology, and sociology—biophysical-psychosocial man. This definition is most often used in nursing texts. Incidentally, some nursing texts do not even define the human being. Generally, biology is the science of living organisms. Biologists define humans as unique living creatures and place them in a taxonomy of all living things. Biologists are concerned with how the body works, and they divide it into systems: circulatory, respiratory, urinary, and so on. Psychology is the science of mind and behavior, and psychologists focus on humans as individuals—behaving, interacting, thinking, and emoting. They classify humans as normal, neurotic, psychotic, depressed, and so forth. Sociology is the science of social institutions and relationships, and sociologists are concerned with humans living in groups, classified according to size, function, and so forth.

In the dictionary, each discipline is defined as a field of study having a particular territory of human knowledge. If one looks up nursing in the dictionary, one will find that nurse means to nourish at the breast or a person who is skilled or trained in caring for the sick or infirm, especially under the supervision of a physician. Nursing is defined as a profession of a nurse, the duties of a nurse.

Among nursing scholars, no generally accepted definition of nursing is available. Orem,[20] as chairman and editor of the Nursing Development Conference Group, presents a detailed analysis of the numerous definitions of nursing in the literature. Many of these definitions are specific to particular theories of nursing. We propose the following definition of nursing to set general boundaries as derived from Donaldson and Crowley's[21] three themes found in nursing history:

> Nursing is the art and science of positive, humanistic intervention in changing health states of human beings interacting in the environment of critical life situations.

In seeking to develop a theory of humanistic nursing, the following concepts should be defined: nursing, human beings, the client, the nurse, the nursing process, health, the environment, critical life situations, and communication, both humanizing and dehumanizing.

Nursing. Nursing is the art and science of positive, humanistic intervention in changing health states of human beings interacting in the environment of critical life situations. A subset of elements of nursing is as follows: communing, caring, and coaching. Communing refers to intimate humanizing communication that occurs "between" people who are aware of each other's presence. It is "being there" and "being with." Communing is the element that makes nursing humanistic. Typically, these people are the nurse and client, but also include the nurse and peers or the nurse and colleagues of other professions.

Caring involves valuing and touching. The nurse values the client and is concerned about the individual's well-being. Caring also involves touching in the sense of providing nursing care—the traditional sense of "laying on of hands." Caring is feeling concerned and responsible for the client's health state.

Coaching refers particularly to the teaching aspect of nursing. The nurse plans and implements the teaching/learning process and provides support and encouragement to clients as they strive to meet health goals.

Client. The client is a human being in a (potentially) critical life situation and is the focus of the nursing process.

Nurse. The nurse is also a human being who practices nursing, intervening through the application of the nursing process. The nurse possesses special educational and licensure credentials to qualify to practice nursing according to the dictates of the society in which one practices.

Human Being. Nursing is concerned about particular human characteristics uniquely relevant to the discipline of nursing. These characteristics may be described as a set of elements that define the whole human being: living, communicating, negativing, inventing, ordering, dreaming, choosing, and self-reflecting. This set of elements is influenced by the work of Kenneth Burke,[22] and each element is defined in the following paragraphs.

Living refers to the ability of a human being to function biologically and physiologically as an animalistic, viable entity. This biologic dimension is shared with other life forms and includes bodily, life-sustaining processes such as reproduction, assimilation, elimination, mobility, oxygenation, and so forth. These processes are susceptible to injury, infection, malfunction, and ultimately death. Similar to other life forms, a human being displays an orderly, sequential process of growth and development (and aging), influenced to some degree by life style and environment, such as quality of nutrition, cleanliness of air, amount of exercise, and so forth. As is true of all mammalian species, a human being's existence depends upon interaction with members of one's own species. Physiologic responses to stimuli, such as flight-or-fight responses to danger or attack, are also shared with other life forms. The human being also tends to share a sign system of nonverbal communication, common to many other life forms, such as sign systems indicating territoriality, rejection, and acceptance. The capability of a person to communicate is of direct concern to nursing care.

Communicating refers to the ability of human beings to label things and to talk about things not present. Human beings are "symbol using, misusing" beings.[23] As a consequence, humans are able to build upon learnings, logic, and perceptions of predecessors and contemporaries through written and spoken language. Using symbols enables one to think abstractly, to use logic and argumentation, to solve problems, and to describe perceptions regarding phenomena observed about the physical environment, about self, and about relationships with others. Humans are particularly capable of expressing feelings arising from within as a response to perceptions. These expressions take many forms, from crying in grief or screaming in terror, to expression through music, paintings, and other art forms.

Negativing refers to the ability of human beings to talk about what is not existing, not happening. People are able to develop moral codes, rules of conduct, and laws governing relationships and functions of individuals as well as of the environment. One can be aware of one's own nonexistence or death and can plan for the implications inherent in this fact. As one develops certain expectations of what can happen in the future, one also can be aware of the expected situation that does not happen. The hospice movement is a recognition of this human characteristic.

Inventing refers to the ability of human beings to invent tools. One extends one's own physical capabilities through the use of these tools, such as transportation (airplanes), communication (radio and television), chemistry (use of chemicals to increase food production), technology (development of atomic energy), and so on. However, a human being risks dangerous side effects in the quest of potential benefits. Some inventions have unanticipated effects, as in the case of insecticides. Thus, the ability to invent has profound implications for human health.

Ordering refers to the ability of human beings to develop categories and hierarchies according to some value or theme. People give structure and system to the environment and tend to organize life, relationships, and the environment according to a particular perspective, goal, or criterion. One tends to practice one-upmanship in relationships, and tends to seek power and status through control of others, of resources, of environment, or of all of these. This sense of hierarchy tends to result in conflict at all levels of human interaction.

Dreaming refers to the ability of humans to consider things as they could be if all were perfect. Each human being has hopes, expectations, and dreams for the future. One tends to work and strive to that end. And human beings are continually experiencing frustration and disappointment as dreams become unattainable.

Choosing refers to the ability of human beings to consider numerous alternatives, compare implications for the future, and select the alternative that tends to be most desirable according to values and criteria. Thus, human beings are able to make choices and control events in their lives. People are also capable of being highly motivated to achieve short-term as well as long-term, even lifelong, goals. And in the choosing, responsibility and accountability for the implications and results are significant factors. Responsibility for making choices regarding one's health can be a matter of life or death.

Self-reflecting refers to the ability of a human being to think and talk about one's own self, one's body, and one's behaviors. Self-reflecting often involves the existentialist elements: being, becoming, choice, freedom, responsibility, solitude, loneliness, pain, struggle, tragedy, meaning, dread, uncertainty, despair, and death. Self-reflecting typically becomes salient during critical life situations.

A significant factor in our concept of a human being is that both client and nurse are human beings first. Both possess, given individual variances, all the characteristics or elements of being human. In this very real sense, they are equal, yet each is unique in individual expression of those characteristics.

Nursing Process. The nursing process involves assessment, planning, implementation, and evaluation. This process is used by the nurse in developing a nursing-care plan, the documented means by which the nurse intervenes favorably to change the client's health.

Health. One's state of being, becoming, and self-awareness is one's state of health. It is indicative of one's adaptation to the environment.

Environment. One's time/space/relationship context is one's environment.

Critical Life Situation. A person's life situation becomes critical when a threat to one's health is perceived; one's existential state of being is in jeopardy. For example, health is threatened in the event of pregnancy, cancer, or accident. Significant changes in personal hygiene and health care are required to cope with such events. Indeed, one's life may be in danger to varying degrees in each of these situations, and the intervention of a nurse is necessary. In a critical life situation, each of the characteristics of being human must be considered by the nurse. The way these characteristics interact with one another, such as self-reflecting, choosing, and communicating, will influence the nursing-care plan. The nurse needs to be aware of the influence of each characteristic.

Communication. Communication—specifically, interpersonal communication—is a dynamic process involving continual adaptation and adjustments between two or more human beings engaged in face-to-face interactions during which each person is continually aware of the other(s); the process is characterized by being existential in nature, and involving an exchange of facts, feelings, and meaning. This theoretical concept specifically refers to communication between the nurse and client(s), the nurse and peers, and the nurse and other professional colleagues.

To be humanistic, then, means to be cognizant of the unique characteristics of being human; to be dehumanizing is to ignore these characteristics. Humanistic nursing denotes the manner and attitude with which interventions are operationalized. Humanizing nursing is communicating and relating interpersonally to clients in such a manner that the client senses warmth and acceptance and can report feeling good about the care. Consequently, humanistic nursing does not occur in just one particular place. It happens *between* human beings, between a nurse and a client. Because nurses are human beings, it would logically follow that nurses themselves would be subject to this definition. Since both clients and nurses share this common bond, then the relationship between clients and nurses would logically be on an equal basis, each respecting the other and showing a concern for the other's individual feelings, needs, worth, and responsibility. We have the beginnings of a theory about how to humanize nursing by Patterson and Zderad[24] which describes this "between" or "in-touchness" experience that happens between a nurse and a client. They have derived this theory from that well-known humanistic philosopher Martin Buber,[25] author of *I and Thou*. Patterson and Zderad focus on the special phenomenon of interpersonal communication between people. This special, warm, genuine, open relationship is positively validating of individual worth. It is believed to be essential to "releasing" people to develop to their fullest potential, that is, "well-being" and "more-being" as Patterson and Zderad phrase it. This relationship may be that special part of nursing that is rewarding to nurses themselves. To feel good about oneself and to feel acceptance, importance, and positive regard "release" clients to heal faster. The concept of humanism thus interacts with nursing. The primary purpose of this book is to give substance to communicating in a humanistic manner—to help nurses deliberately achieve the "I-Thou," the "in-between," or the "in-touchness."

INTERPERSONAL COMMUNICATION

We shall now focus on interpersonal communication to identify important characteristics and to define and describe the communicative processes that we believe are important in operationalizing a humanistic approach in nursing. Interpersonal communication concerns the face-to-face interactions between people who are continually aware of one another. Each person assumes alternately the roles of speaker and receiver of messages. This is a dynamic process that involves continual adaptation and adjustments of each person to the other. The process of relating interpersonally with others is a basic key, not only to coping with reality in order to survive but also to living life to its fullest and most satisfying potentialities. Healthy interpersonal relationships provide for personal growth, development of self-confidence through self-acceptance, and beneficial cooperation through shared responsibility with other individuals. For most persons, it is essential to achieve a deeply satisfying, warm, personal relationship with at least one other person. There is a need to understand processes that provide growth, confidence, and cooperation under normal, healthy circumstances. To understand these processes in the event of illness and the "dis-ease" that accompanies it becomes not only a need but a necessity, particularly for individuals who function as professional health-care providers.

Certain characteristics of interpersonal communication are of particular relevance to being human and establishing satisfying, warm, personal relationships with others. These characteristics are as follows:

1. Interpersonal communication is a *process* that is *existential* in nature.
2. Interpersonal communication involves the generation and exchange of *meaning*, that is, a sense of what is important and what has implications for one's future.
3. Interpersonal communication provides information about "outside the skin" reality or *facts* and about emotions aroused "inside the skin" or *feelings*.
4. Interpersonal communication is a *dialogic* or two-directional process in the sense that one alternately sends and receives messages.

The role interpersonal communication plays in our growth and development is to humanize. Through interpersonal communication processes with significant people, an individual, from infancy, becomes oriented to the physical and social world. Stewart and D'Angelo[26] state:

> The quality of our interpersonal relationships determines who we are becoming as persons. Interpersonal communication is not merely one of many dimensions of human life; it is the defining dimension, the dimension through which we become human.

Thus, this is the basis of our belief that humanistic nursing can be realized through a careful study of interpersonal communication, a humanizing process.

In the next few pages, we shall discuss more fully the key words characterizing interpersonal communication: process, existentialism and meaning, facts and feelings, and dialogic.

PROCESS

Interpersonal communication is characterized above as being a "process" rather than a thing. This distinction is important—nothing is static. Berlo[27] states:

> If we accept the concept of process, we view events and relationships as dynamic, ongoing, ever-changing, continuous. When we label something as a process, we also mean that it does not have a beginning, an end, a fixed

sequence of events. It is not static, at rest. It is moving. The ingredients within a process interact; each affects all of the others.

To analyze interpersonal communication, one has to take a picture, as it were, of a "slice" of time. One can capture the process on film. And even as one looks at the picture—or reads a book or views a movie—one is being changed by the meanings generated in the process. One can talk about process only with certain understandings about the limitations involved. Berlo states the logic of this:

> We have no alternative if we are to analyze and communicate about a process. The important point is that we must remember that we are not including everything in our discussion. The things we talk about do not have to exist in exactly the ways we talk about them, and they certainly do not have to operate in the order in which we talk about them. Objects which we separate may not always be separable, and they never operate independently—each affects and interacts with the others. This may appear obvious, but it is easy to overlook or forget the limitations that are necessarily placed on any discussion of a process.[28]

The interdependency and mutual influence of all ingredients in the process need to be remembered continuously. The process of interpersonal communication is broken down for detailed analysis. The concept of process is not unknown in nursing. Many nursing theorists describe nursing practice as a process and generally discuss it in the manner suggested above by Berlo. More recently, references have been made to general systems theory and to adaptation theories in discussions of processes.[29]

EXISTENTIALISM AND MEANING

We have also characterized interpersonal communication as being existentialist in nature. Existentialism has been defined as focusing on an individual human being and that human's state of "becoming" in the "here and now," that slice of time commonly referred to as the present.[30] Existentialism looks at life as it is and tries to provide meaning to a complicated process of events.

The individual is in a state characterized by finite singularity (solitude, loneliness, and uniqueness), having choice and being responsible for acts. Searching for meaning, struggling to become what they are without rules or structure to point the way, human beings endure uncertainty. One is aware of the *fact* that life can be extinguished by chance at any moment. Coping with choice and struggling with work are persistent. And one is acutely aware of *feelings* of loneliness, dread, and alienation. These facts and feelings are the content of human interpersonal communication. This openness to the unlabeled and unclassified provides potential for greater meaning to be derived through interpersonal communication.

FACTS AND FEELINGS

Facts are one's statements concerning the phenomenologic world; through interpersonal communication, one gains validation of one's perceptions of reality. Feelings come from within the individual and are by nature subjective. Individuals are the only judges of their feelings; no one can dispute one's feelings, and no one can dispute how one feels if, for example, one says one is unhappy. Our definition of existential people includes a humanizing dimension of inner emotions and feelings, in addition to the humanistic emphasis on a person's ability to think, reason, and deal with facts of the world. This dimension emphasizes the following concepts in describing a human being as an individual: existence, becoming, freedom, choice, responsibility, struggle, tragedy, despair, uncertainty, meaning, and dread. The dimension of being human is operationalized in communing, meaning to converse intimately and to exchange thoughts and feelings about facts.

DIALOGUE

We have described the humanizing process as being dialogic in nature, and we define it generally as a two-way interaction in which each person participates by sharing information about oneself and being open to receiving similar information from another. The opposite of dialogic is monologic, or one-way communication—which tends to be didactic and dictatorial in nature, and thus dehumanizing. Dialogic communication is an essential characteristic of interpersonal communication. One existentialist philosopher, Martin Buber,[31] provides a theory of interpersonal communication in his book *I and Thou*.

Generally, Buber's theory assumes human beings to be in an existential state. Not only are human beings seen as symbolic, but communication is also of an immediate, "here and now" nature that involves freedom of choice. And it is assumed there is a difference in relating to an object and to a person; awareness of this difference is necessary to entering into a meaningful interpersonal relationship.

Two types of relationships represent the dehumanizing and humanizing manner of communicating; these are *I-It* and *I-Thou*. *I-It* is a monologic relationship in that *I* speaks to, about, or over an *It*. The *I* usually has some goal, and the communication generally involves strategy, defensiveness, deceptiveness, and evaluation. *I* withholds part of the self from the relationship. The communication concerns a specific time or space, and may involve technical language. Generally, this type of communication is reserved for talking to or about things or objects. When the *I-It* relationship is used for communicating with humans, a great flaw in interpersonal communication occurs. Generally, growth and development are limited when a person is treated as an *It*.

I-Thou is a dialogic relationship in which two human beings stand in relation to one another, experiencing what is between them. This relationship involves meeting, confronting, and encountering with total commitment and genuineness. There is an awareness of the other's being and a readiness to receive the other into one's own experience. Time and space are forgotten as one genuinely listens with the realization that *Thou* is saying something new about the nature of *Thou*. In the *I-Thou* relationship, one can live through an event from the standpoint of another person. If the response becomes calculated, then the relationship becomes an *I-It*. It is through the *I-Thou* relationship that meaningful interpersonal relationships can develop which involve love, not eros (love object) but agape (love relation). The *I-Thou* relationship concerns the spiritual aspect of human beings, that bit of the supremely humanizing being or God residing in each human; it is this spiritual aspect of each one standing in warm, positive regard for another and communing. The effect of the *I-Thou* relationship is to achieve a feeling of rest and peace in being accepted and understood by another without reservation, evaluation, or classification.[32]

Drawing from existentialist thought and from Buber's *I-Thou* theory of interpersonal communication, Patterson and Zderad[33] developed a theory of humanistic nursing practice. Patterson and Zderad note that nurses deliberately approach nursing practice as a short-term, existentialistic experience. They note that nurses experience with clients and patients special existential moments in life that may be labeled peak experiences, such as "creation, birth, winning, nothingness, losing, separations, and death."[34] They emphasize human beings as symbolic beings, noting that words are "the major tools of phenomenological description."[35] The individual can be the only source of self-description "in this situation." They indicate that the purpose and aim of nursing is:

> . . . the ability to struggle with other man through peak experiences related to health and suffering in which the participants in the nursing situation are and become in accordance with their human potential.[36]

The primary relationship statement of humanistic nursing theory is the transaction, the dialogic "reciprocal call and response" interactions occurring between the nurse and client. Both participate in the "lived dialogue" interdependently, yet both are subjects and are independently generators of meaning. The "between" that occurs in this relationship concerns the awareness of meaning generated, and the "being with and doing with the patient." Patterson and Zderad[37] note that this existential involvement is short-lived and suggest that ". . . it is more realistic to think of humanistic nursing as occurring in various degrees."

In summary, Buber's *I-Thou* and Patterson and Zderad's "lived dialogue" occurring in the "between" provide theoretical perspectives and serve to clarify and explain the concept of dialogue as it occurs in and relates to humanistic nursing. These theories also serve to restate important characteristics of interpersonal communication that we have identified thus far, that is, a process, existential in nature, an exchange of meaning, concerning facts and feelings, and dialogic. In the next section, we discuss other aspects of interpersonal communication that are relevant to humanistic nursing.

SUMMARY AND PREVIEW

We are writing from a humanistic point of view, and we make certain assumptions about communicators as people, as human beings. First, we assume that individuals not only receive and interpret stimuli, but also play an active role in selecting stimuli to which they will respond. Humans are born into a "booming, buzzing" world of strange sensations. Visual images, varying pressures and temperatures, degrees of moistness and hardness, and strange sounds impinge upon the sensory system. The early years of life are given to sorting out these sensations. Humans learn that physical needs will be met when certain people are present. Certain pressures, temperatures, and images come to be indicators that certain events are or will be happening. Sounds become meaningful as words are repeated over and over. Humans soon begin to behave in a manner that has an influence on this environment; crying, babbling, and vocalizing tend to elicit signals of warm acceptance from people. As individuals develop, they continue to attach more discriminating meaning to the phenomena they perceive, and they develop greater skills in controlling their interpersonal world. Cultural surroundings and behavior of significant people in their lives enrich individuals' experiences and expectations of interpersonal relationships. Through dialogic communication with others, people learn to adapt to the environment to meet their human needs. Individuals live through interactions with other people. Although humans interact with objects, animals, and other aspects of their total environment, these interactions are relatively unimportant in comparison with the interactions or interpersonal communication experienced with people. It is our belief that the way humans communicate with others is what individuals become. It involves the total being, the whole person.

Second, we believe that the more people can be aware of their own motives and communication patterns, the greater degree of control they can have over them rather than being controlled by them. The nurse calls the pathologist to politely request results of a test and receives a gruff answer. The nurse has a choice: to be angry and upset or to remain polite and pleasant in dealing with the next person. The nurse chooses the latter because the nurse does not want to be controlled. One cannot make the nurse angry unless the nurse allows it. As human beings, it is possible to think and act rather than simply to react.

Third, our humanistic point of view places emphasis on choice and freedom. A person can choose to delay reactions to phenomena or interactions until due consideration has been given and a course of action has been selected. To the extent people can control and select their behavior, to that degree people are free. And this freedom involves a responsibility to oneself and to others for the consequences of one's choices and actions. People so completely take their interpersonal communication for granted that they seldom think of studying it. By the time individuals reach adulthood, communication has become very much like a reflex action, and people simply accept its existence.

Finally, we believe the study of interpersonal communication is necessary to promote awareness of skills as communicators, and it should foster both personal and professional development in at least three areas: knowledge, social decision making, and self-expression. By understanding the interactive-ongoing process of interpersonal communication, it becomes possible to alter certain elements with predictable effects. This requires knowledge of theory and practice: "why" certain behaviors work and "how to" skills in operationalizing the behaviors effectively. Criteria of excellence here are not as well defined as in some fields, and absolute rules are nonexistent. Each individual must make one's own social decisions and choices about communicative behaviors.

We are writing this book because we believe that nursing is an important profession in society. We believe the special services nurses provide inherently are humanizing in nature, and that nursing represents a significant humanizing force within the health-care system. And we believe more emphasis needs to be placed on this seemingly latent asset in the very nature of nursing.

We define humanistic nursing as communicating a concern for the individual's feelings, needs, and self-image, particularly in relation to implications arising from changing health states and coping capabilities. This communication behavior must convey interpersonal warmth, genuineness, and caring. Elements of humanistic nursing include authenticity of feelings as well as facts, validation of the client as a communicator of value, and caring about the client as a person in a manner that promotes coping and independence.

One important aspect of the role of the professional nurse in practicing humanistic nursing is being aware of oneself as a variable in the nurse-client relationship. We believe students and practitioners of nursing need to be sensitive to their own feelings and encouraged in the development of self-awareness. To the extent one is aware of one's own feelings and thoughts, to a greater extent one tends to become sensitive to others. Nurses need to be particularly sensitive to others' feelings and experience; nurses also need to be skillful in communicating this awareness and sensitivity to others. We believe theory and research in interpersonal communication are highly relevant to efforts to operationalize humanistic perspectives in nursing and to humanize health care. To the extent that a humanistic approach occurs in the nurse-client relationship, to that extent health care will tend to be more effective. Studies of primary nursing by Marram and coworkers and by Jones tend to support this belief.[38] We also believe that such health care will tend to cost less, not only in terms of dollars spent, but also in terms of needless repetition of efforts and decreased need for technology. And we believe there will be a greater attentiveness by all concerned to use preventive health-care measures.

We believe nursing to be a discipline and profession at the preconceptual level of development in its theory building. This book is aimed at having influence on moving the nursing profession toward identifying concepts and theories specific to nursing as a discipline. We hope to help students and practitioners to understand the choices available to them as communicators in professional and personal roles. We believe nursing educators, students, and practitioners are seeking ways of combining humanistic beliefs with holistic health practices within the complex, highly structured health-care system that exists today. We offer this text as one way of achieving this goal.

In Chapters 2 through 8, major areas of interpersonal communication theory and research are discussed and related to nursing. Emphasis will be given to the interpersonal communication occurring between the nurse and client, the nurse and peers, and the nurse and colleagues of other health-related professions.

Chapter 9 provides guidelines to assist in the judgments one makes in evaluating interpersonal communication. Some suggestions are given to the reader concerning how one can change behaviors and perhaps improve relationships.

Chapter 10 deals with special communication problems nurses typically encounter today. These include distrust, defensiveness, barriers, and other alienating patterns of communication. Sexual harassment is defined as an alienating communication pattern and is given special emphasis. Recent interpretation of civil rights laws now defines sexual harassment as discriminatory and illegal. Defining and analyzing sexual harassment as an interpersonal communication problem provide a unique view and offers possible remedies. Verbal abuse of nurses is also defined as an alienating communication pattern and analyzed in comparison with the battered wife syndrome.

Chapter 11 discusses interviewing as the means of implementing humanizing interpersonal communication. The interview process is described, and situations are analyzed in which the nurse either interviews or is interviewed.

In Chapter 12, the authors draw upon all preceding chapters to present a new theory, humanistic nursing communication, and look to the future. This theory is discussed according to the major aspects of a theory: assumptions, concepts, relationship statements, and evaluation. Principles are offered to serve as guides to consider in nursing research, education, and practice.

REFERENCES

1. JEAN-PAUL SARTRE: *Existentialism and Humanism*, translation and introduction by Philip Mairet (Brooklyn: Haskell House, 1957).
2. SOREN AABGE KIERKEGAARD: *The Concept of Dread*, translated with introduction and notes by Walter Lowrie, 2nd ed. (Princeton: Princeton University Press, 1957).
3. ABRAHAM H. MASLOW: *Toward a Psychology of Being*, 2nd ed. (New York: D. Van Nostrand Company, 1968), p. 9.
4. H. JACK GEIGER: "The Causes of Dehumanization in Health Care and Prospects for Humanization," in: JAN HOWARD AND AMSEIM STRAUSS, EDS.: *Humanizing Health Care* (New York: John Wiley & Sons, 1975), p. 12.
5. JAN HOWARD: "Humanization and Dehumanization of Health Care: A Conceptual View," in: JAN HOWARD AND AMSEIM STRAUSS, EDS.: *Humanizing Health Care* (New York: John Wiley & Sons, 1975), pp. 57–102.
6. *Ibid.*, p. 89.
7. PHILIP R. LEE: "Epilogue," in: JAN HOWARD AND AMSEIM STRAUSS, EDS.: *Humanizing Health Care* (New York: John Wiley & Sons, 1975), pp. 305–316.
8. LLOYD L. MORAIN: "Humanist Manifesto II: A Time for Reconsideration," *The Humanist*, September/October, 1980, pp. 4–10.
9. HOWARD LEVENTHAL: "The Consequences of Depersonalization During Illness and Treatment: An Information-Processing Model," in: JAN HOWARD AND AMSEIM STRAUSS, EDS.: *Humanizing Health Care* (New York: John Wiley & Sons, 1975), pp. 119–162.
10. *Ibid.*, p. 120.
11. *Ibid.*
12. *Ibid.*, pp. 121–122.
13. LEON FESTINGER: "A Theory of Social Comparison Processes," *Human Relations*, 1954, 7 (2), 117–140.
14. LEVENTHAL: "The Consequences."
15. *Ibid.*, p. 154.
16. SUE K. DONALDSON AND DOROTHY M. CROWLEY: "The Discipline of Nursing," *Nursing Outlook*, 1978, 28 (2), p. 114.
17. MARGARET NEWMAN: *Theory Development in Nursing* (Philadelphia: F. A. Davis Company, 1979), p. 2.
18. DOROTHY E. JOHNSTON: "Development of Theory: A Requisite for Nursing as a Primary Health Profession," *Nursing Research*, 1974, 23 (5), 372–377.

19. BONNIE WEAVER DULDT AND KIM GIFFIN: *Theoretical Perspectives of Nursing* (Boston: Little, Brown & Company, in press).
20. DOROTHEA E. OREM, ED.: *Concept Formulization in Nursing*, 2nd ed. (Boston: Little, Brown and Company, 1979).
21. DONALDSON AND CROWLEY: "Discipline."
22. KENNETH BURKE: *Language as Symbolic Action* (Los Angeles, University of California Press, 1966), pp. 3–24.
23. *Ibid.*
24. JOSEPHINE G. PATTERSON AND LORETTA T. ZDERAD: *Humanistic Nursing* (New York: John Wiley & Sons, 1976).
25. MARTIN BUBER: *I and Thou*, translated by Walter Kaufmann (New York: Charles Scribner's Sons, 1970).
26. JOHN STEWART AND GARY D'ANGELO: *Together: Communicating Interpersonally* (Reading, Mass.: Addison-Wesley Publishing Company, 1975), p. 23.
27. D. K. BERLO: *The Process of Communication* (New York: Holt, Rinehart & Winston, 1960), p. 24.
28. *Ibid.*, p. 26.
29. IDA JEAN ORLANDO: *The Dynamic Nurse-Patient Relationship* (New York: Putnam's, 1961); MARTHA ROGERS: *An Introduction to the Theoretical Basis of Nursing* (Philadelphia: F. A. Davis Company, 1970); ARLENE M. PUTT: *General Systems Theory Applied to Nursing* (Boston: Little, Brown and Company, 1978); and H. YURA AND M. B. WALSH: *The Nursing Process: Assessing, Planning, Implementing and Evaluating*, 2nd ed. (New York: Appleton-Century-Crofts, 1973).
30. RICHARD GILL AND EARNEST SHERMAN: *The Fabric of Existentialism: Philosophical and Literary Sources* (Englewood Cliffs, N.J.: Prentice-Hall Inc., 1973). This text is an excellent reference for the *non*-philosophy major. It summarizes major philosophic perspectives and presents excerpts of most philosophers' writings.
31. BUBER: *I and Thou*.
32. *Ibid.*
33. PATTERSON AND ZDERAD: *Humanistic Nursing*.
34. *Ibid.*, p. 7.
35. *Ibid.*, p. 8.
36. *Ibid.*, p. 7.
37. *Ibid.*, p. 15.
38. GWEN D. MARRAM, ET AL.: *Primary Nursing—A Model for Individualized Care.* (St. Louis: C. V. Mosby Company, 1974); GWEN D. MARRAM, ET AL.: *Cost Effectiveness of Primary and Team Nursing* (Wakefield, Mass.: Contemporary Publishing, Inc., 1976); KATHERINE JONES: "Study Documents Effect of Primary Nursing on Renal Patients," *Hospitals* 49: (December 16, 1975): 85–89.

2
INTERPERSONAL PERCEPTIONS AND ORIENTATIONS

As nurses meet and interact with other persons—physicians, patients, other nurses—they sense certain characteristics that will influence their ways of communicating. Attempts to interact will be guided by what one sees, hears, and feels about the other person.

One's perception of persons (if one perceives them as human beings) differs from one's perception of objects in two ways: Unlike objects, people display behaviors that suggest their attitudes toward one, including ways they are likely to respond to one; also, the person one perceives is simultaneously perceiving one, and how one is perceived will influence the other person's ways of interacting with one. Because of these factors, interpersonal perception is a very important part of the process of interpersonal communication.

This chapter provides an overview of the process of interpersonal perception. Noted are the sources of inaccuracy, the problem of stereotyping, and the danger of selective attention to desirable or undesirable personal characteristics. Special notice is taken of forming impressions of one another—the values and limitations of first impressions. The second section of the chapter describes ways in which people develop habitual modes of generally perceiving other people. If, in general, one tends to see people as harmful or threatening, one may easily develop a habit of responding to people in ways tending toward aggression or withdrawal. On the other hand, if one generally views people as cooperative and helpful, one may develop a habit of responding to people in positive ways. Such habitual ways of viewing other people are called an interpersonal "orientation." Such habits may be very useful or quite self-defeating. For this reason, one needs to evaluate one's own and other persons' interpersonal orientations with great care. They may seriously influence one's interpersonal response style.

THE PROCESS OF PERSON PERCEPTION

As you go down the hallway to look in on "old Mr. Jones," one of the patients, you probably have formed an impression of a nice old man, feeble, lonely, and scared, and you already have a pretty good idea of how you will interact with him. Where did this idea come from? How did it arrive in your consciousness?

By the time people are adults, they tend to take their perceptions of persons pretty much for granted without considering how they were formed or whether they are right. Individuals often find themselves having friends, dates, or work partners, without considering how they formed their impressions of them. To what degree are these perceptions accurate? Why do people think they are correct?

British psychologist Mark Cook has made the following observation:

> People are selected for jobs or higher education, etc., often on the basis of an interview in which the interviewer forms, on the basis of a fifteen-minute encounter, an opinion of the person's suitability, and, in the process, affects that person's life for years to come. Interviewers often never consider whether they are right or not, but rather have a firm belief in their own infallibility.[1]

Are people justified in assuming that their interpersonal perceptions are correct?

All of one's interactions with another person are influenced by one's perceptions of that person. Obtaining and even changing such an impression are preliminary to any given act of communicating with the person. This impression influences how one *initiates* interaction as well as how one *responds* to the individual. And one's responses likewise influence how the person responds to one, and thus, in turn, how one then responds, and again the person's responses, and so on.

Two types of behavior are involved in the process of interpersonal perception:

1. People record the diversity of data they encounter in a form simple enough to be retained by their limited memory; and
2. They mentally go beyond the data given to predict future events, and thereby minimize surprise.

These two behaviors, selective recording and predicting, became the basis for forming impressions of other persons.

To perform the first step, people observe actions, notice voices, consider what persons say and how they respond to them. From such observations, they make *inferences* about the other person's attitudes, needs, goals, habits, and feelings. These inferences or conclusions are then used to predict responses to various alternative behaviors that people may use. Then individuals choose, usually within the limits of their habits, how they will interact with others.

Actions toward another person and expectation of their responses are guided by predictions based on observations. Simultaneously, the other person is making judgments about the first individual that will influence interaction behavior. If both persons' judgments and predictions are correct, genuine communication can be established; even though one may not like what the other person tells one, there will be fewer surprises and misunderstandings. If, however, observations are inaccurate and predictions incorrect, serious difficulties will arise between the two people.

Imagine that the individual described in the following brief case history came to you for treatment. How would you diagnose the ailment, and what therapy would you recommend?

All through childhood, K. was extremely meditative and usually preferred to be alone. He often had mysterious dreams and fits, during which he sometimes fainted. In late puberty, K. experienced elaborate auditory and visual hallucinations, uttered incoherent words, and had recurrent spells of sudden coma. He was frequently found running wildly through the countryside or eating the bark of trees and was known to throw himself with abandon into fire and water. On many occasions, he wounded himself with knives or other weapons. K. believed he could "talk to spirits" and "chase ghosts." He was certain of his power over all sorts of supernatural forces.

Believe it or not, K. was not found insane, nor was he committed to the nearest institution for the mentally ill. Instead, in due course, he became one of the leading and most respected members of his community.

How this strange turn of events could come about may become more plausible to you if an important bit of information is supplied that was purposefully left out of the case history above.

K., we should have told you, was a member of a primitive tribe of fishermen and reindeer herders that inhabits the arctic wilderness of eastern Siberia. In this far-off culture, the same kind of behavior that our society regards as symptomatic of mental illness is considered evidence of an individual's fitness for an important social position—that of medicine man or shaman.

The hallucinations, fits, manic episodes, and periods of almost complete withdrawal that marked K.'s early years were considered signs that he had been chosen by some higher power for an exalted role. His behavioral eccentricities were, in fact, prerequisite to his becoming a shaman, just as balance, solidity, self-confidence, and aggressiveness are prerequisite for the young man who hopes to be successful in American business.[2]

Although occasionally one's first impression of another person may remain essentially intact for a long time, usually the image of a person does not remain static. As with other factors in the process of interpersonal communication, person perceptions repeatedly change in small ways—are modified or re-evaluated. That very nice physician or very grumpy patient may tomorrow be viewed somewhat differently. The loving boyfriend of last week may be today's source of despair. As greater experience with different people is gained, ways of forming impressions become more critical, tentative, and sophisticated.

The process of person perception, broken down into some detail, includes the following elements:

1. Note the available sensory data.
2. Define the other person into one or another stereotyped category.
3. Selectively note further details to create a unified or congruent impression.
4. Predict responses on the basis of the impression—estimate a relationship potential.
5. Behavior often significantly affects the behavior of the other person—setting in motion reciprocal perspectives.

Each of these factors will be examined in some detail.

SENSORY BASES OF PERSON PERCEPTION

Impressions of other people are mainly based on sight, sound, touch, and smell. Each of these is very important in the profession of nursing.

The average American does not rely very heavily on sense of smell in gaining an impression of another person unless body or breath odor is unusually strong. Although persons from other cultures, notably the Near East, are quite conscious of both positive and negative messages through smell, Americans spend many dollars to eliminate personal odors or produce artificial ones—with sprays, soaps, mints, perfumes, and lotions. Although Americans may be influenced more than they know by such artificial odors, a person's "natural" scent seems to have low perceptual value.[3]

Although very little research has been reported on the subject, the smells involved in illness and damaged tissue are quite common to the experience of a nurse. Patients who are in diabetic coma, who have a pressure point under a cast, or who are suffering from uremia or cancer may contribute significantly to your interpersonal impression of them via the sense of smell.

Sight

Whenever two or more people are in each other's presence, visual data about one another are very important. The study of nonverbal communication is much involved with the exchange of visual signals. The first real awareness of the other person may be established via eye contact. George Simmel, an early student of this phenomenon, provides the following observation:

> The union and interaction of individuals is based upon mutual glances. This is perhaps the most direct and purest reciprocity which exists anywhere. . .
> This mutual glance between persons, in distinction from the simple sight or observation of the other, signifies a wholly new and unique union between them. . . . By the very act in which the observer seeks to know the observed, he surrenders himself to be understood by the observer. The eye cannot take unless at the same time it gives.[4]

The dynamic nature of visual contact has generally been experienced by most people even though they may not have speculated on its significance. People have all traded glances with a stranger across a room. Desire for communication will determine whether one seeks or avoids this contact; once made, its nature and consequent feelings or impressions may determine how or if one approaches this other person.

The role of eye contact has been the subject of considerable research in recent years. Mark Knapp, a leading student of such research, summarizes it as follows:

> Eye contact is influenced by a number of different conditions: whether we are seeking feedback, need for certain markers in the conversation, whether we wish to open or close the communication channel, whether the other party is too near or too far, whether we wish to induce anxiety, whether we are rewarded by what we see, whether we are in competition with another or wishing to hide something from him, and whether we are with members of a different sex or status. Personality characteristics such as introversion/extroversion may also influence eye behavior.[5]

If you want to avoid psychologic contact with another person—avoid showing empathy, concern for the person's condition or feelings—start by avoiding eye contact when you are in the person's presence. In this way, you can treat the person as an object and avoid involving your own feelings and emotions. On the other hand, if you want the individual to know you are human and that you are fully with him or her, start by looking directly into the person's eyes. We suggest that the next time you encounter a patient, for whatever reason, you make a point of establishing good eye contact. Look that person directly in the eye and let the person tell you how he or she feels about the condition and feelings. See if this experience is a rewarding one for you.

A second way that sight of another person significantly influences person perception is based on the person's facial features and expression. Various studies show that people tend to agree in correlating certain personality traits with faces and facial expressions. This perceptual behavior amounts to a form of stereotyping that apparently is useful. For example, the use of cosmetics and other grooming aids including hair style has been shown to influence the inferences made, especially about women.[6]

Although most people are unaware of it, they respond subconsciously to fleeting facial expressions. Researchers have labeled these "micromomentary" facial expressions and have studied them on film or videotape run in slow motion. At four frames per second, instead of the usual 24, psychologists have noticed up to 2½ times as many changes of expression as would ordinarily be identified, some lasting only ⅕ of a second. Studies show that these expressions are significant, especially in conflict situations. If a person wishes to appear confident but feels fearful, indications of the fear are shown through these flickering expressions.

It is perhaps small wonder that nurses "see through" people or that they see through nurses' facades more than nurses hope or anticipate. Such research lends support for the basic stance that it is important for nurses to be genuine and avoid artificiality in our efforts at interpersonal communication.

Other visual cues are given in a person's posture, gestures, and other expressive movements. Some cues tend to be tied to certain cultures, but certain actions tend to have near-universal meaning. The highly animated person tends to indicate more openness to your ideas—unless the person is animated and very angry. Stiff, rigid, aloof persons tend to show their lack of likelihood of accepting your ideas by their posture and gestures.

Sound

Let us suppose that there is a new nursing supervisor in a unit where you do part of your work. You call that unit by phone to obtain some needed information. You hear this new supervisor for the first time. Almost immediately, you form some judgments that will influence how you ask for information—even, perhaps, whether you will be satisfied with the information given. Low, resonant voices are perceived as indications of strength, knowledgeability, and maturity. In the American culture, the man with a high-pitched voice has a burden. United States soldiers serving in Vietnam sometimes laughed at orders given in a high-pitched voice by a Vietnamese officer. In one study, 18 male speakers read the same message to an audience of 600 people by a means of audio recordings. The audience did not know the speakers and could not see them. Audience members were asked to match certain personality data of people to the voices they heard. The experimenters concluded that voice alone conveys some correct data in identifying age and some personality characteristics.[8] Even when incorrect in these judgments, audience members tended to respond *in a uniform manner*. When such stereotypes were perceived from the voice alone, other features of that stereotype were attributed to the speakers.

Voices do elicit stereotyped personality judgments as confirmed by a later study. These stereotyped judgments may or may not be accurate. In response to tape-recorded voices, freshman students at the University of Iowa attributed personality characteristics to the speakers in terms of vocal attributes. Among the many findings were:

> Thinness in female voices cued perceptions of increased immaturity on four levels: social, physical, emotional, and mental, while no significant traits were correlated to thinness in the male voice. Males with throaty voices were stereotyped as being older, more realistic, mature, sophisticated, and well adjusted; females with throatiness were perceived as being less intelligent, more masculine, lazier, more boorish, unemotional, ugly, sickly, careless, inartistic, naive, humble, neurotic, quiet, uninteresting, and apathetic.[10]

In the face-to-face encounter, the vocal communication, rather than the fact of being isolated, is but one of the ingredients of the interaction. The question then becomes one of congruency. As with the micromomentary expression studies, unconscious note is taken of whether the words, vocal signals, and movements carry the same message. If there is conflict, the tendency is to put more emphasis on the nonverbal aspects as being more dependable indicators because they are, to a greater degree, unconsciously performed.

Touch

Tactile communication plays an important role in the lives of most people, but it is especially important in the nurse-patient relationship. It is perhaps the most direct way to encourage, support, and show tenderness to a patient.

In a general way, there are widespread reports of positive responses to exercises involving touch in encounter groups and communication-training classes; these reports reflect a rather common yearning to be able to "reach out and touch someone" and to be positively responded to in return. One study controlling the conditions for interaction in groups indicated the following attributions to warm, friendly messages sent by different sensory avenues:

> VERBAL: "distant, noncommunicative, artificial, insensitive, and formal."
> VISUAL: "artificial, childish, arrogant, comic, and cold."
> TACTILE: "trustful, sensitive, natural, mature, serious, and warm."[11]

In this study, as in a number of other reports, touch seems to have greater impact for showing caring and warmth than the other modes of communication.

For many persons, however, touch provokes ambivalent feelings. The American culture places fairly strict limitations on touching another person. Among business associates, a handshake or pat on the back is acceptable. Affectionate pats or embraces are reserved for moments of crisis, or in greeting relatives, or among teammates when a decisive play is made or a game is won. Ashley Montagu suggests, "Perhaps it would be . . . accurate to say that the taboos on interpersonal tactuality grew out of a fear closely associated with the Christian tradition in its various denominations, the fear of bodily pleasure."[12] This attitude restricting touch is a cultural one. Montagu states:

> There are clearly contact people and non-contact people, the Anglo-Saxon peoples being among the latter. Curious ways in which non-contactuality expresses itself are to be seen in the behavior of members of the non-contact cultures in various situations. It has, for example, been observed that the way an Anglo-Saxon shakes hands constitutes a signal to the other to keep his proper distance. In crowds this is also observable. For example, in a crowded vehicle like a subway, the Anglo-Saxon will remain stiff and rigid, with a blank expression on his face which seems to deny the existence of other passengers. The contrast on the French Metro, for example, is striking. Here the passengers will lean and press against others, if not with complete abandon, at least without feeling the necessity either to ignore or apologize to the other against whom they may be leaning or pressing. Often the leaning and lurching will give rise to good-natured laughter and joking, and there will be no attempt to avoid looking at the other passengers.[13]

The environment in which nurses work may be viewed as full of emotional crises, at least from the viewpoint of the patient. The need to reassure patients, their relatives, and even, occasionally, your coworkers may put a heavy strain on your emotional reserves. Consider this pull on your emotions along with cultural pulls to show "proper" restraint; you will need to make wise choices in each situation to provide the best help for patients as well as maintenance of your own sense of well-being. Perhaps a starting point from which to work is to practice a warm, sincere touch on another person's hand or arm. Such an act is quite acceptable between nurse and patient, and is also a warm signal of caring and involvement.

ACCURACY OF INFERENCES

A starting point that should give some indication of the degree of accuracy of perceptions of one another is that two different people may perceive the same third person quite differently. If these perceptions are contradictory, they both cannot be accurate. For example, two nurses may work with the same physician and each perceive that physician in significantly opposite ways. Even so, few people realize that they are constantly drawing conclusions about others, and even fewer consider that they may be wrong much of the time. William V. Haney suggests five sources of differing perceptions: We come from different environments so that we attach importance to differing parts or facets of a person; we note differing actions or behaviors; we use differing sensory receptors so that we notice behavior differently; we may have differing internal states so that we take more or less notice of different features or characteristics of a person; and things we notice may evoke differing attitudes or response patterns. For these reasons we may differ in the way we perceive the same person, noting different feelings, needs, wishes, attitudes, and intentions ot others.[11] This all suggests a large margin for error in perceptions of one another. Even slight errors in correctly perceiving another person may cause difficulties in communicating and working with that person.

How well do you infer what is going on inside another person—feelings, attitudes, intentions, or likelihood of responding in a certain way? Can you always tell when a physician is disgusted with you? When a supervisor thinks poorly of your work? Or when a patient is driven further into despondency? As people observe the behavior of others, they infer only approximately at best what others are thinking or feeling. How well observers do depends on the quality of the cues people give (some give very few), how many times they can be observed, and the observer's capability to "read" these cues. Probably, most people have known co-workers or associates about whom they could not tell in certain situations whether they were serious or joking; with others, it is difficult to determine whether or not they are feeling sad.

Certain motives or intentions of other people are also inferred from observing their behavior. In interactions with nurses and physicians, they may be seen or heard to do certain things. For example, a person may smile and the conclusion drawn that the person is feeling friendly—intends to treat the observer in a warm, positive way. At one major university, the chief of the campus police was known to be able to smile in a warm, friendly manner while he awarded a patrolman two days of extra duty for some rule infraction. At a medical center, a nurse may smile in a warm, friendly manner while telling a young intern a patient fell out of bed and broke a hip; now the intern has all those accident and insurance reports to fill out as soon as the patient comes out of surgery . . . all before the 10 other things the intern has to do. Some nurses and physicians seem to have such discrepancy between their attitudes or intentions and the cues they "give off." This process of inferring traits, attitudes, or intentions of another person by noting the cues provided has become known as the attribution process—the act of attributing to another person certain motives or intentions. This process has recently become the focus of much interest among scholars who study human interaction.

In the development and testing of attribution theory, research has tended to support the following principles: (1) much of the behavior of others that can be observed is trivial or incidental and is not valuable for drawing conclusions regarding personality or intentions—one must be carefully tentative in the attribution process; (2) the observable behavior of others is often neatly designed to mislead or deceive one; and (3) their actions are often determined by external factors beyond their control and not by their internal states, personalities, or intentions. As a result of these limiting factors in the attribution process, one must use it with care; however, experience tells one that in large measure it often works very well. This is essentially true for attribution of general dispositions or intentions on the bases of numerous observations over extended periods of time. Further research has indicated that one can sharpen the use of the attribution process if one pays special attention to two types of behavior: (1) that for which the observed person could have had only one or at most a very few possible reasons (e.g., a young nurse marries a crabby, stupid, ugly, old man who is wealthy), and (2) behavior that deviates markedly from widely accepted social norms (e.g., a nurse-supervisor who cooks all her food over an open hibachi in the middle of her living room).

Recently, at a major university an instructor felt ill and abruptly left class in the middle of a discussion. At the next class meeting, the students were asked by the instructor why they thought he had left. Responses included such reactions as: The instructor was angered over the low quality of the discussion and left in disgust; he had an appointment; he thought he had arrived at a good stopping point; he wanted to give the class more preparation time; he was reacting emotionally to one of the comments made by a member of the class. None of the class guessed the true reason, but all were willing to make inferences concerning the behavior witnessed.

Consider the following situation in which a nurse in a psychiatric hospital made an inference that did not help the patient:

Two days previously, a patient had been transferred from a locked to an open ward. On this particular day, he was walking down the hall when the head nurse said to him, "Your dental appointment is at 10:00 AM." The patient looked startled but he did not speak, blinked his eyes, and then squinted. The head nurse asked, "What's the matter?" but did not pursue questioning and allowed the patient to walk away. At 10:30 AM, the dental clinic notified the nurse that the patient had not kept his appointment. At 3:00 PM, when the patient returned, the head nurse asked, "Where have you been?" The patient did not answer. Later the nurse said to the doctor, "This patient is very confused today, and I'm really concerned about him. He left the ward at 9:45 AM, to go to the dental clinic, but he didn't get there. He wouldn't tell me where he had been when he returned at 3:00 PM. I'm not sure it's safe to keep him on the open ward."

Arrangements were made for the patient to be transferred back to the locked ward. When the patient arrived, he said to the nurse whom he knew, "I don't belong here, I was getting better." "Can you tell me why you think you don't belong?" The patient did not answer. The nurse then said, "Since I don't know why you think you don't belong, I'll tell you what I know. They were concerned about you because they thought you were confused again. You left the ward for the dentist's office but you got lost somewhere, and, to be sure you are protected, they transferred you here. Does any of this make sense to you?" "It makes sense, but I didn't get lost and I wasn't confused. I was scared—afraid of that damn drilling. I was shaking all over and I just couldn't get up nerve enough to go. I sat in the corner of the coffee shop for hours hoping I'd find the courage to go. Finally, about 2:30, I felt better and went to the clinic, but they couldn't take me. They told me they would make another appointment."

As Ida Joan Orlando has observed:

The head nurse's positive feeling of concern for the patient's safety was based on her incorrect thought from observation of the patient, a conclusion she assumed was correct but which was based on insufficient data. The fact that the patient did not answer her questions and did not keep his appointment did not mean that he was confused. As soon as the basis of concern was explored with the patient, he was able to clarify the meaning of what had been observed. Had the head nurse pursued her exploration of the patient's behavior at the onset and learned that the patient was scared, she may still have felt concern, but a different nursing action would have been decided upon. Thus, a positive feeling unexpressed and not explored with the patient did not benefit him. The patient's distress became known when the feeling of concern and its basis were explained, and he in turn was invited to respond with his own meaning.[15]

STEREOTYPING

People's backgrounds and experiences affect the ways in which they collect and arrange or store data about people; this difference in processing observed information thus influences ways individuals respond to others. This process is called stereotyping.

During an active day, a nurse may meet a number of new acquaintances—patients, physicians, other nurses, aides, and others. As a nurse perceives these people, the nurse will attempt to carry certain impressions. There are so many new items of information that it is absolutely necessary to generalize and simplify: Mr. Jones in 407 is an "old man"; the new supervisor is "friendly" but also "firm" in manner; the new surgeon is "very demanding." Walter Lippmann once described such stereotypes as "pictures in the head." All people use them because they permit them to classify people in more or less ready-made compartments; such stored data are used to guide one in initiating interaction or responding to others when they address one.

Use of stereotypes is necessary and useful but imposes a possible communication danger. One may be "biased" or "unjust" if one classifies a person too soon or on too little information or refuses to change an opinion when new, conflicting data become available. The necessary simplification of Mr. Jones as an "old man" may blind one to the innumerable differences between "old men." This blindness is often obvious when categories based on race, national origin, and sex are used. Everyone should realize that this categoric process of perceiving people is not a method used only by prejudiced people. Everyone does it to a greater or lesser degree because everyone has to; it is necessary because of the limits of one's perceptual process. A judgment of the competence of a particular physician, or the capability of a specific nurse, or the willingness to cooperate on the part of a certain patient—each of these is the application of the ability to note certain relevant characteristics, fit them into prelearned categories, and infer additional characteristics of that individual person. In everyday experiences, people must make tentative inferences rather quickly in order to respond in appropriate ways: One sees a long, white coat with a stethoscope hanging out of the pocket and reacts without thinking very carefully: it's a physician. Mostly, such behavior serves fairly well. However, you might want to consider more carefully your reaction to some of these data: a bumper-sticker that says, "I don't get mad—I just get even"; bearded men on a staff-review board; an unmarried physician over age 30; a "no pets" requirement in an advertisement for an apartment for rent; or two female nurses living together.

Data collection and storage are simplified by stereotyping; in this way, individuals can more easily ready themselves for appropriate responses to particular persons. The danger inherent in this process is that one or two aspects of a person (e.g., age and sex) are noted and then this person is assumed to have other characteristics that are associated with this category of persons. Such judgments tend to ignore the differences that all people feel make them unique individuals, especially when they do not have the assumed characteristics—for example, old man, but also (perhaps) assumed aspects such as dirty, cantankerous, senile, and so forth. Actually, an assumed set of *desirable* characteristics such as nice, honest, agreeable, cooperative, and considerate can lead to considerable difficulty for a nurse when an "old man" does not live up to such assumptions.

There is a kind of "probabilities principle" in stereotyping that tends to govern impressions until additional data are available. While all individuals employ the principle, they must be very careful of two serious problems. First, stereotyping tends to diminish the likelihood of noticing gradations of differences among people. People tend to think in "allness" terms. Rather than looking for subtle differences, they try to fit people into general categories, and this guides responses. People may very easily allow one character trait or set of behaviors of which they disapprove—the head nurse is an alcoholic—to keep them from seeing numerous admirable characteristics of that person. Thus, all drinkers may be viewed as degenerates. To some degree, society promotes a two-valued orientation toward other people. Television and movie heroes are often portrayed as all good and the villains without redeeming qualities. People may think they have become too sophisticated to identify with white cowboy hats, but they should think twice: What about Quincy, Luke Skywalker, Johnny Carson, Len Dawson, Martha Rogers, or Richard Nixon? Do you easily categorize such people as good or bad, honest or dishonest, attractive or unattractive? When acquaintances are viewed as American or un-American, saved or damned, wholesome or degenerate, perceptual capabilities are narrowed. To force a person into honest-dishonest, dependable-undependable categories ignores numerous possible degrees between such extremes and limits the likelihood of making an appropriate response to the actual person. How would you perceive Dr. Spock if he were appointed to your state board of nursing?

One should be aware of what is commonly called the "halo effect." It is a special way of perceiving a person in which one very positive characteristic colors one's perception of various other characteristics of that person. As an hypothetical example, suppose you imagine Jane Farber, a nursing supervisor, who works in a hospital with which you are familiar. Nurses and physicians never seem to notice that Jane is sometimes inept, occasionally undependable, once in awhile inaccurate in her reports, and inclined at times to have a snippy, sharp tongue in her discussions with colleagues. Knowing Jane, you probably are pretty much unaware of these less than desirable traits—Jane introduced primary nursing into that hospital and is widely known for improving the quality of nursing care and promoting nursing as a vital service to clients. One physician complained about Jane giving him misinformation about a patient; you thought he was just jealous of Jane's reputation. Everyone should beware of putting haloes on heroes; all relevant information should be included in forming one's image of them—at least, in so far as possible.

A second inherent danger in stereotypes is that they tend to produce self-fulfilling prophecies about people. If a patient is perceived as unable to be cooperative, one tends to treat that person in a way that makes it more difficult for the person to be cooperative. Putting people into erroneous categories tends to perpetuate erroneous myths about them. Suppose that you are a woman, and a physically strong person. But, in your culture, the claim has been made that women are biologically the "weaker sex." Instead of encouraging you to develop and increase your natural strength, people in your culture reinforce your "weakness" by teaching you not to be physically competitive in weight-lifting and track. Political scientist Warren Farrell cites some of the effects:

> To create a myth of weak women when that myth suits economic purposes and destroy it when it does not is a highly cynical use of human potential and aspiration. If this is a form of cynicism, it perpetuates every socializing agent: Television commercials of women with whiter wash for the satisfaction of role number one (woman as a fulfilled washing machine) and soap manufacturer's budget; for role number two (woman as a fulfilled sex object) our woman is transformed into a seductive tigress to be had along with an over-horsepowered, convertible sports car—"a machine made for a man."

Such a self-fulfilling mythic prophecy extends to interpretations of behaviors of men and women even when the behaviors are the same. When a man has a picture of his family on his desk, it is a reflection of a solid family man. A picture on a woman's desk reflects a woman more concerned with her home than her job—"a doting mother at heart." When a man's desk is cluttered, he is thought a busy, overburdened executive; when a woman's desk is cluttered, she is a disorganized, scatterbrained female. And what are the implications when a nurse does not even have a desk? When a man talks about his colleagues, he is engaged in constructive evaluations; when a woman does the same, she is a gossip.

Even women's perceptions of behaviors of other women are influenced by such myths. In a study at the University of Connecticut, 40 college women were given the same writing selection to evaluate, but half of them were told that it was by John T. McKay, while the other half were told it was by Joan T. McKay. John was rated as much more intelligent and persuasive than Joan, even though there was no difference in the material other than the author's name.[17] Because people have a tendency to react on the basis of stereotypes, it is important to recognize the dangers inherent in their use. People should continually remember that their perceptions are thus filtered.

FORMING IMPRESSIONS

As impressions of other people are formed, two very important principles are at work: (1) *selective perception* is used, and (2) *congruence* is sought among the data perceived.

Selective perception is a process whereby choices are made in attributing important meanings of the innumerable items of information available about another person. In an oversimplified way, one can generalize that "we see what we want to see and hear what we want to hear." An important experiment by Solomon Asch attempted to determine how people form impressions of one another. The experimenter read to some college students a number of characteristics that were said to belong to an unknown person. For example, one iist included such adjectives as "energetic," "assured," "cold," "inquisitive," "talkative," "ironical," and "persuasive." After the list was repeated a second time, and the word "warm" was substituted for "cold," the subjects were then instructed to write a description of their impression of this person. One student wrote:

> He impresses people as being more capable than he really is. He is popular and never ill at ease. Easily becomes the center of attraction at any gathering. He is likely to be a jack-of-all-trades. Although his interests are varied, he is not necessarily well versed in any of them. He possesses a sense of humor. His presence stimulates enthusiasm and very often he does arrive at a position of importance.

Another subject reported:

> He is the type of person you meet all too often: Sure of himself, talks too much, always trying to bring you around to his way of thinking, and with not much feeling for the other fellow.

Thus, the discrete terms of the list were organized into a single, unified picture. The subjects even gained impressions about characteristics not mentioned ("He possesses a sense of humor"). Asch summarized his study as follows:

> When a task of this kind is given, a normal adult is capable of responding to the instruction by forming a unified impression. Though he hears a sequence of discrete terms, his resulting impression is not discrete.[18]

When people who are complex are confronted in real life and the observations made of them provide complex and often contradictory data, some people have difficulty in developing a unified impression that reflects all the available data. Individuals seek congruence of the data within their impression, and sometimes achieve it by ignoring some of the data. Another experiment involved a motion picture showing a young woman in five different scenes, each designed to portray divergent aspects of her personality. In the first scene, she is shown being "picked up" in front of a shabby hotel; in the second, she is going to a bar with a man different from the one who had "picked her up"; the third scene shows her giving aid to a woman who has fallen down a public stairway; the fourth shows her giving money to a beggar; and the final scene shows her walking and talking with another young woman. The film was shown to a group of college students, and they were asked to write their impressions of the woman's personality. The investigators then divided the responses into three categories:

1. UNIFIED. The major character qualities of sexual promiscuity and kindness were able to be integrated by 23 percent of the respondents.
2. SIMPLIFIED. Forty-eight percent of the subjects retained only one of the two major character qualities.
3. AGGREGATED. Twenty-nine percent of the subjects kept both major character qualities but failed to unify their impression.

Approximately half of the subjects in this experiment chose to neglect entirely important observations in order to achieve a *congruent* impression of the woman.[19]

The first impression often causes the use of subsequent contradictory data to be ignored. In a study by social psychologist A.S. Luchins, two paragraphs were read separately to different groups of subjects. In one paragraph Jim was portrayed as extroverted, and in the other as introverted. Those who heard the first paragraph pictured Jim as friendly and somewhat extroverted; subjects hearing only the second paragraph correctly viewed Jim as more introverted. To determine the importance of the first impression of a person, the two paragraphs were combined in two patterns—one citing the extrovertive data first and the other citing the introvertive first. Consistently, the data presented first had the greater impact on the subjects' perception of Jim. On the trait of "friendliness," for example, 90 percent of the people who heard the first paragraph noted Jim to be friendly, as did 71 percent of the subjects hearing the combined paragraph with the extrovertive data first. Only 25 percent of the subjects who heard only the second paragraph thought Jim to be friendly; 54 percent of the people who heard the combined paragraph with the introvertive data first considered Jim friendly. Thus, with the only variable being the order of the data presentation, the composite impression of Jim differed markedly.[20]

It appears that a "mental set" is obtained about a person from the first information perceived; it seems hard for some people to change an impression once formed. If in one's mind one initially accepts Jim as friendly, one seems to create special circumstances to account for his later actions. Perhaps he had a bad day at school or is otherwise bothered by something. An attempt is made to fit the conflicting pieces of data together by inferring what is going on inside Jim. On the other hand, if one initially reacts to Jim as unfriendly, one may view his later actions as merely fulfilling some ulterior base motive. Consider how one's impression of Jim would greatly affect one's response to and communication with him.

In an effort to achieve a congruent, simplified impression of a person, one's expectations and later predictions help one to choose to see, internalize, and believe selected data. As everyone knows, upon first contact with another person, a variety of nonverbal and verbal messages are exchanged. The initial moments of contact between strangers tend to be very important. Communication researcher Charles Berger states:

> We believe that the first few minutes of verbal and nonverbal communication between strangers may determine, at least under some conditions, whether persons will be attracted to each other, and by implication, whether the persons involved in the interaction will attempt to communicate at a future time.[21]

When, for example, you meet a client for the first time and you have to work with the client and vice versa, perhaps for years, how long does it take for a first impression to be formed that may have long-lasting influence on your relationship with one another? The first 4 minutes is cited by some researchers as being so crucial that it will determine whether strangers will become coworkers only, good friends, or even lovers. Leonard and Natalie Zunin write:

> Why four minutes? It is not an arbitrary interval. Rather it is the average time, demonstrated by careful observation, during which strangers in a social situation interact before they decide to part or continue their encounter. By watching hundreds of people at parties, offices, schools, homes, and in recreational settings, I discovered that four minutes is approximately the minimum breakaway point—the socially acceptable period that precedes a potential shift of conversational partners.[22]

Berger questions the accuracy of the four-minute estimate, and in a systematic study of initial interaction, he discovers that the content of the first few minutes between strangers is dominated by "demographic" data, that is, information about the backgrounds of the people (home towns, families, academic majors, and so forth). This concern suppresses the opportunity to pass other kinds of information during the first few minutes. After about 5 minutes, these demographic comments decrease and content shifts to topics of attitudes, opinions, and other people. Other topics, such as hobbies, future plans, and personality discussions, are rare during the first 10 minutes of interaction.[23] Although Berger and the Zunins do not agree on the relative importance of the first 4 minutes, they and other researchers generally agree that within a very short part of the first encounter, strangers can form impressions of one another that will significantly influence further interaction between them.

Do you consider yourself to be a reasonably attractive person? Do other people tend to see you as fairly attractive? If you are a woman and find yourself to be seen as quite attractive, you may be feeling quite negative about it, saying that you want people to know you for what you can do (competent, intelligent, skillful nurse, and so forth) rather than "to see only my body."

Everyone can readily sympathize with feelings of resentment toward persons who see you only as a sex object. However, you may be more fortunate than you realize if people see you as an attractive person as well as a nurse. Research has quite clearly shown that the single most important factor in influencing initial positive attitudes between people is perceived physical attractiveness. And people who are seen as attractive are seen as significantly more capable, intelligent, and of good character than persons seen as unattractive. In the research literature, one finds the cliche (not always true but significantly dependable) that persons "seen as good-looking are also seen as smart and good."

Perception of physical appearance has significant impact on first impressions. In many cases, other characteristics are neglected, ignored, or perceptually distorted to accommodate an impression of physical good looks. In this culture, people often try to remind themselves to look beyond this first impression, to give proper consideration to other personal characteristics. Even so, studies tend to indicate that beauty or handsomeness is also perceived as good, intelligent, and worthwhile. Everyone (especially those who do not look like a favorite movie star) should remember, however, that an appearance that is attractive to some people is seen by others as unattractive, and vice versa; thus, there is opportunity for all or most people to be seen as attractive by somebody.

ESTIMATED RELATIONSHIP POTENTIAL

Think for a moment about a new acquaintance you have met in recent days. Focus on a specific person. Would you like to see that person again? Get better acquainted? Would you rather not get involved with that person? To some extent, people are conscious of what they are doing as they meet a new person. Usually, they more or less subconsciously "size the person up," think of what further interaction with the individual would be like, and decide whether it might be an enjoyable or satisfying relationship. In such a case, they are making an estimate of the relationship potential.

What kinds of people are rated high in the estimated relationship potential? Research generally indicates that individuals give higher estimates to persons who are perceived to be more similar to them. Perceptual filters play a role in these estimates. People tend to like persons who have attitudes similar to their own. At the same time, people tend to perceive themselves as being more similar to people they like than they really are—people like what they see and notice those things about themselves that are somewhat similar.[24]

One study attempted to determine why people seek out people like themselves and avoid dissimilar ones.[25] The researchers reasoned that individuals might more often choose to associate with people different from themselves if they were not afraid of being disliked. When the other person is unknown, people are afraid that their behavior will be unacceptable and fear "being themselves." In the study, college students were informed that they had been assigned to one of several groups set up to discuss why people dream. The students could elect to participate in a group of students similar to themselves or in a group composed of such people as psychologists, factory workers, and so on, quite different from the student population. The variable was the information given the students as to whether members of the dissimilar group would probably like or dislike them. As might be guessed, those students who had been assured that everyone would find them likable were more willing to join with dissimilar people, greatly preferring dissimilar groups. Those students who had been told that they would probably not be liked were more anxious to join student groups made up of people like themselves. It was also found that if students were told that it was important to talk with people who would like them, they more often chose to interact with similar than with dissimilar people. Apparently, they assumed that similar people were more likely to like them than were dissimilar people.

As estimates of one another's potential for satisfying needs or desires in a relationship are made, the evident emphasis on physical attractiveness can leave some people seen as less attractive very unhappy. One university coed has stated:

> One of the greatest troubles is that men here, as everywhere, I guess, are easily overwhelmed by physical beauty. Campus glamor girls have countless beaux flocking around them, whereas many companionable, sympathetic girls who want very much to be companions, and eventually wives and mothers, but who are not dazzling physically, go without dates and male companionships. Many who could blossom out and be very charming never have the opportunity. Eventually, they decide that they are unattractive and become discouraged to the point that often they will not attend no-date functions where they have their best (and perhaps only) opportunity to meet men. I will never understand why so many men (even, or maybe particularly, those who are the least personally attractive themselves) seem to think they may degrade themselves by dating or even dancing with a girl who does not measure up to their beauty standards.[27]

Experiences may tell people and they may cognitively agree that there are many facets to a person that matter in a relationship besides physical beauty, but research tends to tell that perceived physical attraction influences people's estimates of the relationship potential of persons they meet.

RECIPROCAL PERSPECTIVES

Suppose you, as a young nurse, and an older nurse-supervisor work together. Let us say that the work requires that she must request from you information needed to do her work, and you feel you must respond. Communication problems can occur when she sees you responding in a way that is different from how you see your responses. Suppose she sees you responding in a way that makes her distrust your information ("These new graduates don't know how to work hard like I did!"); and suppose you see yourself as being absolutely honest and well informed ("I expect overtime pay when I work double shifts"). An additional issue is about to arise: You see her as responding with condescension and suspicion, both undeserved—as you see it. You control your anger—or most of it—but you can't help responding in part to her inappropriate response to you. How do you think she will respond to your response to her response? And what about tomorrow?

Sometimes people respond to others in terms of roles they think deserve certain kinds of behavior; for example, your nurse-supervisor may believe you "should be submissive and respectful," and you may think she should be "helpful and supportive." Betty and Theodore Roszak have depicted in vivid terms the mutually destructive effects of reciprocal responses in terms of masculine-feminine roles:

> He is playing masculine. She is playing feminine. He is playing masculine because she is playing feminine. She is playing feminine because he is playing masculine. He is playing the kind of man that she thinks the kind of woman she is playing ought to admire. She is playing the kind of woman that he thinks the kind of man he is playing ought to desire. If he were not playing masculine, he might well be more feminine than she is—except when she is playing very feminine. If she were not playing feminine, she might well be more masculine than he is—except when he is playing very masculine. So he plays harder. And she plays . . . softer.[28]

This double attempt to play expected roles that are uncomfortable continues until:

> Her femininity, growing more dependently supine, becomes contemptible. His masculinity, growing more oppressively domineering, becomes intolerable. At last she loathes what she has helped his masculinity to become. At last he loathes what he has helped her femininity to become.[29]

These examples have illustrated how the taking of reciprocal roles or perspectives can force either or both parties into behaviors that can destroy a relationship. Physicians may sometimes force nurses into roles that are destructive to an effective nurse-physician relationship. To some extent, nurses may sometimes assume that physicians will "inevitably" play certain roles (e.g., that of a male chauvinist) and even a very well-intentioned man may find his behavior misunderstood or misinterpreted, and an effective working relationship impossible to achieve. Such destructive reciprocal roles between a nurse and a physician may tend to limit the effectiveness of each. One woman perceived her role as nurse in a physician's office as being very formal, distant, and subordinate yet dignified. The way she played the role of office nurse included all of the stuffiness of an English butler. She responded to directions, asked the physician's preferences, and blandly said "Yes sir, Doctor," similar to classic English butlers. At first, the physician was delighted to have the services of such an attentive nurse who took directions so well. But within a few weeks, he found himself developing numerous preferences. Soon he kept forgetting today what he had liked yesterday: The nurse blandly responded to whatever he said. This was annoying. He found himself giving more detailed directions, and the nurse blandly began to wait for directions rather than take any initiative. That was infuriating. The office routine slowed, and the waiting room became crowded. Some patients left to go elsewhere. That was disastrous. He fired her; she couldn't understand why. After all, she was an excellent nurse and hadn't made any errors.

Taking a very positive and hopeful attitude toward another person is not easy to do in situations like these. It is even more difficult to change your behavior so that the other person may respond to you in a different way. You may need to try to talk over the situation with the other person so that together you can help one another change. Of course, you may simply get a rebuff, being told that you have to grow up and get on with your job. Jack Gibb's research has provided some bases for hope. Gibb has studied climates in small groups; in some cases, the climate was negative and defensive; in other cases, positive and supportive. He found that negative, defensive behaviors tend to produce defensive, negative responses that hurt the accuracy of interpersonal perceptions. As people become angry or anxious, they tend to lose their objectivity—their "perspective." On the other hand, Gibb found:

> The more "supportive" or defense reductive the climate, the less the receiver reads into the communication distorted loadings which arise from projections of his own anxieties, motives, and concerns. As defenses are reduced, the receivers become better able to concentrate upon the structure, the content and the cognitive meanings of the message.[30]

Thus, to a very great extent, each person has a possible opportunity to create the "other person" in one's work relationships. Of course, this will not be true in every case, but it can be true in some. People should challenge themselves to see what can be done in any case.

ORIENTATIONS TOWARD PEOPLE

Most people develop fairly habitual ways of responding to other people. For anyone, this may be a habit of being friendly, even though one does not respond to everyone in this way. This section discusses ways a person responds to others as a general rule. This is called one's interpersonal orientation. This response pattern is closely related to one's typical perception of other people.

In the nursing profession, as for most people in general, many actions immediately or ultimately consist of responses to other people. Nurses must be able to respond to the way a physician views the physician's responsibility—how symptoms or test results of a patient will be interpreted by the physician, how the physician will develop the plan of medical care, and what will be expected of the nurse. The purpose of this section is to review systematically various interpersonal orientations. As the discussion proceeds, you may see yourself falling into one or another category or perhaps somewhere between two polar categories. Certainly, you should be able to think of colleagues or clients who fit one or another of the polar extremes, as well as many who are somewhere in the middle or "gray" areas; even so, you will want to think about those who fit the polar categories—they are most often the ones with whom you are most congenial or with whom you have the most difficulty.

Scholars have developed several different systematic approaches to this issue. Each is slightly different, indicating that this field of study is in the process of being explored but has not become well stabilized. Each approach provides some additional insight into possible understanding and improvement of ways of relating to one another.

OPEN-CLOSED

Milton Rokeach theorized one framework for examining a given person's interpersonal orientation—a continuum extending from closed-mindedness to open-mindedness, depending on the characteristic way in which an individual receives and processes messages from others.[31] The general degree to which a person will change one's attitude toward an object or concept after hearing another person's orientation toward that object or concept is the basis of a scale from open- to closed-mindedness. Extreme closed-mindedness is identified as dogmatism. A dogmatic person is described as follows:

1. Likely to evaluate messages on the basis of irrelevant inner drives or arbitrary reinforcements from external authority, rather than on the basis of considerations of logic; for example, the client who will listen only to the physicians and not the nurses.

2. Primarily seeking information from sources within one's own belief system—for example, "the more closed-minded a Baptist, the more likely it is that one will know what one knows about Catholicism or Judaism through Baptist sources";
3. Less likely to differentiate among various messages coming from belief systems other than one's own—for example, an "extremely radical rightist may perceive all nonrightists as communist sympathizers";
4. Less likely to distinguish between information and the source of the information and likely to evaluate the message in terms of one's perceptions of the belief system of the other person—for example, the young mother who quotes Aunt Minnie, not the nurse, as an authority on bathing babies.

Essentially, the "closed" person is one who rejects any ideas or information from you in an attempt to maintain a rigid system of beliefs. Such a person sees a wide difference between your ideas and the person's own, even though you may see the difference as rather small.

The openness or closedness of a person thus can be an index to the way the person will want you to respond to him or her (agree) and the way the person will respond to you (agree or disagree), depending on how your ideas or behavior are seen as fitting into the person's belief system.

COOPERATIVE-UNCOOPERATIVE

A characteristic response of some people is to be generally cooperative; for some others, to be generally uncooperative; for many people, of course, to be somewhere in between, sometimes one and sometimes the other.

Many situations call for cooperation, for example, when a doctor and nurse are each carrying out their responsibilities in providing care to a client in a hospital operating room. The gain is for the third party, the client. When one is engaged in purchasing an automobile, one is in effect competing to maximize one's purchasing power and to reduce the margin of potential profit for the salesperson. In such situations, one's gain is at the expense of the other party. Other situations, however, involve the potential for mutual gain since all are seeking compatible goals; for example, planning a vacation with the family may involve conflicting ideas, but the outcome of the best possible trip for all is shared mutually. Regardless of situation, some people display orientations of willingness to cooperate or an inherent tendency to compete.

A general attitude of cooperation with other people is significantly influenced by the degree of trust felt toward them. If others and their motives are feared, a defensive, uncooperative response is likely. Only when people trust—are willing to rely on people to achieve a desired objective in a risky situation—is cooperation possible.[32] Such trust can be shown from a classic example that has been labeled "the prisoner's dilemma":

> Two suspects are taken into custody and separated. The district attorney . . . points out to each that he has two alternatives: to confess to the crime the police are sure they have done or not to confess. If they both do not confess then the district attorney states that he will book them on some trumped-up charge . . . if they both confess, they will be prosecuted, but he will recommend less than the most severe sentence; but if one confesses and the other does not, then the confessor will receive lenient treatment for turning state's evidence, whereas the latter will get the "book" slapped at him.[33]

The situation described above might be compared with disarmament talks between nations, or with the willingness to cooperate requested of a diabetic patient working with you in learning to take care of the patient's own health-care needs.

It is necessary to realize that some people are very competitive and tend to view all interpersonal relationships as situations in which they either win or lose; obviously, they individually wish to win. Perhaps the saddest cases in this domain are those persons who have concluded that "It is not enough that I should win, but all my friends must fail."

A classic body of research on cooperation/competition was compiled by Morton Deutsch.[34] He studied human behavior in gaming situations in which subjects could win or lose, but possibly win most by mutually cooperating; thus, to cooperate meant mutual gain for both parties in the game, while individual gains could be made by being competitive at the other person's expense. From Deutsch's work and that of his students and associates, the following inferences can be drawn concerning interpersonal cooperation:

1. A cooperative (or noncooperative) orientation on the part of the individual will influence his tendency toward actual cooperative behavior.[35]
2. Communication between the speaker and listener will tend to increase the likelihood of cooperation between them, especially if they express their intentions and expectations of each other and indicate their plan of reacting to violations of their expectations.[36]
3. Increased social power over another person increases the likelihood of the powerful person cooperating with the person over whom he has power.[37]
4. A person will tend to cooperate with another person if he knows they both dislike a specified third person.[38]

5. Cooperative persons tend to have personalities which can be characterized as below average in authoritative or dogmatic orientations.[39]

A further inference can be drawn regarding the interpersonal behavior of nurses. Your work with clients, as well as with peers and colleagues of other health-care professions, requires that you be cooperative much of the time. For them to be cooperative with you and not surprise you with fits of defensiveness or sudden attacks designed to "beat" you in some competitive orientation, you will need to gain and hold their trust.

MOVING TOWARD, AWAY, OR AGAINST

A very useful classification of interpersonal styles was developed by the well-known psychiatrist Karen Horney.[40] She classified people into three types according to their interpersonal response traits: (1) moving toward others, (2) moving against others, and (3) moving away from others. According to Horney's system, *going toward* others ranges from mild attraction to affiliation, trust, and love. Such a person shows a marked need for affection and approval and a special need for a partner, that is, a friend, lover, husband, or wife who is to fulfill all expectations of life and to take responsibility for good and evil. This person "needs to be liked, wanted, desired, loved; to feel accepted, welcome, approved of, appreciated; to be needed, to be of importance to others, especially to one particular person; to be helped, protected, taken care of, guided."[41]

Behavior identified as *going against* others ranges from mild antagonism to hostility, anger, and hate. Such a person perceives that the world is an arena where, in the Darwinian sense, only the fittest survive and the strong overcome the weak. Such behavior is typified by a callous pursuit of self-interest. The person with this interpersonal orientation needs to excel, to achieve success, prestige, or recognition in any form. According to Horney, such a person has "a strong need to exploit others, to outsmart them, to make them of use to himself." Any situation or relationship is viewed from the standpoint of "what can I get out of it?"[42]

Behavior characterized as *going away* from others ranges from mild alienation to suspicion, withdrawal, and fear. With this orientation, the underlying principle is that one never becomes so attached to anybody or anything that the person or thing becomes indispensable. There is a pronounced need for privacy. At a hotel, such a person rarely removes the "Do Not Disturb" sign from outside the door. Self-sufficiency and privacy both serve the outstanding need, the need for utter independence. The person's independence and detachment have a negative orientation, aimed at not being influenced, coerced, tied, or obligated. To such a person, according to Horney, "to conform with accepted rules of behavior or to additional sets of values is repellant. . . . He will conform outwardly in order to avoid friction, but in his own mind he stubbornly rejects all conventional rules and standards."[43]

Horney summarizes the three types as follows:

Where the compliant type looks at his fellow men with a silent question, "Will he like me?"—and the aggressive type wants to know, "How strong an adversary is he?" or "Can he be useful to me?"—the detached person's concern is "Will he interfere with me? Will he want to influence me or (will he) leave me alone?"[44]

It is quite clear that most people display more than one of these three interpersonal response patterns at different times toward different people. However, it is quite surprising how easily acquaintances can be classified. Some of them seem to be clearly giving primary consideration to one of the following questions:

1. "Will they like me?"
2. "How can I beat (or use) her or him?"
3. "Will they bother me?"

MEETING ONE'S INTERPERSONAL NEEDS

Perhaps you have realized that each of the previously discussed orientations toward people is, in one way or another, related to the personal needs of the people who hold them: Uncooperative people are fearful and defensive because they need to preserve status, face, reputation, gain, "winning," and so forth.

Considering directly people's needs as a possible source of interaction style or orientation toward other people, William Schutz advanced a more elaborate systematic approach.[45] The major premise of his theory is that people need people; and each person, from childhood on, develops a fundamental interpersonal relations orientation. Schutz posited three fundamental dimensions of interpersonal behavior: inclusion, control, and affection. His analysis of the results of a large number of research studies—parental, clinical, small-group—shows convergence in their discovery of the importance of these three areas and demonstrates how a measure of these three variables can be used both to test a variety of hypotheses about interpersonal relations and to understand and predict communication behavior.

Each of these three areas can be divided into two parts: the behavioral characteristics that the individual actively expresses toward others and the degree to which the individual wishes such behavior to be directed toward oneself.

INTERPERSONAL COMMUNICATION IN NURSING

Inclusion concerns the entrance into associations with others. The need for inclusion involves being interested in other people to a sufficient degree that others are satisfactorily interested in oneself. Behavior aimed at gaining inclusion is seen as an attempt to attract the attention and interest of others.

The need to control includes the ability to respect the competence of others and the need to be respected by others. It is the need to feel adequate and reliable. Control behavior implies decision-making and is identified by such terms as "authority," "influence," "dominance," "submission," and "leadership."

Affection, unlike inclusion and control, occurs primarily between two people (at a time). It includes the need to love and to be loved. Degrees of affectionate behavior are implied in the terms "friendliness," "caring," "liking," "hate," "loving," and "emotional involvement."

To have satisfactory interpersonal relationships, according to Schutz, in each of these three areas the individual must establish a balance between the amount of behavior actively expressed and the amount that is desired to be received from others.

Schutz's theory has been shown to be significant in efforts to help people understand the basis of their current relationships with others. From this theory, they can infer that others respond to them within the framework of the role they indicate others should take. For example, a nurse-supervisor may indicate to others that she wishes from others (especially nurses) little inclusion, no control over her, and very little affection. Within this framework you are supposed to respond to her. What about *your* interpersonal needs, that is, personal needs you want to have met by others? Who will satisfy them? When? Just in passing, this conclusion might be suggested: Organizations (especially hospitals) are not equipped ordinarily to supply love. Your affection needs may have to be met elsewhere.

SUMMARY

People meet and become newly acquainted with different persons. As individuals come into contact with one another, they receive sensory signals that establish the basis for their communication. Attempts at communication will be guided by individuals' interpretation of these signals, "interpersonal perceptions," the way individuals view and evaluate each other in direct interaction.

While all the sense receptions form the basis for a variety of perceptual cues, interpersonal perception differs from perception of objects in at least two ways: First, unlike objects, other people are perceived as having motives that influence their behaviors; second, the person being perceived is simultaneously perceiving the other person and may alter his or her behaviors accordingly.

When one person responds in a specific way to another person, this manner of response might be termed a type of interpersonal orientation. However, the concern of this chapter has been with the way in which a person or persons generally respond to other people—an interpersonal lifestyle. This interest might be seen as on the wholesale, rather than the retail, level. Sets of typical interpersonal responses may be identified, classified, observed, and analyzed. Basic classifications of interpersonal response sets are commonly recognized by everyone: People note that a person is generally cooperative or competitive, generally open to new friends and ideas, or usually closed to these situations. Individuals may orient themselves toward other people to satisfy interpersonal needs identified as inclusion, control, and affection. A case is made for the proposition that these needs, as described, constitute a conceptual system that is helpful in the prediction and explanation of interpersonal behavior. And it is proposed further that the interpersonal perception and orientation of the nurse will influence the way others interact with the nurse; it will influence the degree to which one is able to practice humanistic nursing.

REFERENCES

1. M. COOK: *Interpersonal Perception* (Middlesex, England: Penguin, 1971), pp. 13–14.
2. *State of Mind*, published by Ciba Pharmaceutical Products, Inc., Summit, N.J., Vol. I, No. 1 (January, 1957). Reprinted by permission.
3. M. L. KNAPP: *Nonverbal Communication in Human Interaction* (New York: Holt, Rinehart & Winston, 1972), p. 76.
4. G. SIMMEL: "Sociology of the Senses: Visual Interaction," in R. E. PARK AND E. W. BURGESS, EDS.: *Introduction to the Science of Sociology* (Chicago: University of Chicago Press, 1921), p. 358.
5. KNAPP: *Nonverbal Communication*, p. 138.
6. P. F. SECORD: "Facial Features and Inference Perception," in R. TAGIURI AND L. PETRULLO, EDS.: *Person Perception and Interpersonal Behavior* (Stanford, Calif.: Stanford University Press, 1958), pp. 300–318.
7. E. A. HAGGARD AND K. S. ISAACS: "Micromomentary Facial Expressions as Indicators of Ego Mechanisms in Psychotherapy," in L. A. GOTTSCHALK AND A. H. AUERBACK, EDS.: *Methods of Research in Psychotherapy* (New York: Appleton-Century-Crofts, 1966).
8. G. W. ALLPORT AND H. CANTRIL: "Judging Personality from Voice," *Journal of Social Psychology*, 5 (1934), 37–55.
9. *Ibid.*, pp. 52–54.
10. D. W. ADDINGTON: "The Relationships of Selected Vocal Characteristics to Personality Perception," *Speech Monographs*, 35 (1968), 499–502.
11. J. P. BARDEEN: "Interpersonal Perception Through the Tactile, Verbal and Visual Modes," paper presented to the International Communication Association, Phoenix, Ariz., 1971.

12. A. MONTAGU: *Touching: The Human Significance of the Skin* (New York: Perennial Library, 1972), p. 273.
13. *Ibid.*, pp. 303–304.
14. W. V. HANEY: "Perception and Communication," *Communication and Organization Behavior*, rev. ed. (Homewood, Ill: Irwin, 1967), pp. 51–77.
15. I. J. ORLANDO: *The Dynamic Nurse-Patient Relationship* (New York: G. P. Putnam's Sons, 1961), pp. 52–58.
16. W. T. FARRELL: "The Resocialization of Men's Attitudes Toward Women's Role in Society," paper presented to the American Political Science Association, Los Angeles, September 9, 1970.
17. P. A. GOLDBERG: "Are Women Prejudiced Against Women?" *Transaction*, April 1968, pp. 28–30.
18. S. E. ASCH: "Forming Impressions of Personality," *Journal of Abnormal and Social Psychology*, 41 (1946): 256–290.
19. E. S. GOLLIN: "Forming Impressions of Personality," *Journal of Personality*, 23 (1954): 65–76.
20. ABRAHAM S. LUCHINS: "Primacy-Recency in Impression Formation," in CARL HOVLAND, ET AL.: *Order of Presentation in Persuasion* (New Haven: Yale University Press, 1957).
21. C. R. BERGER: "The Acquaintance Process Revisited: Explorations in Initial Interaction." Paper presented to the International Communication Association, April, 1974.
22. L. ZUNIN AND N. ZUNIN: *Contact: The First Four Minutes* (New York: Ballantine, 1973), p. 6.
23. BERGER: "Acquaintance Process."
24. E. BERSCHEID AND E. H. WALSTER: *Interpersonal Attraction* (Reading, Mass.: Addison-Wesley Publishing Company, 1969), pp. 69–70.
25. E. WALSTER AND G. W. WALSTER, "Effect of Expecting to Be Liked on Choice of Associates," *Journal of Abnormal and Social Psychology*, 67 (1963): 402–404.
26. S. B. KIESLER AND R. L. BARAL: "The Search for a Romantic Partner: The Effects of Self-Esteem and Physical Attractiveness on Romantic Behavior," in K. GERGEN AND D. MARLOW, EDS.: *Personality and Social Psychology* (Reading, Mass.: Addison-Wesley Publishing Company, 1970).
27. Quoted in E. W. BURGESS, P. WALLIN, AND G. D. SCHULTZ: *Courtship, Engagement and Marriage* (Philadelphia: J. B. Lippincott, 1953), pp. 63–64.
28. B. ROSZAK AND T. ROSZAK: *Masculine/Feminine* (New York: Harper & Row, 1969), p. vii.
29. *Ibid.*, p. viii.
30. J. R. GIBB: "Defensive Communication," *Journal of Communication*, 11, No. 3 (September, 1961): 142.
31. MILTON ROKEACH: *The Open and Closed Mind* (New York: Basic Books, 1960).
32. For a detailed discussion of the dimensions of trust, see K. GIFFIN: "Interpersonal Trust in Small Group Communication," *Quarterly Journal of Speech*, 53 (1967): 224–234.
33. R. D. LUCE AND H. RAIFFA: *Games and Decisions: Introduction and Critical Survey* (New York: John Wiley & Sons, 1957), p. 95.
34. M. A. DEUTSCH: "Trust and Suspicion," *Journal of Conflict Resolution*, 2 (1958): 265–279.
35. M. A. DEUTSCH, "The Effect of Motivational Orientation upon Trust and Suspicion," *Human Relations*, 13 (1960): 123–139.

36. J. LOOMIS: "Communication, the Development of Trust, and Cooperative Behavior," *Human Relations,* 12 (1959): 305–315.
37. L. SOLOMON: "The Influence of Some Types of Power Relationships and Game Strategies upon the Development of Interpersonal Trust," *Journal of Abnormal and Social Psychology,* 61 (1960): 223–230.
38. J. N. FARR: "The Effects of a Disliked Third Person upon the Development of Mutual Trust," paper presented to the American Psychological Association Annual Conference, New York, 1957.
39. M. DEUTSCH: "Trust, Trustworthiness, and the F Scale," *Journal of Abnormal and Social Psychology,* 61 (1960): 138–140.
40. K. HORNEY: *Our Inner Conflicts* (New York: Norton, 1945).
41. *Ibid.,* pp. 50–51.
42. *Ibid.,* p. 65.
43. *Ibid.,* p. 78.
44. *Ibid.,* pp. 80–81.
45. W. C. SCHUTZ: *FIRO: A Three-Dimensional Theory of Interpersonal Behavior* (New York: Holt, Rinehart & Winston, 1958).

3
RESPONDING TO ENVIRONMENTAL FACTORS

In one's daily routine as a health-care professional, one meets a person with whom one would like to spend some time, get better acquainted. Or one may wish to talk things over regarding work or the organization of which one is a member. Or one may need to have a conference to discuss more serious problems involved in the job.

As one contacts such another person and feels the need to have a more or less private talk, one looks at the surroundings and seeks a place that is suitable. One also notes or asks about momentary commitments to others: is one person due to be in another place now or soon? This questioning goes on without thinking much about it because, as adults, people are accustomed to meeting limitations on opportunities to talk with others; people have developed habits of accommodating the physical and social environments.

The aim of this chapter is not to recount the obvious, nor is it to provide a complete catalog of environmental factors that may inhibit or promote interpersonal communication for nurses. The purpose is to identify factors that most severely influence the communication process, calling attention primarily to those that, because they are so obvious or commonplace, may have been overlooked or given too little consideration. The objective is to assist in the understanding of the process of humanistic interpersonal communication, by suggesting ways environmental problems may be handled with greater effectiveness.

PHYSICAL SETTINGS

Certain physical environmental factors obviously influence the process of interpersonal communication. Suppose you wish to "talk things over" with a physician. The question arises: How can you best use the available environment? How can conditions be selected or arranged to serve your purpose best?

ROOMS AND PLACES

As you walk around through almost any hospital or health-care facility, various rooms have ways of giving messages. Some places seem to say, "Sit down and relax; talk things over if you wish." Other places are cold, formal, or barren, and contribute to difficulties in overcoming psychologic distance between people. In many ways, the physical elements influence the behaviors that can be expected in such a place.

When one wishes to talk things over privately with another person, the size and shape of the room selected (or available) exercise significant influence. A large lobby in a hospital suggests that strangers may meet, pass by each other, perhaps smile or nod, but in general exchange only minimum courtesies—what Erving Goffman calls "civil inattention."[1] Here acquaintances may pause briefly for a greeting; friends may greet and show each other calm affection. Lovers warmly embracing appear out of place.

Interpersonal face-to-face interaction is facilitated by a small room, one no larger than necessary to provide a feeling of comfort for a few persons. A larger room tends to suggest that other persons foreign to this particular grouping might enter and diminish the atmosphere of privacy, as in the case of a semiprivate room. To some extent, people tend to feel that if there are only two or three individuals, they should not "tie up" the amount of space afforded by a large room.[2] Mark Knapp has called special attention to the significance of room furnishings, carpeting, and draperies.[3] There is some evidence that interpersonal communication is facilitated in rooms thought to be attractive; pleasing colors can enhance the effect of social interaction. The usual behavior that occurs in many hospital rooms tends to provide an atmosphere that distracts attention, making it more difficult for people to note carefully both the verbal and nonverbal cues necessary for them to consider as they try to understand each other on something more than a surface level.[4] Relatives meeting in a time of crisis at a hospital need a place where private, solemn thoughts can be exchanged.

By their very nature, rooms and places tend to imply a social contract between all persons who enter, a contract regarding the kind of interaction that is supposed to take place within their walls. Thus, semipublic (or semiprivate) places, such as hospital lounges, have a special tone or atmosphere that suggests you may talk to your friends. But there is also a kind of piquant loneliness felt, such that if you have no friends, or none are present, you may talk to others who are similarly lonely. In such a place, some persons are clearly observing the surface rule—talking with friends; others are more or less involved in hopes, fears, and actions that go beyond the surface rule—looking for a stranger with whom to be friendly.[5] In semiprivate hospital rooms, strangers put together by chance occasionally become close friends.

One of the advantages of being in the "management" class of persons working in many hospitals is that for such people interpersonal communication is allowed, sometimes even encouraged.[6] If a nurse is seen chatting, it is supposed that the nurse is doing part of the job—"getting to know" the person, perceiving the other person's problems, gaining insight into the person's needs. An important status line in organizations can be drawn on the basis of who may be allowed to "talk things over with others" or told to "get back to work." Persons who may be told to "get to work" may provide an outward show of activity while surreptitiously attempting to chat with other employees.[7]

In most rooms or places in which nurses work, interpersonal communication possibilities are institutionalized, that is, regulated and understood as conventional for that spot. Even if persons present are not quite aware of these conventions, they will sense something is amiss if norms are violated. For optimal use of the process of interpersonal communication, one should find a place where face-to-face encounters without interruptions or distractions are common occurrences. Perhaps the best place of all is the living room in your home. For a student nurse away from home, a dormitory room may have to suffice. However, the dormitory lobby is equally unsatisfactory in other ways. Most professional practices have private offices; nurses do not, often even head nurses and supervisors. It is probably true that part of the loneliness expressed by many nurses and the feeling of being continuously "on display" are caused by lack of a place for personal, private communication. One nurse led a grieving teenaged boy to a room so he could cry over his father's death without having to stand in the hallway. He sobbed uncontrollably for a few minutes, leaning his 6-foot-high head on the nurses' 5-foot-high shoulder. Soon, he wiped his face with a cool washcloth the nurse offered, composed himself, and marched out to be a strong support to his mother. But he had to have his private time first. Generally, for nurses, there is no equivalent of a private office, especially in a hospital.[8]

There is a vast amount of literature on the alienation of young people, particularly students who have a sense of loneliness and separation.[9] Little information is available about the impact on nursing students or visitors of ill clients of the unavailability of an equivalent of their living room at home—a place that offers a sense of appropriateness for interpersonal communication of a private or semipersonal nature. Their usual available spaces are a lobby or their sleeping-study room. Of even less attraction are semipublic places such as cafeterias, empty classrooms, or lawns.

Small wonder that people away from home are lonely; they have no home, no place suitable for interpersonal communication. Lobbies, as suggested earlier, are characterized by the interruptions of others walking by, coupled with a sense of a lack of privacy. If something important and personal is said in a low voice so that others nearby can't hear, the simple act of leaning forward to hear produces a feeling that others will interpret this closeness as out-of-place intimacy, inappropriate behavior in a semi-public lobby. Yet this need for intimacy is salient for family and friends of clients and for nurses, too, in relating to them. Few patients can afford private rooms in hospitals, and in many areas only curtains and 6 feet separate patients' beds. For those relatives who stay in the client's room, their very private behaviors—sleeping, changing clothes, and private body functions—are difficult to accomplish. Body odors are often offensive. This is hardly the place to encourage relatives to stay for long periods, yet closeness of the relationship requires this physical proximity in times of stress. The available alternatives—lobby, hallway, or the client's room—tend to provide little privacy or too much too near the client. In part, it appears that many people are distressed covertly because they have no place to overcome their loneliness and to talk things over.

CHAIRS AND TABLES

Whether one is sharply aware of it or not, chairs and tables have a significant influence on the way people interact in face-to-face communication. Chairs have an effect in two respects: physical comfort and psychologic relationship to each other. In a similar fashion, tables (including desks) provide physical convenience as well as psychologic distance between people.

Chairs may be arranged in such a way that they encourage interpersonal communication, if that is the goal desired. They may be placed so that participants face each other and can easily see each other's eyes. An interpersonal encounter starts with the eyes. The eyes provide information to the important first impression and can indicate answers to such questions as, "Does he or she really want to talk to me?" "Is his or her intention friendly, serious, sincere?"

There is a kind of "I-am-willing-to-talk-with-you" ritual that people use to start interpersonal communication. First they come into each other's presence. As they approach, their eyes are scanning the territory—the room, chairs, tables, and places where they may easily talk. When within a few paces of each other, their eyes connect. In the first flash of eye contact, they recognize each other and *show this recognition*. Goffman, perhaps modern sociology's best-known "people watcher," thus describes the ritual for starting interaction:

An encounter is initiated by someone making an opening move, typically by means of a special expression of the eyes. . . . The engagement properly begins when this overture is acknowledged by the other, who signals back with his eyes, voice or stance that he has placed himself at the disposal of the other for purposes of eye-to-eye activity. . . . There is a tendency for the initial move and responding "clearance" sign to be exchanged almost simultaneously.[10]

In another of his writings, Goffman suggests that "when one individual meets the eyes of another he can indicate a position (attitude), perceive the other's response to his taking this position, and show his own response to the other's response all in a brief moment."[11]

The importance of eye contact in interpersonal communication can hardly be overemphasized. It is so significant that if held slightly too long at a time, it can be taken as an intrusion on another's privacy. Staring or glaring can easily be taken as an offense.[12] Additional evidence of the importance of eye contact for personal interaction may be obtained by observing persons who are alienated from those around them, particularly persons who are mentally ill; they commonly express their alienation through avoidance of eye contact.[13]

For interpersonal communication to become optimal, the eye contact used at the beginning of the encounter *must* be maintained. The persons involved *must* have full access to each other's feelings as expressed in visual contact. Studies have shown that the arrangement of chairs in a discussion circle influences interaction; persons sitting side by side tend not to address each other except for side comments, but tend to direct their remarks to persons whose eyes they can see.[14] In conducting health assessment interviews, the nurse whose chair is facing the client, but slightly to one side, can maintain good eye contact and will not convey an overpowering presence; the client can choose to look at the nurse or easily look to the side to "escape" momentarily. In any interpersonal encounter, the arrangement of chairs can have either a damaging or an enhancing effect.

The *distance* between participants in interpersonal communication is also of special significance. Perhaps there is no specific optimal distance; it will likely vary with the participants' attitudes and roles toward each other. If convenient or appropriate, a nurse may move a chair close enough to the patient to feel comfortable while talking with each other; the distance thus chosen may define their perceptions of their relationship, a point to be considered in more detail later. If the available chairs are not easily moved, the distance thus dictated will have subtle influence on the participants' interaction.

Edward and Mildred Hall have carefully observed the distances commonly used for different kinds of human interaction.[15] The Halls divide interaction space into four distances: intimate, personal, social, and public.[16]

Intimate distance, close phase (touching), is the distance for love-making, comforting, and protecting (also struggling or fighting). Intimate distance, far phase (6 to 18 inches), is too close for interaction unless the participants have an intimate relationship; it serves well for those who wish to comfort each other or get to know each other well.[17] It is thus limited to the interpersonal communication of those who wish to become psychologically close—at least for most middle-class Americans.[18] In health care, there is a "permission" granted to nurses and some other professionals to enter this area to provide care, to touch, and to comfort. The fact that nurses are allowed to come so close probably contributes to the belief by many that nurses are "special people."

Personal distance ranges from 18 to 30 inches (close phase) and from 30 to 48 inches (far phase). These distances are used for interpersonal communication by persons who are friendly and favorably inclined toward each other.[19] The far-phase limit (48 inches) is the distance used to keep another person "at arm's length away" and marks the distance at which the dominance of one person by another is less effective. Those who are not afraid of being dominated may move within this range; those who are afraid will not.[20]

Social distance, according to the Halls, ranges from 4 to 7 feet (close phase) and 7 to 12 feet (far phase). Close phase is the distance at which *interpersonal* interaction generally occurs. It is commonly used by acquaintances attending an informal social gathering and is the usual distance maintained by those who work together at impersonal tasks—executives and their secretaries, teachers and their students. Social distance, far phase, is ordinarily used for formal business or social interactions.[21] Incidentally, at this distance, two people may work separately at different tables or desks in a nursing station.

Public distances, close phase (12 to 25 feet) and far phase (more than 25 feet), are used on formal occasions involving public ceremonies. Public figures—kings, presidents, governors, celebrities—may occasionally maintain this noninvolvement distance.[22] Conversely, politicians try to move in closer when seeking votes.

The Halls' analysis of interaction distances provides special insight into the subtle influence of chairs and tables, particularly desks, on interpersonal communication. The uses of personal and social distances tend to vary from culture to culture, to some extent in a rather arbitrary fashion.[23] However, tables and desks almost universally provide distances that separate people psychologically and interfere with personal interaction. People ordinarily thought to be important usually have desks that keep visitors at the far phase (7 to 12 feet) of social distance. People talking across desks in modest offices are 9 to 10 feet apart. At this distance, feedback from each other's eyes is significantly lost.[24] Not lost, however, is the impression of social distance separating the participants—a feeling that closeness, personal involvement, and a sense of interpersonal solidarity might be achieved only with special effort, if at all.[25] As a nurse, you will be accustomed to working at intimate distance; yet recognize that some patients may be initially bothered by such closeness.

Some chairs and tables (or desks) are personal territories, staked and claimed by an individual for one's personal use. They may be the legal property of a hospital or institution; but they are personal territory from 7:00 AM to 3:30 PM, assigned to an individual for one's use. If an acquaintance drops by, even an older personal friend, across that desk that person is a "visitor" no matter how warmly the friend is greeted. The flow of interpersonal communication is subtly influenced by such environmental conditions.[26] A physician may come out from behind the desk to meet patients and talk with them in a "conference corner" equipped with easy chairs, coffee table, side tables, and rug. Such practices are not unknown in industrial circles.[27]

For the typical charge nurse, there is seldom a specific desk or territory that can be claimed as one's own. Typically the desk area, often a long counter, is the place where clients' charts are located, along with all requisition forms, Kardex, telephone, intercom, and the like. The area may seem to "belong" to the head nurse, but usually anyone on the nursing staff may enter the area, particularly other nurses, the unit secretary, the physicians, and others who need access to charts, phone, and so forth. To a great extent, the nurse's work area is similar to that of a gas station attendant—open to the public and easily invaded by all. Many head nurses cannot even claim a chair as their own. Few head nurses and even fewer nursing staff have offices; those who do tend to share the space with another, or it is blatantly a closet. This may covertly communicate a sense of tentativeness to nurses, indicating there really is no "place" for them, and contributes to nurses' feelings of alienation and dissatisfaction and high turnover rates.

TIME

Perhaps you have not thought of time as part of your physical environment. In this culture, however, people are quite accustomed to regulating their behavior in terms of the relative amounts of time required. For example, work crews avoid starting a new task in the late afternoon if it cannot be completed that day. People tend to schedule the day's events with full attention to the time available and the time required. Similarly, use of the process of interpersonal communication is influenced by the sense of available time. Nurses must be aware of the way in which their use of time is likely to be interpreted.

An event such as a team conference regarding a medical patient may serve a special purpose and involve use of special language; such an occasion is essentially a "time-person-space" event, entailing special consideration of *when* certain persons are brought together to use designated space in a certain way. It will not serve your purposes for achieving interpersonal communication to violate the norms connected with such an occasion; in effect, the purposes of the occasion will take precedence over your personal purposes. For example, smiling and exchanging confidences during such a conference would defeat such purposes.

Many occasions involve primarily public communication, and the point is that violating the protocol involved in any specific situation is usually to defeat the purposes of interpersonal communication.

People tend to "tell time"—note its passage—in three ways: by use of clocks; by events that transpire (e.g., before or after lunch); and by the way people act. In an interpersonal encounter, the time available is frequently indicated by the way a person behaves. If one feels one's time is being used for interaction that one doesn't desire, one's hands may clasp and unclasp; one's eyes may wander to "not here, out there" distances; and one's voice may diminish in interest-value cues. In nonverbal ways, the other person is being told to move along. Consumers of health care frequently complain about nurses and others who seem to be in a hurry and who do not seem to listen. And nurses tend to have so many tasks to accomplish that they tend to feel pressured by time passing too quickly.

The influence of the passing or availability of time on interpersonal communication has not received great attention from scholars. Nurses are aware of the importance of talking with people "in time," meeting people "on time," giving medications "on time," and being careful of the ways they "spend their time." They avoid "wasting time" unduly.

When one wishes to engage a person in conversation, there is a kind of "access ritual" used to establish that each is open to the other for at least a brief interchange.[28] Typically, the two persons face each other and their eyes lock for a brief moment. Usually, there is a smile of recognition, perhaps their eyes glisten or crinkle at the corners, and mutual pleasure is shown in some way. As they continue to show mutual willingness to talk with each other, a kind of "time-person-space" contract is subtly understood. If either "lacks the time at this time," a different agreement is necessary if further interaction is to take place.

The practical point to be made on the basis of these observations is that when you desire to talk to someone in particular, you may easily overlook the fact that the other person may be viewing his or her time quite differently from the way you are viewing yours. Patients may be quite anxious to know the outcome of tests that to you are unimportant. A patient may wish to talk with you, but you have other commitments and needs for use of time right now. It is recommended that as soon as the access ritual has taken place, you might well avoid misunderstanding and needless feelings of personal neglect or rejection if you courteously ask, "Are you taking enough time to talk with me? Perhaps you can spend more time with me?"

SOCIAL FACTORS

There are people as well as things in the environment of nurses. Much of your interpersonal communication will take place in the presence of persons other than the one or more persons with whom you wish to talk. For example, you may need to talk to a physician and find difficulty in doing so except in the presence of other nurses or even patients. Such people often can *overhear* what is said. Often, you will be unable to talk with one person alone but only in the presence of a group where that person is in attendance—for example, you may wish to talk with a physician but be able to do so only at the nurses' station where other members of a nursing team, students, or visitors are present. The presence of others, either persons who overhear you or members of a group with whom you interact, can have significant influence on your interpersonal communication behavior.

Almost all interpersonal communication is influenced to some extent by the fact that people are members of various organizations. When two people belonging to the same organization attempt to interact, the norms and regulations of that organization have impact on the behavior of both people. The same is essentially true regarding the influence of a culture, although such influence may be relatively unnoticeable until one meets someone from a culture different from one's own.

This section discusses the influence of those who overhear as well as the influence of membership in groups, organizations, and cultures. The objective is not to review the nature of groups, organizations, or different cultures, but to focus on primary ways they influence interpersonal communication.

WHEN OTHERS ARE PRESENT

Interpersonal communication is a clear-cut form of behavior, such that a third person who is present must be either *within* the interaction or *outside* it.[29] Imagine yourself with a close friend, lying on a beach, gazing at the water, and intermittently chatting with one another. A kind of bond of mutual trust and obligation has been established. You have laid yourself open to confidences and special privileges. In so doing, you have made yourself available, to some extent, to special requests or expectations. In addition, although you may feel quite secure that they won't occur, there is the possibility—though faint—of demands, threats, insults, and false information. In this kind of situation, your openness or availability will change considerably if an unknown person sits down near you and your friend. Perhaps you will feel like leaving the beach, hoping your friend will go along. Such feelings will likely be subtly conveyed to your friend even though not verbalized; in turn, however, the friend may not understand their source and suspect that you do not enjoy the conversation. In this way, your interpersonal communication can be influenced by the presence of others not participating; unless such influences are well understood by both you and your friend, miscommunication and misunderstanding may occur.

The primary effect of the presence of persons who may *overhear* interpersonal communication is inhibition of openness. Individuals may conduct business in the presence of others as long as it does not involve personal affairs, but a great portion of conversations in nursing are personal. People may exchange greetings and impersonal information if it does not impinge on private feelings. In a word, people may be courteous but not personal when persons are present with whom they cannot trust their personal views or feelings. The usual resolution to this problem, of course, is to find a "private space," a room where nonparticipants in the interpersonal exchange can be excluded. Walls, even though sometimes very thin, are a social convention that provide a necessary feeling of privacy and are felt by most people to exclude fairly effectively the influence of those who may be on the other side.[30] Screens in a hospital may partially serve this purpose.

There is a considerable body of experimental research to show that people tend to behave differently in the presence of even passive other persons.[31] Their presence tends to *impair* the learning of new material[32] but *facilitates* the performance of well-learned patterns of behavior.[33] In the presence of passive others, the motivation to do well or "look good" is increased,[34] and the exposure of ideas or feelings that might make one "look bad" is inhibited.[35] In addition, there is significant evidence that behavior that is ordinary or habitual is much more likely to occur in the presence of others than is behavior that is used only rarely or on special occasions.[36] Thus, a quite reasonable conclusion is that making new friendships, exchanging information about our private thoughts, and, in general, opening up selves to others will likely be inhibited if people attempt interpersonal communication in the presence of persons not included in the interaction. This tends to be particularly true in the nurse-client relationship from the client's perspective.

BEING A MEMBER OF A GROUP

Professional nurses very frequently find themselves working in groups or teams whose members together must confront a mutual problem and develop a group solution—make a group decision that the members can cooperatively implement. Such a group may consist entirely of nurses—peers of essentially equal influence in the group. However, very often, various members of such a policy-making group will consist of professionals who are not of equal status or influence: physicians, nurses, psychiatrists, social workers, and sometimes government officials. How does interaction in groups, or even just membership in one or more related groups, influence one's interpersonal communication?

Probably no phase of human behavior has received more study and careful research than human interaction in small groups.[37] Literally thousands of experimental studies have been reported[38] and their results compared.[39] Chapter 7 discusses the dynamics of group interaction. This section focuses on those particular ways interpersonal communication is influenced by groups of which a participant is a member. In this focus, such groups are being viewed as part of the social environment. Actually, a group's influence may be felt by persons engaging in interpersonal communication even though other members of the group are not present, that is, if one or both of the participants are members of the group.

Perhaps before progressing further a brief definition should be given of "group" as it is being used here. The most common definition of "small group" used today in research studies and sociopsychologic literature involves two factors: (1) a small number of persons in interdependent role relations who (2) have a set of values or norms that regulate behavior of members in matters of concern to each other.[10] Thus, in a group, as the term is used, each member is aware of each other member's belonging to the group and is concerned to some extent about one's own behavior as it affects the group.

Two major factors of group membership influence the interpersonal communication of nurses: (1) *conformity* to the norms of behavior established by and for the group members and (2) *task or goal commitments* made by the group members. These factors tend to influence the interpersonal communication of a group member even if one is talking with another person who is not a member of that group.

On the other hand, when a nurse is engaged in discussion with members of one's own group, these two factors—conformity and goal commitments—exercise even greater influence. In such a circumstance, a third factor also has considerable influence on interpersonal communication: the size of the group, that is, the number of group members present. These three factors are discussed briefly in this section—with due apology to the thousands of researchers who have devoted extensive time and energy to many other variables shown to have some relevance. This selection has been made in recognition of the time available to the readers; for those who have greater need or interest, we have prepared another book devoted to a detailed discussion of group interaction.[41]

Two other variables exercise great influence on the interpersonal behavior of nurses in groups: (1) the *power* of one person over another, and (2) *personal attitudes* involving affection or hostility. However, these two variables are not in any sense uniquely a property of group interaction; they are the basic dimensions of any interpersonal relationship and may be easily observed in operation as two persons engage each other in interaction. They are a significant influence on the way a wife interacts with her husband or a nurse with a physician. They are, in fact, those primary variables that determine the specific nature of any interpersonal relationship. There is a vast amount of literature on these two factors in reported studies of small groups. *Power* or influence is frequently discussed as a function of difference in social status, and personal attitudes are often discussed under the rubric of *group cohesiveness,* sometimes that of *interpersonal attraction.* Because these two variables are not unique properties of groups and are pervasive in all interpersonal communication, they are discussed in Chapter 6, "Building Relationships."

Long ago, casual observation suggested that "birds of a feather flock together." However, the degree to which people *change* to be like others with whom they associate was only conjectured. In 1952, Solomon Asch experimentally derived solid evidence for one of the most disturbing of all facets of human behavior.[42] In Asch's primary experiment, college students were asked to look at a black line on a white card, then look at three other lines, and then pick the one of the three that was the *same length* as the first one shown. *One* of the "comparison" lines was *exactly the same length* as the original one. All lines were held in plain sight of the subjects. However, when the subject entered the experimental room, several other students were already present, and the subject was told that all present were there to perform the same task. Unknown to the "naive" subject, the other students present were Asch's confederates, "planted" there to lead the subject astray. The experimental session consisted of 12 trials. In each trial, the confederates were asked to make their judgments *first;* they unanimously selected an incorrect line, erroneous by as much as 1¾ inches. All choices were given orally, *and after the others had individually voiced the unanimous but incorrect opinion,* the naive subject gave an opinion.

Asch's results were astounding. Control subjects working alone achieved about 93 percent accuracy on the same-line judgments. However, naive subjects exposed to erroneous social influence achieved only 67 percent accuracy, a drop of 26 percent. In further experiments, confederates were instructed to give answers incorrect by as much as 7 inches, the original line being 10 inches and the confederates' "choice" being only 3 inches. The results were almost the same. Control subjects were 98 percent accurate. Naive subjects were 72 percent accurate—again a drop of 26 percent! Asch's comment was rather poignant:

> We are appalled by the spectacle of the pitiful women of the Middle Ages who, accused of being witches by authorities they never questioned, confessed in bewilderment to unthought-of crimes. But in lesser measure we have each faced denials of our own feelings or needs.[43]

The work of Asch and others confirms the principle of social conformity in dramatic ways. The essential principle is that subjects agree to, or go along with, the conclusions of others—even decide to act upon them—*even when such decisions are contrary to evidence staring them in the face*. There is really no way of estimating how many people conform to others' decisions that are contrary to their own beliefs and values *if no clear evidence is available*. Additional experiments have shown that conformity tends to increase as the topic for judgment becomes more difficult.[44] As few as three confederates giving unanimous but incorrect answers can produce this effect. And experimental evidence is in no way limited to American college sophomores. Studies have shown that American military officers "yielded" (conformed to incorrect conclusions of experiment confederates) 37 percent; engineers, writers, scientists, and architects did about the same.[45] Norwegian students "yielded" 50 to 75 percent, and French students between 34 and 59 percent.[46] To what extent do you guess that nurses would "yield"?

It should be pointed out that in these studies, the "groups" formed were not bound together by group norms or very much psychologic cohesiveness; they were strangers prior to the experiments. Also, no attempts were made to use personal power or influence; no "leaders" or status persons were identified or chosen. *Under conditions where group norms, cohesiveness, status persons, or leaders are involved, one could expect even greater degrees of social conformity* on the part of the group members. Some support for this conclusion is given in experiments where the experimenter (a sort of leader or status person) also made his or her choice known; when the experimenter chose the erroneous stimulus picked by confederates, the naive subjects yielded about 60 percent![47] Studies of leadership and status influence support this line of reasoning.

Conforming to the behavior of other members of a group is not necessarily undesirable, even when such behavior violates evidence in front of you; when people start to rush out of a building, you may not see the fire but you may save your life if you leave rather than decide they are crazy. "Blind conformity" can sometimes have survival value, and its practice can easily be observed in the animal world: One dog barks at a stranger in the dark, and dogs blocks away pick up the cry. However, in many cases, *blind* conformity to group norms can be less than a proper use of one's intelligence.

If a collection of people can be characterized as a group, certain *norms* and conformity behavior may be identified. The concept of group norms was derived from long usage in sociopsychologic studies. It identifies the ways members of a group behave and ways that are thought by them to be proper. Norms may be viewed as a set of directions bestowed by the group on all its members concerning their behavior. Through interaction, members find out the group's standards. For example, a nurse may be asked to become a member of a case-team: the nurse may find that such membership is important because it improves status and provides opportunities for influence. To be an effective member of the team, the nurse must first determine *what is expected* of members. Such a "period of adjustment" accounts for the fact that freshman Senators in the United States Senate are seen but rarely heard.[48]

The relationship between norms and communication has received considerable attention by students of group communication. Members who do not conform to group norms are initially the targets of greater amounts of communication, usually of an instructional nature; if they continue as nonconformists, the tendency is to give them rejecting communication and eventually little or none. The degree of rejection is a direct function of the cohesiveness of the group and the degree to which the nonconformist is deviant.[49] These results do not hold for just any collection of people, but for groups where belonging is attractive to its members. In some tightly knit, highly cohesive groups, a nonconformist is almost immediately rejected upon detection, in which case communication is both minimal and rejective.

Conformity to group norms is in actuality a yielding to group pressures, explicit or implicit. Conflict arises when the individual tends to react or respond in one way, but group pressures force the individual in another direction. Thus, when a nurse has to express an opinion to peers or colleagues of other professions, or to a group that determines aspects of a plan of care or makes policy in a health-care institution, the nurse may have an opinion that is at variance with other members of the group; the nurse may choose to remain independent of group consensus, and possibly suffer the consequences. Indeed, this is seen as the nurse's professional role—advocate of the client, change agent, and supporter of humanistic values in health-care matters. For example, in some regions it is common today for obstetric services to offer only natural childbirth as an option for care, particularly in public hospitals. With less medication, a small number of nursing staff is required to care for alert clients. This care is less expensive and thus a preferred type of service for welfare and nonpaying clients. Maternal-child bonding and parenting classes are becoming typically the "in" thing. However, as a board member of a home for unwed and rejected teenagers, one of the authors was appalled to learn that the teenaged clients who had decided to give up the baby for adoption were being forced to go through natural childbirth procedures involving the mother-child bonding process. The teenagers were not able to support the child and would be psychologically tied for life to a child that was the result of rape or incest. It seems to be rather cruel to observe societal or community norms that force a child-mother to go through the process of bonding and then have to give up the baby. At the minimum, the humanistic thing to do, it seems, would be to give the teenager the informed choice of natural childbirth or a light anesthesia doing minimal harm to mother or child. Hospital and agency norms cannot cover all situations; the nonconforming nurse can signal needs for change and flexibility. The other option is to conform and watch the pain continue.

When a collection of people systematically meets as a group, there is usually some common goal or task to be accomplished. If communication is poor within the group, there is no effective way of working toward the agreed-on task. A person will work for a group goal only if one believes that its achievement will satisfy one's own wants. Individual studies of the relationship between worker morale and productivity emphasize the importance of the acceptance of group goals and the *perceived relevance* of group goals to individual wants. For example, if a nurse is to be comfortable with one's job on a nursing staff, the nurse must see the philosophy and goals of the nursing department as personally satisfying, that is, congruent or compatible with one's personal goals. Groups in such organizations as health agencies are constantly challenged by problems of task or goal commitment. The feeling that members have toward their goals will not only affect their interaction with each other, but also their interpersonal communication with persons outside the group.

Roles or role functions are commonly conceptualized in the literature on small groups as a set of behaviors related functionally to the goals of the group. Research on experimental groups has demonstrated that roles tend to appear in a relatively short time, require different but specifiable sets of behaviors, and have performance criteria set up by the group members. Factor analysis of a large number of alleged role functions has revealed three major factors:

1. *Individual prominence*—that is, giving and receiving a higher amount of communication;
2. *Aiding group goal attainment*—that is, presentation of "best ideas" and general suggestions for guidance of group thinking; and
3. *Sociability*—that is, the characteristics of being well liked by members demonstrating emotional stability.[50]

The relationship of these roles to communication is quite clear. The role of "prominent individual" correlates with the amount of talking and being talked to by other group members.[51] The amount of verbalization is also correlated with offering best ideas and guidance. However, individuals who achieve the sociability role (i.e., those who are well liked) generally do not give or receive as much verbalization and ordinarily do not present the best ideas for guidance of the thinking of the group.

Role behaviors customarily performed by a member in a group are frequently observed in one's communication behavior with persons outside the group. This is especially true whenever the goals of the group are relevant to the outside interaction.[52]

The variable of group size, that is, the number of members present, may not have much effect on members' interaction outside the group; however, as members engage in interpersonal communication within the group, it has significant influences. Researchers have typically found that as the size of the group increases, the most active participant becomes more and more communicative, identifiable as both a communication initiator and receiver; less participative group members become even less communicative.[53] As size increases, the degree of feedback decreases, producing loss of communication accuracy and increased hostility.[54]

One study examined some correlates of group size in a sample of groups ranging from two to seven members. These groups met four times to discuss problems in human relations. After each meeting, members were asked to evaluate group size as it influenced group effectiveness. Members of five-person groups expressed most satisfaction; members of larger groups felt their groups wasted time and that members were disorderly, aggressive, too pushy, and competitive; members of groups with fewer than five members complained that they avoided expressing their ideas freely through fear of alienating one another.[55]

These studies were limited to decision-making task groups. However, other studies with "opinion" problems tended to confirm these results; they also showed communication behaviors different for odd-numbered versus even-numbered groups in degrees of disagreement and antagonism. An even-numbered opinion split in a small group of two, four, or six members may produce impasse, frustration, and unwarranted hostility. This difficulty was most marked in groups of only two members, a fact that should have relevance for marriage partners as well as continuing medical teams.[56]

How does group size influence productivity in creative groups? One researcher found that larger groups produced a greater number of ideas, though not in proportion to the number of members; that is, there were eventually diminishing returns from the addition of members. Perhaps as the size of the group increased, a larger and larger proportion of the group members experienced inhibitions that blocked participation. The researcher also noted that if he deliberately undertook to increase inhibitions by formalizing group procedures, the number of ideas contributed was reduced.[57] Additional information on discussion in small groups is provided in Chapter 7.

INFLUENCE OF THE ORGANIZATION

There are many similarities between the ways a nurse's communication is influenced by a being member of a group and being a member of an organization. This discussion uses the term *organization* to denote a combination of interrelated groups comprising an integrated social unity such as a total hospital. This unit, like a group, has norms and conformity influence. In most organizations, those factors providing greatest impact on the communication behavior of their members are similar to those factors most influential in small groups: conformity and goal commitments. In actual operation, they take these forms: (1) an emphasis on achieving the organization's goals—"getting the job done"; (2) suppression of discussion of interpersonal problems; (3) insensitivity regarding one's impact on the feelings of those around oneself; (4) avoidance of taboo topics; and (5) creation of a climate of distrust. Perhaps these concepts can be made less abstract by reporting an interview held recently with a former student. Ten years ago, Phyllis was hired as a supervisory trainee by a large hospital. She was interviewed recently by one of the authors who later visited Phyllis's hospital at her invitation and surveyed conditions there.

In Phyllis's hospital, it is believed that important communication is concerned with the primary objective: *getting the job done*. Phyllis's communication is designed to be rational, objective, unemotional. She believes that her personal effectiveness will decrease if interpersonal attitudes are exposed and discussed; the keynote is, "Let's keep feelings out of our discussions." Phyllis keeps her communication with others impersonal through the use of informal suggestions and little penalties.

The hospital's suppression of discussion of interpersonal problems has influenced Phyllis's interpersonal behavior. She has learned to hide, suppress, and disown her own interpersonal attitudes: "I didn't really mean it to sound that way." She has developed ways of keeping other people from discussing interpersonal problems: "Let's not get into personalities." Phyllis has difficulty in handling situations in which personal attitudes are expressed; afterward, she asks herself, "I wonder what he meant by that?" Phyllis avoids or refuses to consider new ideas involving human values: "I wouldn't want to get into that sort of thing." She tends to avoid *any* new idea for fear personal attitudes *might* become involved: "I never like to rock the boat." She avoids experimentation and risk-taking with new ideas that might involve value judgments: "Let's do it the safe way." She has become unaware of the impact on other people of her own inner feelings: "I wonder why he thinks I don't like him." In Phyllis's unit, most interpersonal problems go unresolved; they tend to recur and have been increasing over time. One of Phyllis's employees said, "Those people at the front office certainly don't like each other."

Phyllis is quite unaware of the impact of her personal attitudes toward other persons; she is also poor at predicting the impact on herself of the personal attitudes of others toward her. Thus, she occasionally shows the following:

1. Surprised confusion: "Why did she get sore over that?"
2. Frustration: "How can you talk with a guy like that?"
3. Heroic attempts at "objectivity": "My plan is really very simple."
4. Mistrust of others: "You just can't trust people like that."

Phyllis has adopted certain "play it safe" behaviors. She avoids intentional communication of her personal attitudes toward others. She ignores (or frowns at) communication of interpersonal attitudes by others. She tries to communicate "very clearly"; this means that she discusses only those ideas for which there is a clear hospital policy. She affirms values thought to be held by her superiors: "Yes, I think Mr. _____ would see it that way." She gives only tentative commitments to any direct question, especially one involving a new idea. She has gathered around her a group of employees whose communication behavior is similar to her own. Her support of her superiors lacks "commitment from within," which might involve personal warmth. As you can see, Phyllis is not winning personal regard or trust for herself.

In Phyllis's situation, mistrust, conformity, conditional commitment, and dependence have operated in a circular fashion and now feed on themselves. The presentation of technical data is being substituted for the exploration of interpersonal problems. Careful, close supervision and "sticking to the rules" have replaced any real attempts at teamwork on decisions and policies. Phyllis resists any suggestion of organizational change unless it is proposed by a superior; in such a case, she gives an indefinite, "sir, I believe so." Phyllis makes no decisions or changes until absolutely necessary, that is, only when a crisis occurs. In such cases (two witnessed), Phyllis's communication of emotion is high—too high for the situations; Phyllis's emotional outbursts are only temporarily fruitful. Phyllis mistrusts her superiors and peers, and her *modus operandi* has become defensive behavior designed to avoid any possible crisis.

Perhaps you may think that Phyllis's organization and its influence on her interpersonal behavior are unique or unusual. Our observation, as well as careful studies, shows that it is rather ordinary for older, established organizations.[58] Many points could be emphasized about organizational impact on interpersonal communication; however, it is felt that they have been adequately identified in the description of Phyllis's hospital and her behavior. If you believe you need further evidence of these influences, look closely at your health agency and nursing service department. The odds are you will see supportive evidence all around you, with the exception of rare and special individuals—perhaps some of your nurses.

A DIFFERENCE THAT MAKES A DIFFERENCE: CULTURE

For many years, American nurses have often worked side by side with nurses and physicians from other cultures and have provided health services to clients of many nationalities. In some cases, the differences between members from various subcultures (city-country, black-white, north-south) have posed problems. Significant problems have been encountered as large groups of citizens of one country have migrated to the United States and have been "stationed" suddenly in a circumscribed area. For example, the placement of Cuban refugees in Fort Chaffee, Arkansas, and the Vietnam "boat people" taken in by well-intentioned, sympathetic Americans have had a significant impact on people accustomed to southern American culture only.

The norms and traditions of a culture not only influence the way people behave, but they affect the use of space, rooms, and chairs. In addition, viewpoints may differ regarding the use of time. Thus, a consideration of cultural differences could have been included in the discussion of the physical environment. We chose to discuss the cultural use of these variables in this section because the *use* of space and time are *behaviors*, "people variables" more than "object variables." People from one culture can move into another, and even if their cultural objects are left behind and they are confronted with new ones, they tend to *use* them according to old ways. In effect, they carry their cultural use of physical items around with them.

Perhaps culture is, in the long run, the most important environmental factor influencing interpersonal communication. Like clothing, people tend to carry their culture around on their backs. As long as they interact only with persons from their own culture, this influence may pass unnoticed; however, when they attempt interpersonal communication with persons from Europe, the Near East, or the Orient, they usually notice important differences. Today, many nurses become personal acquaintances of people from other cultures, and many visit foreign places. Cross-cultural differences have become—for many people—not just an item of romantic interest, but a part of the immediate interpersonal communication environment.

It seems that the most important aspect of cultural influences on interaction is behavior of persons from other cultures that may surprise one or make one feel awkward. Similarly, one's own usual, habitual behaviors that may be misinterpreted by, or prove embarrassing to, persons from foreign lands should be identified. For these reasons, we believe that your interests can best be served in this section by focusing on those cultural differences that relate directly to interpersonal communication. E. T. Hall, author of *The Hidden Dimension*, is the outstanding authority on this topic, and to a large extent this review relies on his careful observations.[59]

Probably the most important cultural differences regarding the use of environmental factors are in the way people from Europe, the Orient, and America tend to use space.[60] Each individual surrounds oneself with a "bubble of privacy," a small space that one feels is one's own little territory; others must gain permission to enter unless they are willing to be perceived as intruding. To an American, a short distance is necessary for this "bubble"—perhaps 2 to 3 feet.[61] To a German, this distance must be much greater. Space is felt as an extension of the ego and is implicit in a German's use of the term *lebensraum*, a concept almost impossible to translate directly because of the emotional feelings implied. Hitler was able to use this feeling as a lever to move the Germans to combat. If an American pokes one's head into an office or inside the screen door of a home to chat briefly, the individual is considered still "outside"; not so to a German—privacy has been intruded upon if you can *see* inside the room.[62]

The German's ego is, by American standards, quite tender, and the individual will preserve privacy with great effort. During World War II, German prisoners were housed four to a small hut in one prison camp in the Midwest. Out of any materials they could scrounge, they each built internal partitions so that each could have his own tiny private space.[63] During the Allied occupation a few years later, when Berlin was in ruins and the housing shortage was indescribably acute, occupation authorities ordered Berliners with kitchens and baths to share them with neighbors. This arrangement had worked fairly well in Italy and France. The order had to be withdrawn in Germany when neighbors started killing each other over shared space.[64]

Americans keep the doors of office buildings open; Germans keep them closed. German doors are very important; they are usually quite solid, fit well, and are often double in public buildings. To a German, a closed door does not mean that the person behind it is doing something one shouldn't; it is one's way of protecting the privacy of the individual. Hall describes the problem in one American overseas company where the use of doors had created a situation severe enough to have Hall brought in as a consultant: The Americans wanted the office doors open, and the Germans wanted them closed. Hall reports that "the open doors were making the Germans feel exposed . . . closed doors . . . gave the Americans the feeling that there was a conspiratorial air about the place and that they were being left out."[65] The point is that if you want to get to know a client or colleague from Germany, don't try to hold interpersonal communication with the person in a crowded room or cafeteria; find a room and close the door! Similarly, recognize the orientations of patients of German origin.

In this context, the English are quite different (as they are regarding other factors). To an American, space is a way of classifying people; large homes and yards indicate important owners. The English person is born into a social class, and space has nothing to do with it; a lord is a lord even if he lives in a one-room apartment.

An English person may never have a "room of one's own." As a child, one will likely live with siblings in a "nursery"; in school, one may live in a dormitory having large communal eating and sleeping rooms; as a professional person, one will likely share office space with numerous colleagues. Even members of Parliament have no offices and often conduct their interviews in foyers or on terraces.[66] The English are often puzzled by an American's need for enclosed private space; the English need no such device to protect their egos. Their social status bequeathed by their parents is their permanent birthright.

The typical English attitude toward personal space is significant for interpersonal communication. An American who wants to be alone goes into some room and shuts the door; to refuse to respond to someone else in the same room is to render the "silent treatment," implying displeasure or lack of regard. An English person who wants to be alone simply quits talking. In so doing, no interpersonal disrespect is meant; the person simply wants to be alone with one's thoughts. Having never in one's life used enclosed space or distance for this purpose, the English person is surprised when an American fails to understand this "common social convention." This factor holds much meaning for Americans wishing to hold interpersonal communication with the English: The more quiet or withdrawn the English person is, the more the American thinks something is wrong in the relationship, and the more the American will press for assurances that all is well. The more one presses, the more one *intrudes* upon the English person's sense of privacy! Consequent tension will likely increase, lasting until one perceives the other's true intentions.[67] Thus, in relating to an English client, nurse, or colleague, one need not suspect depression, grief, pouting, or plotting. One more appropriately should remain quiet until the person begins to talk again. Or, if one must ask something, it would be appropriate to say, "Excuse me, please. I need some information. Would you talk to me now?"

To many Americans, the French appear to be from a world of their own, but they are fairly representative of that complex of cultures bordering the Mediterranean. In ways quite unlike the English and especially unlike Germans, they live, breathe, and eat in crowds. Crowded living is exemplified in their buses, trains, and cafes. They crowd themselves into small cars that contrast sharply in size with Detroit models. Their personal spheres of ego protection are relatively small.

In contrast to the Germans, their neighbors, the French hold their conversations outdoors. Their homes are for the family and are usually quite crowded. Their cafes are for socializing, and here also are quite crowded; the French are sensually very much involved with one another. If you wish to enjoy interpersonal communication with a client, colleague, or a nurse from France or Italy, you can expect the person to stand or sit quite close, to touch you from time to time,[68] and to expect your full attention.[69] This means avoiding backing away, maintaining eye contact, and leaning forward almost with one's own face very near the other's.

The Arabic culture of the Near East provides some contrasts of a paradoxic nature with respect to the use of space. In their public places, Arabs are compressed and almost overwhelmed with crowding, pushing, and shoving; however, inside their homes—at least in the upper and some middle classes—they rattle around in what suburban Americans would call too much space. The Arab's dream is of a home with unlimited internal space, high vaulted ceilings, few items of furniture to obstruct one's "moving around," and a limitless view *from a balcony*. This home, however, is simply a protective wall to shield the family from the outside world.[70]

Among Arab people in public, there is no privacy as Americans know it; in fact, Arabs do not even have a word for privacy.[71] In public, it is quite acceptable to push, shove, and intrude on what Americans and Europeans regard as their "bubble," or personal sphere. An American "pardon me" is surprising and confusing to an Arab and, if meant as a request, is usually ignored. Hall describes a personal experience of having his privacy violated in a public place; later, in his discussion of the incident with an Arabic friend, the Arab regarded Hall's feelings as strange and puzzling. His conclusive comment to Hall was, "After all, it's a public place, isn't it?"[72]

Where, then, is the Arab's sense of privacy—the spatial shield for one's ego? It is somewhere inside the body. This may partially explain why severing of a thief's hand is standard punishment in Saudi Arabia.[73] Arabic dance is focused on expressing feelings from the stomach or middle of the gut rather than from the heart as tends to be true of Western dances. Arabic and many middle Eastern dress covers all of the body, but exposes the midriff area. Paradoxically, although an Arab's ego is not violated by touching and pushing, it is not thus protected from words; a verbal insult is not something taken lightly.[74]

Arabs tend to breathe on each other when they talk; this is not accidental, but a cultural pattern. To Arabs, smelling each other is a desirable way of being involved; good smells are pleasing and to smell one's friend, particularly the friend's breath, is desirable. Arabs are careful about the way they smell; they take special pains to enhance body odors and to use them in building human relationships.[75] This is significant for Americans who want to achieve satisfactory interpersonal relations with persons from the Near East. Even more important, however, is that to "deny one's breath" (i.e., to refuse to interact closely enough so that your breath can be smelled) is to act as if you are ashamed! Arabs are quite willing to tell each other when their breath smells bad, but to avoid letting a friend smell your breath is to deny friendship![76] Can you imagine, then, that you, having been taught in America not to breathe in people's faces, are overtly denying your acceptance of an Arab client, nurse, or colleague, communicating shame to this person when you are trying to be polite? If you really wish to be successful in relating interpersonally, perhaps you might discuss these cultural differences with the Arab person.

At no time, in either public or private places, does an Arab like to be left alone. The person is used to crowds of people and a lack of physical privacy. How, then, does the individual achieve personal privacy, a sense of the integrity of oneself as a person? Actually, it is easy: Like the

Englishmen, one just quits talking. If you inquire about one's thoughts at this time, you will be regarded as a "pushy American"! Sometimes a member of an Arabic family may go for hours without saying a word, and no one in the family will think anything about it. Now imagine an Arab exchange student who visited a Kansas farm family; his hosts became angry at a long silence and withdrew—gave him the silent treatment. He was actually unaware of their anger until they took him to town and forcibly put him on a bus. He was on his way back to the university before he knew there was anything wrong![77]

Probably those representatives of the Orient most often encountered by American nurses are the Japanese. Sitting closely together has special warm connotations to the Japanese. Deeply imbedded in their culture is the feeling of a family sitting closely together around the *hibachi*, the "fireplace." This feeling has even stronger emotional overtones than the American concept of the hearth.[78] Hall quotes an old Japanese priest:

> To really know the Japanese you have to have spent some cold winter evenings snuggled around the *hibachi*. Everybody sits together. A common quilt covers not only the *hibachi* but everyone's lap as well. In this way the heat is held in. It's when your hands touch and you feel the warmth of their bodies and everyone feels *together*—that's when you get to know the Japanese. That's the real Japan.[79]

An American student nurse may be surprised, even confused, by the emotional show of warmth on the part of a friendly Japanese patient. In such a situation you may wish to take extra pains to overcome what, to a Japanese, may appear to be cold disinterest—the usual American use of interpersonal distance. But by the time these two persons get this spatial distance worked out to their satisfaction, a paradoxic problem may arise. It has to do partially with the Japanese way of regarding space and objects, but it realizes its full potential in the way the Japanese approach topics of special interest.

There is an ethic in the Japanese culture that encourages people *to help a friend discover something for oneself* rather than tell one bluntly something one should know. This leads the Japanese to approach a subject *indirectly* rather than head-on. One American banker who had spent years in Japan voiced his greatest sense of frustration with the Japanese: "They talk around and around and around a point and never get to it."[80] They behave somewhat like a rancher "rounding up" cattle; the Japanese round up more or less related ideas until this "herd," with its size, shape, and related proportions, is obvious to you or anybody—but this takes some time and patience. This way of behaving is illustrated dramatically in the way they treat space: they name intersections (growth centers) rather than the streets leading to them; and houses are numbered in the order they are built (grow) rather than along a linear distance.[81] These factors cause travelers inestimable problems, but very well illustrate the way Japanese feel about relationships among objects, people, and ideas. People in close contact get to know each other well; peripheral areas relate somewhat. An area of concentration on the periphery will have *its own center* and focus; thus, each "center" will have its own sense of unity and integrity. Similarly, with ideas, the circle or area is of greater importance than the linear or logical relationship between concepts. And the *feeling* one has about ideas is of greater value than the logical connections between ideas.

In talking with a Japanese patient, exercise time and patience; look for the feeling tones expressed rather than the logical rationale. Don't worry about "coming to the point," but sense your feelings and the patient's about the general area of discussion as well as your feelings toward each other. And don't be surprised if you seem to sense an unexpected feeling of warmth and closeness. As the old priest said, "This is the real Japan!"

This section on foreign cultures would be remiss if only space and interpersonal distance were discussed and eye contact not mentioned. One's way of using the eyes in interpersonal communication is one of the most dramatic differences between cultures and carries considerable impact.

To get along without private rooms and offices, the English have developed skill in paying strict attention, listening carefully, and, from about a distance of 6 to 8 feet, looking you directly in one eye—or so it will feel to you.[82] In fact, an English person will likely fix an unwavering gaze on you—*and blink his or her eyes to let you know he or she has heard you!* Once you have come to understand these social conventions, their meaning, and source or derivation, you may come to use them—even appreciate their value in a crowded room. To misunderstand them is to increase confusion and minimize interpersonal understanding.

In like manner, as a French person talks with you, he or she really looks at you—in one eye, then the other eye, and then up and down. All French, especially the women, have grown accustomed to being looked at and will feel you are being cold and distant if you don't look at them in a direct manner.[83]

Arabs seem to be *unable* to talk without *facing* you at close range (1 to 2 feet); to talk to a person while viewing him or her peripherally is regarded as impolite.[84] While talking, Arabs will look at you in a way that may seem to approach a stare or glare; sometimes this searching gaze appears to beseech or demand more attention than you wish to give. Arabs frequently complain that Americans are aloof, "don't care."[85] Their searching gaze may at times seem hostile or challenging; some Arabs barely avoid fights with Americans because of the intensity and possible implications of this behavior.[86] If you have a patient from the Near East, think carefully before you take offense at one's close and intense look into your eyes as the patient talks with you; show that you mean to be friendly by looking the patient directly in the eye even though such behavior may seem awkward or uncomfortable to you at first. If you really want to be friendly and make the patient feel "at home" with you, this effort will have its reward.

Although differences between the American culture and those of Europe, the Near East, and the Orient have been stressed, another purpose has been to give you some appreciation of the way your own American culture has conditioned you to the use of physical space in interpersonal behavior. From this discussion, you should have gained some deeper understanding of the influence of your own culture on the use of the environment in interpersonal communication.

As you can easily see from your observations of Americans, not all of them are alike; neither are *all* English, French, Arabs, or Japanese. The behaviors described apply in a general way but will not be depicted by each individual. Even so, they apply well enough to be of value in your attempts to improve your interpersonal communication with persons from various cultures.

SUMMARY

This chapter has discussed environmental factors, physical and social, that have particular influence on interpersonal communication.

An enclosed space, a hospital room or place where an atmosphere of privacy prevails, can favorably influence interpersonal communication. A room of modest size and pleasant furnishings and attractive colors can have a positive effect. Tables and chairs can be helpful in terms of personal comfort and convenience, but they can have a deleterious effect as psychological barriers. Chairs and tables must not be allowed to interfere with eye contact as people attempt to engage others in interaction. Messages carried by perceiving each other's eyes are perhaps almost as important as the verbal interchange; certainly these messages influence the interpretation of relationships between people. In the discussion of chairs and tables, the four "interaction distances" identified by the Halls were noted.

The way participants feel about the passage of time can significantly influence interpersonal communication; feelings of limited time or time poorly spent can subtly demolish the anticipated value of such interaction. Special occasions are essentially "time-person-place" arrangements wherein these environmental factors are controlled for specific purposes.

The social environment influences interpersonal communication in terms of four social contexts: the presence of other persons not currently engaged in the interaction, participants who are members of certain groups, interaction within an organization, and interpersonal customs within a culture.

Interaction within the presence of others who are not involved will likely be inhibited or limited; this will be particularly true if the participants hold allegiance of some sort to those who overhear.

Membership in groups tends to influence the interaction of members both in and out of the group. Members tend to conform to group norms and adhere to group goal commitments; these factors may severely limit the interpersonal communication behavior of group members, even when talking with nonmembers. Within the group itself, interaction is significantly influenced by the size of the group (i.e., the number of persons attempting to interact).

Interaction within the boundaries of most older, established organizations will likely be influenced by the following norms or practices: an emphasis on achieving the organization's goals, suppression of discussion of interpersonal problems, insensitivity to one's influence on the feelings of others, avoidance of taboo topics, and creation of a climate of distrust.

There are significant cultural differences among Americans, Europeans, Arabs, and Japanese. Those cultural differences having the most significant influence on interpersonal communication are social customs regarding use of space, interpersonal distance (sense of physical closeness), and the use of eye contact. These customs are not uniform for all members of these cultures; but the degree of difference among cultures is stable enough to be important as you try to improve your interpersonal communication with persons from other cultures, whether clients, other nurses, or colleagues of other professions.

REFERENCES

1. E. GOFFMAN: *Relations in Public* (New York: Basic Books, 1971), p. 209.
2. Cf. A. H. MASLOW AND N. L. MINTZ: "Effects of Esthetic Surroundings: I. Initial Effects of Three Esthetic Conditions Upon Perceiving 'Energy' and 'Well-being' in Faces," *Journal of Psychology,* 41 (1956): 247–254.
3. M. KNAPP: "The Effects of Environment and Space on Human Communication," *Nonverbal Communication and Human Interaction* (New York: Holt, Rinehart & Winston, 1972), pp. 25–62.
4. B. H. WESTLEY AND M. S. McLEAN emphasize the use of all sense modalities in "A Conceptual Model for Communications Research," *Journalism Quarterly,* 34 (1957): 31.
5. Cf. GOFFMAN: *Relations in Public,* pp. 106–107.
6. Cf. E. GOFFMAN: *Behavior in Public Places* (New York: Free Press, 1963), p. 52.
7. *Ibid.,* p. 56.
8. See N. SANFORD: *Self and Society* (New York: Atherton, 1966), pp. 48–51.

9. See, for example, K. KENISTON: *Young Radicals: Notes on Committed Youth* (New York: Harcourt Brace Jovanovich, 1968); see also G. B. BLAINE, JR., ET AL.: *Emotional Problems of the Student* (Garden City, N.Y.: Doubleday, 1966).

10. GOFFMAN: *Behavior in Public Places*, pp. 91–92.

11. GOFFMAN: *Relations in Public*, p. 18 (fn.).

12. For a detailed treatment of such effect, see *Ibid.*, pp. 45–46, 59–60, 126–132.

13. See, for example, M. D. RIEMER: "The Averted Gaze," *Psychiatric Quarterly*, 23 (1949): 108–115.

14. For a report of experimental evidence, see B. STEINZER: "The Spatial Factor in Face-to-Face Discussion Groups," *Journal of Abnormal and Social Psychology*, 45 (1950): 552–555.

15. See also E. T. HALL: *The Hidden Dimension* (Garden City, N.Y.: Doubleday, 1969), pp. 113–129.

16. E. HALL AND M. HALL: "The Sounds of Silence," *Playboy*, 18, No. 6 (June 1971).

17. HALL: *Hidden Dimension*, pp. 117–118.

18. Hall's studies deal primarily with middle-class subjects living in the northeastern United States. He suggests that great care should be exercised in any attempt to generalize his findings to other geographic areas or ethnic groups.

19. HALL: *Hidden Dimension*, pp. 119–120.

20. *Ibid.*, p. 121.

21. *Ibid.*, pp. 121–123.

22. *Ibid.*, pp. 123–124.

23. See *Ibid.*, pp. 128–164. See also Birdwhistell's comments cited in a symposium reported in B. SCHAFFNER, ED.: *Group Processes* (New York: J. Macy, 1959), pp. 184–185.

24. HALL: *Hidden Dimension*, p. 122.

25. Cf. A. G. WHITE: "The Patient Sits Down: A Clinical Note," *Psychosomatic Medicine*, 15 (1953): 256–257. See also K. B. LITTLE: "Personal Space," *Journal of Experimental and Social Psychology*, 1 (1965): 237–247.

26. Cf. GOFFMAN: *Relations in Public*, p. 28–32.

27. Cf. KNAPP: *Nonverbal Communication and Human Interaction*, pp. 25–36.

28. Cf. GOFFMAN: *Relations in Public*, pp. 73–90.

29. Cf. GOFFMAN: *Behavior in Public Places*, pp. 102–104.

30. Goffman suggests that "the work walls do, they do in part because they are honored or socially recognized as communication barriers," even though they may not actually deter others from overhearing conversations. See GOFFMAN: *Behavior in Public Places*, pp. 152–153.

31. For a review of this literature, see R. B. ZAJONC: *Social Psychology: An Experimental Approach* (Belmont, Calif.: Wadsworth, 1966), pp. 10–15.

32. J. PESSIN: "The Comparative Effects of Social and Mechanical Stimulation on Memorizing," *American Journal of Psychology*, 45 (1933): 263–270.

33. B. O. BERGUM AND D. J. LEHR: "Effects of Authoritarianism on Vigilance Performance," *Journal of Applied Psychology*, 47 (1963): 75–77.

34. See R. B. ZAJONC: "Social Facilitation," *Science*, 149 (1965): 269–274.

35. Cf. D. SEIDMAN, ET AL.: "Influence of a Partner on Tolerance for Self-Administered Electric Shock," *Journal of Abnormal and Social Psychology*, 54 (1957): 210–212.

36. See K. W. SPENCE: *Behavior Theory and Conditioning* (New Haven, Conn.: Yale University Press, 1956).
37. See, for example, D. CARTWRIGHT AND A. ZANDER, EDS.: *Group Dynamics*, 3rd ed. (New York: Harper & Row, 1968).
38. For a review, see J. E. McGRATH AND I. ALTMAN: *Small Group Research* (New York: Harper & Row, 1968).
39. For a critical synthesis of this research, see G. LINDZEY AND E. ARONSON, EDS.: *The Handbook of Social Psychology*, Vol. 4 (Reading, Mass.: Addison-Wesley Publishing Company, 1969), especially pp. 1–283.
40. Cf. K. GIFFIN: "The Study of Speech Communication in Small-Group Research," in J. AKIN, ET AL., EDS.: *Language Behavior* (The Hague: Mouton Press, 1970), pp. 138–162.
41. B. R. PATTON AND K. GIFFIN: *Decision-Making Group Interaction* (New York: Harper & Row, 1978).
42. S. ASCH: *Social Psychology* (Englewood Cliffs, NJ: Prentice-Hall Inc., 1952).
43. *Ibid.*, pp. 450–451.
44. P. SUPPES AND M. SCHLAG-REY: "Analysis of Social Conformity in Terms of Generalized Conditioning Models," in J. CRISWELL, H. SOLOMON, AND P. SUPPES, EDS.: *Mathematical Methods in Small Group Processes* (Stanford, Calif.: Stanford University Press, 1962), pp. 334–361.
45. R. S. CRUTCHFIELD: "The Measurement of Individual Conformity to Group Opinion Among Officer Personnel," *Research Bulletin* (Berkeley: Institute of Personality Assessment and Research, University of California). See also R. S. CRUTCHFIELD: "Conformity and Character," *American Psychologist* 10 (1955): 191–198.
46. S. MILGRAM: "Nationality and Conformity," *Scientific American*, 205 (1961): 45–51.
47. E. E. JONES, H. H. WELLS, AND R. TORREY: "Some Effects of Feedback from the Experimenter on Conformity Behavior," *Journal of Abnormal and Social Psychology*, 57 (1958): 207–213.
48. For a detailed review of these studies, see B. E. COLLINS AND B. H. RAVEN: "Group Structure: Attraction, Coalitions, Communication, and Power," in LINDZEY AND ARONSON, pp. 102–205; see especially pp. 168–174.
49. S. SCHACTER: "Deviation, Rejection, and Communication," *Journal of Abnormal and Social Psychology*, 46 (1951): 190–207.
50. L. G. WISPE: "A Sociometric Analysis of Conflicting Role-Expectation," *American Journal of Sociology*, 61 (1955): 134–137.
51. R. F. BALES AND P. E. SLATER: "Role Differentiation in Small Decision-Making Groups" in R. F. BALES, ET AL.: *Family Socialization and Interaction Process* (New York: Free Press, 1955), pp. 259–306.
52. See, for example, W. H. CROCKETT: "Emergent Leadership in Small Decision-Making Groups," *Journal of Abnormal and Social Psychology*, 51 (1955): 378–383.
53. R. F. BALES: "The Equilibrium Problem in Small Groups," in T. PARSONS, R. F. BALES, AND E. A. SHILS, EDS.: *Working Papers in the Theory of Action* (New York: Free Press, 1953), pp. 11–161; and P. A. HARE: "Interaction and Consensus in Different Sized Groups," *American Sociological Review*, 17 (1952): 261–267.
54. H. J. LEAVITT AND R. A. MUELLER: "Some Effects of Feedback on Communication," *Human Relations*, 4 (1951): 401–410.

55. P. E. SLATER: "Contrasting Correlates of Group Size," *Sociometry*, 21 (1958): 129–139.
56. R. F. BALES AND E. BORGATTA: "Size of Group as a Factor in the Interaction Profile," in P. A. HARE, E. F. BORGATTA, AND R. F. BALES, EDS.: *Small Groups: Studies in Social Interaction* (New York: Knopf, 1955), pp. 396–413.
57. C. A. GIBB: "Effects of Group Size and Threat Reduction upon Creativity in a Problem-Solving Situation," *American Psychologist*, 6 (1951): 324.
58. Cf. C. ARGYRIS: *Interpersonal Competence and Organizational Effectiveness* (Homewood, Ill.: Irwin, 1962), pp. 27–50.
59. E. T. HALL: *Hidden Dimension*.
60. See E. T. HALL AND M. HALL: "Sounds of Silence."
61. GOFFMAN: *Behavior in Public Places*, pp. 98–99.
62. HALL: *Hidden Dimension*, pp. 133–134.
63. *Ibid.*, p. 135.
64. *Ibid.*, pp. 135–136.
65. *Ibid.*, p. 136.
66. *Ibid.*, p. 139.
67. Cf. *Ibid.*, pp. 139–140.
68. See GOFFMAN: *Behavior in Public Places*, p. 101.
69. Cf. SCHAFFNER, ED.: *Group Processes*, p. 184.
70. HALL: *Hidden Dimension*, pp. 158–162.
71. *Ibid.*, p. 159.
72. *Ibid.*, p. 156.
73. *Ibid.*, p. 157.
74. *Ibid.*, pp. 158–158.
75. *Ibid.*, pp. 159–160.
76. *Ibid.*, p. 160.
77. *Ibid.*, p. 159.
78. *Ibid.*, p. 150.
79. *Ibid.*, pp. 150–151.
80. *Ibid.*, p. 151.
81. *Ibid.*, pp. 149–150.
82. *Ibid.*, pp. 142–143.
83. *Ibid.*, p. 145.
84. *Ibid.*, pp. 160–161.
85. *Ibid.*, p. 161.
86. *Ibid.*, pp. 161–162.

4
VERBAL MESSAGES

If you were asked what behaviors are included in nurses talking to one another or to clients and colleagues, you would very likely picture two or more persons using words. Communication behavior in the overall sense ordinarily includes many elements: perceiving one another; considering and using space, rooms, furniture, and time; and interacting with both nonverbal and verbal behavior. For purposes of studying these factors, they are considered one at a time. The order in which they are studied is quite arbitrary. They usually occur in sets, all at once. This book discusses them in the order in which they come to one's attention upon meeting someone for the first time: Individuals may have, at that time, thoughts and/or feelings that they need to express; people meet in a physical setting; people are more or less aware of their social environment; as individuals meet, nonverbal behavior that carries meaning inevitably occurs; also, people may employ verbal behavior involving a linguistic code. Previous chapters have discussed personal needs to communicate, the person perception process, and the use and influences of environmental factors. The next two chapters consider interpersonal behaviors that aid individuals in expressing themselves to one another.

In the nursing profession, as in most other social interactions, people gather, share, give, and receive information through words. They establish, continue, or terminate relationships by words. The process by which people arbitrarily make certain sounds or symbols stand for ideas is societal in essence. By mutual agreement, any word can be made to stand for anything. This chapter examines some of the problem areas involved in people's attempts to communicate by words. Since interpersonal communication relies partly on words, individuals must be satisfied with degrees of mutual understanding.

CHARACTERISTICS OF LANGUAGE

The first fragmentary utterances of a small child who is just learning to speak indicate the interpersonal nature of human language. Swiss psychologist Jean Piaget distinguished two functions of speech for the child: the social and the egocentric. In social speech, "the child addresses his hearer, considers his point of view, tries to influence him or actually exchanges ideas with him." In egocentric speech, "the child does not bother to know to whom he is speaking, nor whether he is being listened to. He talks either to himself or for the pleasure of associating anyone who happens to be there with the activity of the moment."[1] Other investigations have concluded that the bulk of the child's speech, approximately 90 percent, is social.[2] The work of the Russian psychiatrist L. S. Vigotsky suggests that even the monologues labeled by Piaget as "egocentric" are actually directed toward others. When Vigotsky placed a child who demonstrated the characteristics of "egocentric" speech (babblings, incomplete sentences) in isolation, in a very noisy room, or among deaf-and-mute children, the child's speech dropped off considerably. Vigotsky concluded that the child believes the speech is being understood by others, and when external conditions make speaking difficult or when feedback is lacking, the child stops speaking.[3] The child does not initially clearly differentiate one's perception of the world from the world as perceived by others. The child seems to believe that everyone else perceives and understands the world just as the child perceives and understands it; thus, others must understand the child's highly idiosyncratic language. This tendency, as shall be shown, is not completely restricted to the child, and it lies at the heart of many communication problems. The most important point, however, is that according to available experimental data, all speech is a form of interpersonal behavior.

The child attaches meanings to visual and verbal phenomena and, in effect, works to "break the code." As noted, however, all language and symbols are entirely by agreement and consent. There is usually no connection between the sound or series of letters in a word and the "thing" in reality except what is arbitrarily attached by human beings. Semanticists have used the analogy of a *map* and the *territory* it represents to describe the relationship between our verbal symbols and the reality for which they stand. Those characteristics of language that potentially cause problems in interpersonal communication will be examined in some detail below.

WORDS HAVE DIFFERENT MEANINGS
FOR DIFFERENT PEOPLE

Generally, words are thought of as having two kinds of meaning or two kinds of definition. One is the connotative, or associative, definition. The other is the denotative, or operational, definition. The latter kind of meaning refers to the thing or event, a phenomenon to which the word refers. This denotative definition is what one would point to if asked to define a word without being able to speak or use any other words. Such denotative meanings are reasonably stable; they are common to science (H_2O), business (debit), industry (arbitration), and to nursing (S.O.A.P.). They mean about the same to everyone, but problems can develop if agreements are not reached. Even in as restricted an area as parliamentary procedure, to "table" a motion in the United States means to put it aside, whereas in England it means "Let's bring it up for discussion."

Consider numerous possible meanings in the following story:

> Struck by a sign in a plumber's window ("struck"?) reading "Iron Sinks," a wag went inside to inform the merchant that he was fully aware that "iron sinks." The storekeeper, ready to play the game, inquired, "And do you know that time flies, sulphur springs, jam rolls, music stands, Niagara Falls, concrete walks, wood fences, sheep run, holiday trips, rubber tires, the organ stops . . .?" But by then the wag had had enough and fled.

Such multiple meanings inherent in language force people to consider context and nonverbal cues to give more exact meaning. The educated adult uses, in daily conversation, only about 2,000 of the more than 600,000 words in the English language. Of these 2,000, the 500 most frequently used words have more than 14,000 dictionary definitions. Even the term *meaning*, which we have attempted to define, has 18 groups of meanings in one dictionary. Further, language is constantly changing, adding new words, and modifying definitions as usage changes. It may be of some interest to look at Figure 4-1, in which the dictionary meanings of the word "nurse" are provided. All people know what "nurse" means—or do they?

Even greater problems result from the connotative meaning of a word or expression than from the denotative. While the denotation gives sharpness and accuracy to a word, its connotations give it power. The most familiar words are rich with connotations—doctor, cancer, heart. The connotation may even be so strong that it erases the denotation, and, for the individual, only the connotation then has significance.

The connotative meaning of a word is the thought, feeling, or ideas that people have about the word, the things they say about the word

Nurse (nurs)., n., v., nursed, nursing—n. 1. a person (woman or man) who has the care of the sick or infirm. 2. a woman who has the general care of a child or children. 3. a woman employed to suckle an infant; wet nurse. 4. any fostering agency or influence. 5. a worker that attends the young in a colony of social insects. 6. Billiards, act of nursing the balls. —v.t. 7. to tend in sickness or infirmity. 8. to seek to cure (a cold, etc.) by taking care of oneself. 9. to look after carefully so as to promote growth, development, etc.; foster, cherish (a feeling, etc.). 10. to treat or handle with adroit care in order to further one's own interests. 11. to bring up, train, or nurture. 12. to clasp or handle as if fondly or tenderly. 13. to suckle (an infant). 14. to feed and tend in infancy. 15. Billiards, to gather and keep (the balls) together for a series of caroms. —v.i. 16. to act as nurse, tend the sick or infirm. 17. to suckle a child. 18. (of a child) to take the breast.
—Syn. 14. Nurse, nourish, nurture may be used practically interchangeably to refer to bringing up the young. Nurse, however, suggests particularly attendance and service; nourish emphasizes providing whatever is needful for development and nurture suggests tenderness and solitude in training mind and manners.

FIGURE 4-1. Definition of "nurse." (From *The American College Dictionary*, p. 832. Copyright © 1958 by Random House, Inc. Reprinted by permission of the publisher.)

when asked what it means to them. The words "factory worker" denote a person who earns a living by performing productive tasks in a building where many persons are organized to produce a product at a cost below what other people will pay for it. However, the words connote certain feelings and emotions. To some people, "factory worker" may mean a lazy, irresponsible, and apathetic person hostile to management. To others, it may connote an honest, good person who is exploited, unjustly treated, and deprived of any freedom and opportunity to exercise responsibility and judgment. In the course of a lifetime, the denotations of words change but little, while their connotations alter with one's experience.

To some extent, the individual experiences of each of the approximately 300 million English-speaking people differ from all others. Every second of one's life one is experiencing something that is not exactly the same experience as any other one has had before, or that anyone else has had. Each individual has certain personal connotations derived from one's experience with objects, persons, or ideas that are the referents of the words one uses. General connotations are those accepted as the typical reaction of a majority of people; thus, most people in our society regard "war" with fear and abhorrence. Being able to anticipate a person's reaction to a word allows some people to manipulate another by the simple use of that word.

Virtually all words have both denotative and connotative dimensions. The type and degree of reaction to words will vary from person to person. Meanings reside not in the words, but in the minds of people using them. One might consider the following example:

> For the first time, the nursing students appeared in the clinical areas of the hospital in full uniform—even white hose, caps, and bandage scissors. Looking fresh and crisp in comparison with the senior students with the faded and patched uniforms, one new student was invited to watch an intern start a blood transfusion. Unfortunately, the procedure did not go well and the blood began to infiltrate into the client's tissue. The young intern cried out, "Cut it off—cut it off!," meaning to clamp off the plastic tubing and stop the flow of blood. Whereupon the new nursing student whipped out new bandage scissors and cut the plastic tubing off! As the blood ran out on the floor and the intern glowered, the student said, "Well, you said to *cut it off!*"

WORDS VARY IN DEGREE OF ABSTRACTNESS

A second major aspect of words and language is that words, like thoughts and conceptions, vary in degree of abstractness; words are symbols used to represent a generalized category of things, experiences, or ideas. The degree of abstractness varies from indicating a total class ("foreigners"), to a particular class ("Spaniards"), to a specific member of the class ("Juan Martinez"). S. I. Hayakawa depicted the principle of abstracting with his story of "Bessie," a cow. If persons perceive in front of them a living organism, they respond, based on their previous experiences with other similar animals, by labeling the creature they are seeing a "cow." The cow is at the same time unique (different from all other living creatures in certain respects) as well as a member of a class ("cows").[5]

This characteristic of language permits people to avoid one another in arguments by retreating from one level of abstraction to another. Teachers and politicians are often adept at handling difficult questions by changing the level of abstraction when pushed as to specifics. The more abstract people become, the more they are relying on "what is in their heads" rather than any sort of denotative reality.

When dealing with concrete empirical references (denotative definitions)—such as "hospitals," "prescription," "Illinois"—people have generally agreed-on referents; highly abstract terms such as "humanistic," "holistic," and "public welfare" are less likely to have common referents.

In general, the more abstract a word, the greater the ambiguity and the greater the chances of misunderstanding.

Hayakawa cites a course in aesthetics in a large midwestern university in which an entire semester was devoted to Art and Beauty and the principles underlying them, and during which the professor, even when asked by students, persistently declined to name specific paintings, symphonies, sculptures, or objects of beauty to which the instructor's principles might apply. "We are interested," the professor would say, "in principle, not in particulars."[6]

Wendell Johnson labeled the linguistic phenomenon of a person's remaining more or less stuck at a certain level of abstraction "dead-level abstracting." As an example of a persistent low-level abstracting, he cites the following:

> Probably all of us know certain people who seem able to talk on and on without ever drawing any very general conclusions. For example, there is the back-fence chatter that is made up of he said and then I said and then she said and I said and then he said, far into the afternoon, ending with, "Well, that's just what I told him!" Letters describing vacation trips frequently illustrate this language, detailing places seen, times of arrival and departure, the foods eaten and the prices paid, whether the beds were hard or soft, etc.[7]

This example contrasts sharply with the persistent, high level of abstraction of the professor cited by Hayakawa. Usually, speech demonstrates a constant interplay of higher- and lower-level abstraction, as people adapt quickly up and down the abstraction ladder.

High-level abstractions are quite useful when they are related to sensory experience and demonstrate relationships and order. On the other hand, these abstractions can be dangerous as merely evocative terms standing for anything or nothing. The most highly valued terms in the language (love, beauty, truth, rights, choice, and so forth) can either be maps without territories or can point to specific experiences and feelings. Stuart Chase summarizes the point as follows:

> When we use words as symbols for the abstraction that we "see," they are an abstraction of an abstraction. When we use generalizations like chairs-in-general or "household furniture," we abstract again. The semantic moral is to be conscious of these abstraction levels, and not to lose sight of the original chair.[8]

Harry Truman was never a man to mince words. A constituent once wrote him about the postmen's motto "Neither snow, nor rain, nor heat, nor gloom of night stays these couriers from the swift completion of their appointed rounds" and asked what it meant. "It means," replied Truman, "they deliver the mail in the wintertime."

LANGUAGE IS, BY ITS NATURE, INCOMPLETE

Millions of people, when reporting their experiences, use the same meager store of accepted words. Each common word must, therefore, be used to cover a wide range of "meanings." Obviously, such categoric symbols omit details.

Chapter 2 discussed people's perceptual tendency to simplify by the use of black-and-white categories and stereotyping. This characteristic of perception is reflected in language. People are ill equipped linguistically to describe gradations of differences, so they describe someone as either lazy or industrious, unable to categorize the individual in any unique fashion.

To be of any value, language must categorize and omit unique details, but this characteristic forces people to overgeneralize. If individuals fail to recognize that words are only generalized symbols, they are in danger of making certain invalid assumptions:

1. They may assume that one instance is a universal example: "Nobody likes me." "All men are . . ." "This always happens to me." "Nothing ever turns out right."
2. They may assume that their perceptions are complete: "Yes, I already know about that."
3. They may assume that everyone shares their feelings and perceptions: "Why didn't you do it the right way?" "Why would anyone eat in that hospital cafeteria?"
4. They may assume that people and things don't change: "That's the way she is!"
5. They may assume that characteristics they attribute to people or things are truly inherent: "That picture is ugly." "He's a selfish person."
6. They may assume that their message is totally clear to someone else: "You know perfectly well what I mean." "You heard me!"

Although generalizations are potentially dangerous, they cannot be avoided because language is a body of generalizations. Absolutely perfect interpersonal communication is impossible to achieve because language is inherently incomplete. Yet there are degrees of incompleteness, and communicators should recognize that they are always functioning at levels of probability of understanding. The incomplete nature of language makes it easy for people to misunderstand one another. Consider the following example:

> As she begrudgingly told her story, sixty-seven-year-old blind woman
> sat in her street clothes on the edge of one of the eight med-surg beds

crammed into one ward of a large metropolitan hospital . . . Her shoes were on the bedside table. She refused to let go of anything else.

Her version of what had happened to her was that strangers had broken into her apartment last night and forcibly dragged her to this place. She did not want to be here; she was not sick; she just wanted to go home. . . .

The house staff on call the night before claimed that she had been left by the police in the Emergency Room. On examination, they could find nothing wrong. But the old woman was blind and they could not send her home alone in the middle of the night. They kept her in the emergency room, not knowing what else to do. . . .

The police account of the events was that they had been summoned to Ida's apartment by concerned neighbors. There they found her with another old woman who had apparently died of natural causes some time ago. The old woman was Ida's aunt. The two had lived together for about twenty years—ever since Ida had begun to lose her sight.

Once the body of Ida's aunt had been taken to the morgue, the police decided that the best thing to do with Ida would be to take her to the nearest hospital. That done, their job was ended; they had no further responsibility in the matter.

The nursing staff on the unit was enraged.

So was Ida.

The nurses were enraged mostly because . . . Ida refused to undress . . . also enraged because there was nothing wrong with her, and she was being pushed to undress. The symbolic meaning of that act was the same for everyone; if Ida relinquished her clothes for a hospital gown, she would become a patient. So she refused as adamantly as the staff insisted.[9]

LANGUAGE REFLECTS PERSONALITY AND CULTURE

It has been noted that an individual's language behavior necessarily reflects basic features of one's personality and that individual experiences and attitudes contribute to different reactions to words. Language, having developed in the context of a certain culture, of necessity reflects that particular culture. As a derived system of human interpretations of recurring events, experiences, and conditions, culture constitutes a system of social organization that differentitates and integrates human interaction and provides guides to behavior and motives to conform.

Language gives innumerable insights into a culture. As an example of how language mirrors a culture, a study was made of the figures of speech in the language of the Palaun people of the western Pacific. Because figures of speech are a means of making the abstract concrete, such an analysis provides unique insights into a culture. To Palauns, a beautiful woman is a "comet." Because maternal descent is more greatly valued than paternal descent, superlative expressions reflect this organizational bias. "Largest" is *delad a klou* ("mother of large") and "highest" is *delad a ngarabub* ("mother of up").[10]

Even subcultures have language behaviors that distinguish one from another. Although Americans tend to discount class differences in this society, a team of investigators examined social-class speech differences of people surviving an Arkansas tornado. Ten people were classified as middle class by virtue of 1 or more years of college education and a moderate income. Ten other respondents were matched with them on such factors as age, race, and residence, but were able to be classified as lower class on the basis of income and education (no schooling beyond elementary school). Analyses of the transcribed tape-recorded interviews revealed the following differences:

1. Almost without exception, descriptions of the tornado and its aftermath by lower-class participants were given as seen through their own eyes; middle-class respondents, however, described the actions of others as the others saw them.
2. Lower-class respondents demonstrated a relative insensitivity to differences between their perspective and that of the interviewer. For example, surnames were used without identification, and pronouns like "we" and "they" had no clear referents. By comparison, middle-class respondents used contextual clarification of their perspective in an attempt to consider the listener's role.
3. Whereas middle-class respondents used overall frames to organize their entire account, lower-class respondents were basically disorganized, giving segmental, limited accounts. Connections between incidents were obscure because respondents tended to wander from one incident to another.

It could be concluded that lower-class respondents perceive in more concrete terms and that their speech reflects these more concrete cognitions. However, as the investigators ask:

Does his (the lower-class person's) speech accurately reflect customary "concrete" modes of thought and perception, or is it that he . . . is unable to convey his perception? . . . One concludes that speech does in some sense reflect thought. The reader is perhaps best left at this point to draw his own conclusions. . . .[11]

There is the great temptation to render value judgments on the language development and behavior of various subgroups, instead of viewing language differences as merely reflections of cultural differences. The imposition of linguistic rules to formulate language into predictable sound patterns and a well-ordered grammatical structure and formal vocabulary facilitates analysis and description of the language, but does not provide a basis for qualitative judgments. A case of such a linguistic assumption can be noted in the following:

The syntax of low-income Negro children differs from standard English in many ways, but it has its own internal consistency. Unfortunately, the psychologist, not knowing the rules of Negro non-standard English, has interpreted these differences not as the result of well-learned rules but as evidence of "linguistic underdevelopment." He has concluded that if black children do not speak like white children they are deficient. One of the most blatant errors has been a confusion between hypotheses concerning language and hypotheses concerning cognition. For this reason, superficial differences in language structures and language styles have been taken as manifestations of underlying differences in learning ability. To give one example, a child in class was asked, in a test of simple contrasts, "Why do you say they are different?" He could not answer. Then it was discovered that the use of "do you say," though grammatically correct, was inappropriate to this culture. When he was asked instead, "Why are they different?" he answered without any hesitation at all.[12]

Such assumptions evolve because of misconceptions of what language is and how it functions.

Because language thus reflects a particular culture, problems abound when cross-cultural communication is attempted. Although words may mean different things to different people within a cultural grouping, at least some consensus and predictability are possible. The predictability is far less and the potential for misunderstanding is far greater in dealing with nonnative speakers. A young mother from the Middle East, for example, phoned a friend in extreme distress: Something must be wrong with her child because her two usual babysitters were *afraid* of her baby. She had called the sitters and both had told her, "I'm sorry, but I'm afraid I can't sit with your child tonight." If the diverse ways in which the different peoples of the world have attempted to cope with the universal problems of adapting to their environment are not recognized, the groundwork is laid for misunderstanding and conflict.

LANGUAGE CREATES A "SOCIAL REALITY"

It is ridiculous to consider language a neutral medium of exchange. Specific words are selected for use because they do affect behavior. Words call forth internal experiences as if by hypnotic suggestion. The role of language in contributing to people's (clients and health-care professionals) problems and potential solutions can be shown to contribute to dangerous misconceptions and prejudices.

The color of a person's skin, for example, is tied to plus-or-minus words that inevitably condition people's attitudes. The words "black" and "white" in Western culture are heavily loaded—"black" with unfavorable connotations and "white" with positive values. Ossie Davis, black actor and author, concluded after a detailed study of dictionaries and Roget's *Thesaurus* that the English language was his enemy. In the *Thesaurus,* he counted 120 synonyms for "blackness" and noted that most of them had unpleasant connotations: "blot, blotch, blight, smut, smudge, sully, soot, becloud, obscure, dingy, murky, threatening, frowning, foreboding, forbidden, sinister, baneful, dismal, evil, wicked, malignant, deadly, secretive, unclear, unwashed, foul, blacklist, black book, black-hearted," and so on, as well as such words as "Negro, nigger, and darky."[13]

In the same book, 134 synonyms for the word "white" are cited; they have such positive connotations as "purity, cleanliness, birth, shining, fair, blonde, stainless, chaste, unblemished, unsullied, innocent, honorable, upright, just, straightforward, genuine, trustworthy, honest," and so on. Orientals fare little better than blacks because "yellow" calls forth such associative words as "coward, conniver, baseness, fear, effeminacy, fast, spiritless, timid, sneak, lily-livered," and so on.

Because colors are not truly descriptive of races, color designations are more symbolic than descriptive. It seems reasonable and likely that Americans' racial attitudes have been affected by the language. This culture is not unique in this regard. In the Chinese language, "yellow" is associated with "beauty, openness, flowering, and sunshine," whereas "white" connotes "coldness, frigidity, bloodlessness, absence of feeling, and weakness." Similarly, in many African tongues, "black" has associations of "strength, certainty, and integrity," whereas "white" is associated with "pale, anemic, untrustworthy, and devious."

Language can also be shown to be sexist in nature. Feminist writer Jean Faust observes:

> All the titles, all the professions, all the occupations are masculine. They are weakened when they are made feminine by the addition of ess, ette. And man insists that these suffixes be used; he knows the power of language. He knows that language can control not only behavior, but thought itself. Words can determine the function, the very being of a person. Hence the awkwardness of lady novelist, sculptress, authoress, etc. *The New York Times* reached a low in its history when, on January 15, 1969, in the heat of the Great Jockey Controversy, it referred to girls who wish to ride horses in races as "jockettes."[14]

Note the exception to the rule: nursing—and note the history of discrimination nurses have endured as documented by Joan Ashley in her book, *Hospitals, Paternalism and the Role of the Nurse* (New York: Teachers College Press, 1976). A problem with "reverse English" (to pun a point) is that encountered by a male who enters the nursing profession. Are there now two categories: nurses and "male nurses"? Society has hardly gone so far as to call males in the nursing profession such degrading terms as "nursettes" or some equivalent. Perhaps the reason people have not done so illustrates the point: Women currently suffer in linguistic status by the way language customarily is used in Western culture.

One indication of the sexism of the language is in the grammatical use of personal pronouns. In most cases when the pronoun "he" is used, "he or she" is actually meant. To repeat the referent (e.g., "the speaker recited the speaker's speech") is extremely awkward; further, to state "The speaker recited his or her speech" is confusing.

The point is, the lack of a single pronoun for "he or she" forces a distinction in the case of an individual whose sex is not known and makes no difference. It forces emphasis on differences between the sexes, instead of similarities, and instead of accepting one common humanity (huwoman/manity? or huwomanity?).

UNDERSTANDING ONE ANOTHER

As individuals attempt to elicit responses from other people, they seek to describe or "display" their thoughts in such ways that the receiver is able to identify with their thoughts. This process depends on both effective transmission and effective reception of the messages.

SPEAKING

As the encoder of the message, the speaker has certain responsibilities. Implicit in this discussion has been the assumption that words matter; the choice of words in the interpersonal relationship makes a difference to the people involved. If one wants a child to move from a particular chair, one asks the child to move. If at first words and vocal emphasis do not impress the child, an attempt may be made to cajole the child out of the chair or, as a last resort, threaten or physically remove the child. In the adult world, because most of the action people desire from others cannot be induced by the direct threat of force, they must rely on words and nonverbal communication to achieve any change in others.

Any attempt to manipulate people must be considered on ethical as well as pragmatic grounds. Interpersonal behavior depends to a great extent on persuasive symbol manipulation designed to achieve certain actions from others, based on some kind of psychologic consent. Such efforts might be viewed as unethical if the action called for is judged to be advantageous to the persuader at the expense of the other person. The information, if deliberately distorted, can be viewed as constituting unethical behavior.

Skilled salesmen become adept at selecting the key words that appeal to people's motives, fears, and desires. Motivational selling has progressed to a fine art with its near-scientific procedures. The encyclopedia salesman may induce individuals to buy because they think they are getting something for nothing, because they want an educated environment for their children, or because the product will make a significant contribution to their lives.

Word association is a common device in eliciting a desired response. A brewer was considering using the word "lagered" to describe his beer and conducted a word-association test. Only one-third of the people tested gave such responses as "ale," "beer," or "stout." Another third gave such responses as "tired," "drunk," "slow," and "dizzy," while the remaining participants had no response to the word. Thus the word was discarded.

The "social reality" created by words can be used to control the minds of people. For example, a Soviet dictionary is reported to define "religion" as:

> a fantastic faith in gods, angels and spirits . . . a faith without any scientific foundations. Religion is being supported and maintained by the reactionary circles. It serves for the subjugation of the working people and for building up the power of the exploiting bourgeois classes . . . The superstitition of outlived religion has been surmounted by the Communist education of the working class. . . .[15]

In a similar vein, Hungarian Communists are reported to have taught their children the following Sovietized version of the Nativity:

> There was once a poor married couple who had nothing to eat or dress in. They asked the rich people for help but the rich people sent them away. Their baby was born in a stable and covered with rags in a manger. The day after the baby was born, some shepherds who had come from Russia brought the baby some gifts. "We come from a country where poverty and misery are unknown," said the shepherds. "In Russia the babies grow in liberty because there is no unemployment or suffering." Joseph, the unemployed worker, asked the shepherds how they had found the house. The shepherds replied that a red star had guided them. Then the poor family took to the road. The shepherds covered the little baby with furs, and they all set out for the Soviet paradise.[16]

Are any persons so very different from the Soviet propagandist as they entice, seduce, and coerce (all "loaded" words) others to view the world as they want them to see it? As individual senders of messages, people select the words designed to have the greatest desired effect on the listener. When they want to make a side trip, they tell their fellow traveler that the trip is "only about 100 miles"; but if the idea comes from their companion and they oppose it, they protest, "Why, that trip is over 100 miles!" When the nurse is instructing the patient with newly diagnosed diabetes about taking insulin injections, the nurse tells the client that the injection will "only have to be taken in the morning," but the client usually retorts, "that's a shot every morning for the rest of my life!" Virtually every utterance that one makes reflects a coloring of reality to reflect one's feelings, attitudes, and values.

Language usage creates attitudes and behaviors that would not otherwise occur. The exact words used at any particular time reflect people's attitudes, feelings, and desires at that time. The same woman may be referred to as "young woman," "young lady," "miss," "hey-you," "girl," even "broad," or worse, depending on the feeling and intent of the speaker.

Columnist Sydney Harris has frequently used what he labeled "antics with semantics" to demonstrate how attitudes determine the words selected:

> I lost the match because I was "off my form"; you lost because you were "over-confident"; he lost because he was "too cocky." The academic expert I agree with is a "scholar"; the academic expert I disagree with is a "pedant." When our statesmen say what they do not really mean, they are exercising "diplomacy"; when their statesmen say what they do not really mean, they are engaging in "guile."[17]

One of the cruelest practices in the labeling process is the "tag" that follows a person—sometimes for life. Putting a label on a child can influence the child's entire life; for example, "porky," "shorty," or "fatty" can have the effect of encouraging the victim either to live up to the label or to try to overcome it by changes in behavior. "Clumsy" may be awkward for years unless the child is able to forget the label. The labels "juvenile delinquent" and "ex-con" may brand people for life.

LISTENING

The nursing profession, as in most areas of professional endeavor, spends far more time as receivers of messages than as senders. Just as the sender attempts to elicit a response from the receiver, the receiver must attempt to interpret the genuine meaning in the message. In the interpersonal verbal transaction, the receiver fulfills the role of listener.

People have become quite adept at not listening. In a society in which they are constantly bombarded with noise, they learn to close their minds to such distortions. The brain picks and selects those cues having genuine significance. This capacity to shut out and ignore insignificant noise is a genuine blessing, but it can lead to listening habits that can adversely affect the capability for interpersonal communication. The listener actually determines whether communication will take place. For any reason, receivers can shut the speaker off mentally.

Part of the problem can be attributed to the disparity between a person's thought speed and the rate of a speaker. Whereas people speak in the vicinity of 125 to 175 words per minute, people's thought rate is far greater. They may use this spare time to "detour," or make brief excursions away from the subject, then come back to listen. Unlike the reader who loses one's chain of concentration and rereads the section missed, however, the listener may have no opportunity for reiteration. The differential between thought speed and speech rate tempts one into the bad habits of daydreaming, shutting out the speaker, and impairing the flow of communication.

A leading authority on listening believes that much bad listening results from an emotional reaction to certain words or ideas that blots out the rest of the message. Consciously watch for the times when you tend to tune out a speaker because you fail to like the speaker's personality or ideas. Even if one's goal is to argue the speaker down, one owes it to oneself to listen fully. Notice the words or thoughts that make you stop listening. Today, some people develop static when hearing such words as "pot," "chauvinist," "degree," "liberated," or others. And there are special terms that jar persons involved in certain fields and distort their listening judgment. A man who has been having trouble with a newly purchased house may go "deaf" at the mention of leaks, termites, or contractors; his interest perks up, but he hears mainly his own jangled thoughts. Similarly, a person who has been speculating in the stock market may tune out anyone who mentions losses, sharp drop, or sell-off.[18] Thus, people filter incoming stimuli and perceive only those parts of the total pattern that fit their general or specific orientations (biases).

An additional problem for the listener is to distinguish between observational statements and statements of inference. A speaker may be reporting one's own perception of reality ("That man lives in a brown house") or drawing inferences ("That man is proud of his house"). Observational and inferential statements are extremely difficult to distinguish because grammar, syntax, and pronunciation offer no clues to the differences. Likewise, the inference may be made with such vocal dynamics and certainty that the "truth" of the statement may go unquestioned. Previously noted was the willingness of students to infer motives for the instructor's departure from the classroom ("He had another meeting"), all of which were wrong. Inferences are necessary for behavior and communication, but problems may develop when people tacitly assume that statements of inference are totally factual.

FEEDBACK

The accomplishment of mutual understanding between encoder and decoder can be determined only by feedback. Because of the numerous sources of error and distortion in the message, it is often valuable to check back to see if understandings exist. Among the possible problems are the following:

1. The encoded message may not be the same as the message intended by the speaker, or it may be garbled or unclear.
2. The receiver's perception of the speaker's motives or goals may influence the way the message is interpreted.
3. The words in the message may have different meanings to the receiver than to the sender, or they may have no meaning at all for the receiver.
4. The listener's attention might be diverted at a crucial time during transmission.
5. Expectations of the relationship may be confused.

You can probably add to this list. The point is that there are so many pitfalls that people owe it to themselves to provide adequate feedback to one another if they are to have any hope of gaining understanding and rapport.

SUMMARY

This chapter discussed the characteristics of language that make effective communication difficult to achieve. Words have different meanings to different people; words vary in their degree of abstraction; and language is by nature incomplete, reflects the culture of a person's society, and creates a "social reality." These factors all contribute to misunderstandings between people, so they must be satisfied with degrees of mutual understanding.

Words play an important part in every human relationship. They are among the tools used to establish bonds between people and may clarify or obscure ideas, and may unify or alienate people. As senders and receivers of verbal messages, individuals must be aware of the potential problems and be constantly on guard to ensure understanding.

REFERENCES

1. JEAN PIAGET: *The Language and Thought of the Child* (New York: Harcourt Brace Jovanovich, 1926), p. 26.
2. G. A. MILLER: *Language and Communication* (New York: McGraw-Hill, 1951), pp. 155–156.
3. L. S. VIGOTSKY: "Thought and Speech," *Psychiatry*, 2 (1939): 29–54.
4. J. A. M. MEERLOO: *Conversation and Communication* (New York: International Universities, 1952), p. 83.

5. S. I. Hayakawa: *Language in Thought and Action* (New York: Harcourt Brace Jovanovich, 1964), pp. 173–180.
6. *Ibid.*, p. 189.
7. W. Johnson: *People in Quandaries* (New York: Harper & Row, 1946), p. 270.
8. S. Chase: *Power of Words* (New York: Harcourt Brace Jovanovich, 1954), p. 55.
9. Penny A. McCarthy: "Blind Ida and the Dilemma of Disposition," *Nursing Outlook*, February, 1981, p. 91.
10. R. W. Force and M. Force: "Keys to Cultural Understanding," *Science*, 133 (1961): 1202–1206.
11. L. Schatzman and A. L. Strauss: "Social Class and Modes of Communication," *American Journal of Sociology*, 60 (1955): 329–338.
12. J. C. Baratz: "The Language of the Ghetto Child," *The Center Magazine*, 1 (1969): 32.
13. This study of the effect of language on our prejudices was conducted at Pro Deo University in Rome. It is reported and evaluated by N. Cousins: "The Environment of Language," *Saturday Review*, April 8, 1967, p. 36.
14. Jean Faust: "Words That Oppress," *Women Speaking*, April, 1970.
15. *Time*, January 29, 1951, p. 62.
16. *Newsweek*, September 21, 1953, p. 62.
17. Sydney Harris: "Last Things First," syndicated column appearing in the *Chicago Daily News*, December 18, 1962.
18. R. G. Nichols and L. A. Stevens: *Are You Listening?* (New York: McGraw-Hill, 1957), pp. 90–94.

5
NONVERBAL
MESSAGES

Of all the various ways of communicating with patients, other nurses, administrators, and physicians, there is probably no means at your disposal more important than nonverbal behavior. The chances of improving interpersonal communication in this domain are fairly good—and extremely valuable.

If you and one of the authors were to meet and talk, you would notice sights and sounds that in your mind would have certain meanings. The nonverbal and verbal behavior you observed would be a series of events. Based on your awareness of these events, you would interpret them in terms of various possible messages. In essence, interpersonal communication consists of making meaning out of events. People seek to make sense out of what they see and hear.

Communication without words makes up a large part of the meanings shared between nurses. Sometimes, patients are unwilling or unable to express their true feelings and desires in words, or they may even be unaware of these feelings. Yet all people convey messages by the way they use their bodies and through their facial expressions, gestures, touch, and tone of voice.

We distrust much of the recent writing on "body language" that has attempted to assign psychodynamic meanings to particular facial expressions or explain what a woman's crossing her legs "means." We are not concerned with simplistic views of using nonverbal communication, or with suggestions of ways of using it to manipulate another person, to gain popularity, or to be able to "read a person like a book." Instead, we are concerned with nonverbal communication in the context of the total relationship between people.

The perceptual channels of sight, sound, and touch have been discussed previously. Although scholars disagree on the definitional limits of verbal and nonverbal communication, the distinction is made to indicate that communication in addition to words occurs and has profound effects on nurses and patients.

The interlacing of fingers, twist of a foot, slump of a shoulder, curl of a lip, direction of a gaze, or tilt of the head are instances of what is called nonverbal behavior. All can occur simultaneously or separately, with or without words, spontaneously or by contrivance, during an interaction or when an individual is alone. The nurse's concern is with the communicative functions of nonverbal behavior in the nurse's environment.

THE VERBAL/NONVERBAL INTERFACE

You may say the sentence "I don't know where I'm going to have dinner tonight" in a variety of ways. You may be seeking information on good restaurants, or you might be angling for an invitation to dinner. By your intonation, the context, the relationship between you and your listener, and the various nonverbal cues you are providing, one may infer what you mean. Even "good morning" can convey a number of meanings. A "good morning" to a physician may indicate timidity, awareness of subordinate status, anxiety as to how the greeting will be received, and so on. Another may convey condescension, awareness of power position, rejection, hostility, and the like. The key is to make sense out of the verbal and nonverbal messages, to arrive at a congruent perception of a transaction.

Congruent messages contain information from a number of channels to be combined harmoniously, agreeably, and consistently into one clear meaning. Messages from both verbal and nonverbal cues form complete statements; clusters of behaviors reinforce and complement one another. For example, after a difficult task is completed, a nurse might express a congruent message of relief by saying, "Thank heaven that's done," relaxing the body as the nurse eases into a chair, exhaling a full, audible sigh, and resting the arms lightly beside the body.

When the verbal and nonverbal aspects of the message do not fit, the receiver must somehow translate the data into a single message. A physician—for example, one who has had a heavy surgery schedule—comes into the nurses' station and says in an irritable tone of voice, "Damn it, the suture broke!" The nurse must then, with great agility and skill, go through the following mental process:

1. He is reporting on the condition of the suture.
2. I know he is irritated. His "Damn it" and the tone of his voice make this clear.

3. Is he blaming me for the condition of the suture? If he is criticizing me, what does he think I should do—apologize, help him, or what?
4. Maybe he is criticizing himself and is frustrated by the broken suture. If so, what is he asking me to do—sympathize, just listen, or what?
5. Since I know from working with him that he has little patience with malfunctions, he is probably just irritated at the situation and is asking me primarily to sympathize with him.
6. Now how can I communicate that I am genuinely sympathetic—listen quietly, offer to help, offer suggestions? How can I best communicate my conscious concern and interest?

Had the physician merely said, "I'm having a hard time today; I need a cup of coffee," the nurse would have had little difficulty assessing the message. The nurse would still be in the position of deciding what to say about the physician's request, but at least the nurse would not be in doubt about what the physician wants.[1]

Nonverbal behavior in an interpersonal situation speaks as effectively as words and usually is more readily accepted. Nonverbal communication establishes the basis for interaction in the animal world and for animal interaction with humans. In research with bottle-nosed porpoises, investigators have noted the unique way the porpoise attempts to establish a relationship with humans. The animal tries to take a person's hand in its mouth and gently squeeze the hand in its powerful jaws, which contain razor-sharp teeth. If the human will submit to this demonstration, the porpoise seems to accept the act as a message of complete trust. Its next move is to reciprocate by placing the forward, bent portion of its body, roughly equivalent to the human throat—its most vulnerable area—on the person's hand, foot, or leg, thereby signaling its trust in the friendly intentions of the person. Similarly, a cat routinely establishes a demonstration of trust through the ritual of throwing itself on its back, exposing its jugular vein to younger cats or cats from outside its own territory. The taking of the jugular vein in the jaw of the other cat establishes an "I-shall-not-attack-you" message that serves to define the relationship.[2]

While language can be used to communicate almost anything, however abstract, nonverbal behavior is rather limited in range. It is usually used to communicate feelings, liking, and preferences and to reinforce or contradict the verbal message. It may also add a new dimension to the verbal message, such as when a patient describes the illness to a nurse and simultaneously conveys, nonverbally, the impression of liking the nurse.[3]

Nonverbal messages can, like linguistic ones, be misinterpreted. For example, a nurse may find oneself suspected of an unconfessed guilt if one spontaneously presents one's supervisor with a gift. In another kind of situation, a nurse may be confused in trying to interpret the meaning of a patient's growing pale, trembling, sweating, or stammering, perhaps when being interviewed. Such behavior can be interpreted as unmistakable proof of illness, or it may merely be the behavior of a person going through the experience of being interviewed and realizing that anxiety may be interpreted as illness. People add to the potential confusion by their propensity to "play games" with their outward manifestations of feelings. Some people have become good "poker faces" and are temporarily able to conceal their genuine feelings.

The ways of interpreting another nurse's reactions to oneself in the form of nonverbal messages will determine one's relationship with that nurse. This person's acceptance of one can, in turn, cause one to accept the person. The cues are constantly being reinterpreted and reanalyzed at the subconscious level as the basis for future interaction. Because the nonverbal behaviors tend to be less conscious, people tend to believe them even more than the linguistic messages if the two are incongruent. Recent work with lie detectors shows the impact of unconscious nonverbal communication behaviors. These detectors record physiologic changes, such as pulse and perspiration changes, that cannot be controlled by the person being tested.

It is important to note that communication by use of words is usually more or less conscious; often, use of words is not deliberate, but it usually involves conscious cognitive effort. On the other hand, nonverbal communication may be either conscious or unconscious. When people are conscious of their nonverbal communication, they deliberately use signs to signify their intended meaning. Artful use of posture, gestures, tones, and body language may assist others to interpret meaning from their actions. Unconscious behavior of a nonverbal kind ordinarily operates whether people want it to or not—in fact, frequently in spite of their wishes. For the most part, it serves very well in helping others to interpret meanings, motives, and intentions in limited circumstances. Ordinarily, you should not have to worry about your unconscious nonverbal behavior so long as you wish to be honest with others. In such cases, it will tend to take care of itself and serve its purposes well in helping others to understand you. For most people, it does not serve well when they are dishonest, dissembling, and trying to deceive one another. Most patients seem to be able to discern deceit—unless you have consummate skill in "acting."

As people meet and interact, they are constantly interpreting each other's actions, both verbal and nonverbal, to help them make judgments about what the other person is thinking, feeling, wanting, or intending. People interpret the other's actions by ascribing meaning that "makes sense." Certain acts are taken to signify certain attitudes, motives, or feelings. In passing, it should be pointed out that the "meaning" of such acts is in the observer's head, not in the acts as such, although it may appear that certain acts have "certain meanings." The study of this process has recently become an important interest of communication scholars. This interest has come to be called *semiology*, the science of signs.

THE SCIENCE OF SIGNS: SEMIOLOGY

In human interaction, acts can be taken to signify events, thoughts, attitudes, motives, intentions, and feelings. As a nurse, you must be interested in the nature of this process—how it works. Such study is relatively new to students of communication, having been developed in the last 15 years. Semiology as a science is rather less than exact, although it has a long tradition in the medical profession: the diagnosis of diseases from *symptoms.*

If you have ever been diagnosed as having any disease other than the "flu," you know that a symptom or sign stands for or refers to something else, usually something more important than the symptom itself. Thus, a basic concept of semiology is the idea of the *sign.* Very simply, a sign stands for something other than what it is. A complicating factor is that any specific sign can signify more than one thing. Students of semiotics are interested in three broad questions: (1) How does the use of signs affect or influence perceivers *(pragmatics);* (2) what is the system of the code employed—the form of statements received by observers of signs *(syntactics);* and (3) how are signs interpreted to mean specific things or sets of things—ideas, events, attitudes, and so on *(semantics)?* Each of these branches of semiology will be discussed very briefly. It should be understood that each of them refers both to nonverbal and verbal communicative acts. Although the primary interest of this chapter is in nonverbal communication, this discussion of semiology is clearly related to the discussion of verbal communication in Chapter 4.

PRAGMATICS

As the name of this approach to the study of semiology would indicate, a very practical (or pragmatic) question is this: How does the use of signs influence people to do, think, or feel certain ways? Scholars who pursue this issue are concerned with the results of the use of signs—their effect on people. How and to what extent do people respond to symbol systems? For example, what effects do advertising, news releases, slogans, and television have on people? What are their effects on children? Can the use of words, symbolic actions, and slogans seriously influence public opinion? Government officials? Nurses? Patients? As shown in a later section of this chapter, nonverbal behavior in the forms of personal appearance, vocal tones, facial expressions, eye contact, and "body language" can have important influences on nurses as they engage in interpersonal communication.

In hospitals, what clothing people wear is often a sign of their role and status in the hospital hierarchy. Most housekeeping staff wear colored uniforms, such as blue or gray. Most medical nursing staff members wear white, and volunteers often wear pink or perhaps pink and white stripes. In hospitals in which nursing staff began wearing colored uniforms or street clothes with laboratory coats in pediatrics or psychiatric nursing areas so that clients would be more comfortable, the pragmatic sign system fell apart. There are even more minute signs. Women who are nurses and women who are medical interns often dress in white blouses, skirts, and short jackets, so that it is difficult to distinguish which woman is the nurse and which is the medical intern. The distinguishing sign more recently seems to be where the stethoscope is carried: the medical intern carries it in the jacket pocket, and the nurse drapes it around the neck. These signs lead people to expect certain behaviors or services from the individuals according to the costume.

SYNTACTICS

The format of a statement that is perceived as being made by another person can make a difference to one's ability to interpret such signs. People are most easily made aware of complexity and awkward word order (as illustrated in the preceding sentence). However, nonverbal communication also employs a format in the use of signs that, if violated, can lead to misinterpretation or confusion. For example, suppose you and another nurse are going to the theater; you drive by to pick her up and she is dressed in a track suit, athletic socks, and jogging shoes. Obviously, she isn't ready, and you infer it will be at least a few minutes before you can depart together. Now, if she were in an evening dress, hair neatly combed, with athletic socks and jogging shoes on her feet, the message you infer is not so clear. Is she ready to go that way? How well do you feel you really know this woman? The *format* of her nonverbal behavior causes you to be confused, or at least to hesitate in ascribing meaning to what you see.

A more matronly, conservative nursing supervisor will hesitate turning a very ill client's care over to a young intern on call who arrives dressed in dirty lab coat, sneakers, blue jeans, and a T-shirt with "Jesus is coming and is He pissed!" printed across the front. The interaction of a free generation, humanitarian roles, and mockery of Christianity may be too much to many midwestern matronly women—including patients. And this leads to a question of semantics.

SEMANTICS

The third question asked by students of semiology is: What does a specific sign refer to? What is the nature of the meaning intended by the person who chose to use such a sign? How can you be sure?

The answers to these questions of semantics lie in three more or less separate areas. In the first place, a sign can signify something because it resembles it. We call such a signifier an *icon* (from the Greek word for simile) because the sign is *like* something else. It can look like it, smell like it, feel like it, or taste like it. For example, suppose you meet another nurse wearing a T-shirt with a drawing of your school symbol on it—perhaps a wildcat, tiger, or lion. There are numerous inferences you might draw about the wearer of such a shirt, many of which are interesting and useful to you for further interaction, but mostly tenuous. Icon signs often cannot be taken at face value; the intended meaning (if any) and the inferred meaning may not match.

A second way in which semantic meanings may be inferred from signs is when the signifying event or circumstance was *caused by* another event or circumstance. We call such an *index* of the event or situation thus signified. For example, suppose you come into the nurses' station holding your nose, which is bleeding profusely. One would tend to infer that you had had an accident. As you can see, *indexical* signs are somewhat tenuous—not certain, but frequently very useful.

A third way in which semantic meanings may be inferred, and by far the most often used in human communication, is from *symbolic* signs. Symbol systems do not work by resembling something (although sometimes this occurs as an additional factor), or by being caused by an event or circumstance; they work simply by arbitrary agreement or social custom. The word "woman" does not look like a woman, is not caused by a woman, but by social agreement has come to stand for or refer to (in English) an adult female human being. *Symbols* are the essence of natural human languages, and their essential use has been demonstrated in Chapter 4 in the discussion of verbal communication. However, nonverbal symbols can help people infer meaning through arbitrary use of social conventions. Traffic signs may provide an interpretation of their meaning even if snow has covered the verbal (words) on them; uniforms may be taken to provide meaning about those who wear them; by agreement (social convention), even a "meaningless grunt" can be taken as a sign of recognition when given by a hard-shelled, mean, old physician (sometimes that's all the affection for another human such a person ever shows—at least, in front of nurses).

The unlimited opportunity to invent and use arbitrary symbols is uniquely human; it has allowed people to communicate meaning far beyond rudimentary limits. Humans can speak of ideals, fantasies, unrealized hopes, and even unrealistic fears through the use of arbitrary symbol systems. They have helped people develop statistics, calculus, chemistry, history, religion, physics, astronomy, stocks and bonds, organizations, nations, governments, laws, and even mythology; the list is endless.

Perhaps human beings owe their greatest of all debts to those who have, before and along with them, developed symbol systems. Even so, ascribing meaning to symbols as people see or hear them used in their presence carries inherent risks and problems. Symbols can refer to things that are thought to exist but cannot be found; people can think they know their meaning when they do not; and people can use such symbols as if they meant one thing when, in fact, they mean something else. In addition, individuals can use words as if they signified something when, in fact, they are meaningless, "full of sound and fury, signifying nothing." Languages may thus be viewed as a special kind of sign system, and other sign systems, in part, may be used in place of language.

Both nonverbal and verbal (word) communications employ all three types of semantic use of signs: iconic, indexical, and symbolic. All three are useful in nonverbal communication, but the first two are of primary utility. Thus, there is an inherent risk in signs employed in nonverbal communication because iconic and indexical signs are less definite, more ambiguous, and more subject to erroneous interpretation than symbolic systems. On the other hand, they are often viewed as more dependable because they are less easily manipulated; it is more difficult to communicate deceitful or artificial iconic and indexical signs than it is to use dishonest words.

Students of communication should be interested in how the total process of communication works and should be especially interested in codes and symbol systems. When one tries to determine what a sign means, one should try to discover all of its meanings—iconic, indexical, and symbolic. One should be aware of all that is happening when one hears a friend say, "The Minnesota North Stars put out the Atlanta Flames last night, 4 to 3."

Nurses should be careful not to interpret an *icon* on a T-shirt worn by a teen-aged patient as an *index* (caused by some underlying motive or emotion). They should not attribute to a *symbol* that they hear the same strong value they might attribute to an *icon* or *index*. Is a woman on television beautiful *because* she uses Revlon (or Kinney shoes, Regal cookware, Salem Lights, and so forth)? Is a presidential candidate handsome *because* he is a Democrat? Or is he honest *because* he has an innocent smile? What, if anything, is the meaning of a woman with a stethoscope around her neck, a nurse's cap, a soft smile, a trim figure, a strong handshake, a slumping posture, twisting fingers, a firm step, or eyes that are wide open? In essence, what are the various meanings that can reasonably be attributed to nonverbal behaviors?

NONVERBAL COMMUNICATION BEHAVIORS

There are many nonverbal actions to which one might attribute meaning as one meets and interacts with another person. When people talk, they rarely trust the words alone. People shift their weight, wave their arms, frown or smile, and convey their words in varying tones. When individuals are in the presence of other people, they *cannot not* communicate. Meanings may be attributed to the ways people straighten their clothing, read a magazine, or hold a cigarette or a coffee cup. Interest in such nonverbal behavior has increased greatly in the past several years. As yet, however, there are varying opinions concerning the classification of nonverbal behaviors and the generalizations that may be made about them.

Chapter 3 noted that Edward and Mildred Hall identify different nonverbal behaviors with the "distance zones" involved. At close or "intimate" zones, the head, pelvis, eyes, and trunk can be brought into actual contact; there is also an exchange of heat and body odors and an ability to see sensitive shifts in eye movements and facial expressions. As the distance increases into the "public" zones, nonverbal communication plays a less precise role.

How do these classifications of the Halls relate to an interpersonal relationship? Obviously, in a love or friendship relationship, the intimate distances are far more likely to be experienced. In such relationships, greater reciprocity is desirable. Close contact with another person who is physically passive or rigid, who avoids eye contact, who turns one's head away, and who does not reciprocate certainly cannot be identified as a relationship of intimacy or responsiveness.

In another analytic study, Paul Ekman and Wallace V. Friesen developed a classification of nonverbal behaviors based on origin, circumstances of usage, and interpersonal significance or coding.[4] They describe five generic classes of nonverbal behavior: (1) emblems, (2) illustrators, (3) affect displays, (4) regulators, and (5) adaptors.

Ekman and Friesen's classification helps people to understand and identify certain types of nonverbal coding. Good friends, lovers, and spouses may be able to communicate on an intuitive or subliminal level with a flick of the head, an eye glance, or a special movement that conveys great meaning to the partner. As the relationship grows, all facets of nonverbal communication become more synchronized and more concrete in their meanings. Whether one's partner is upset, detached, or "with one," one is able to notice this without using words.

In another attempt at classification, Mehrabian identified three dimensions of nonverbal behavior: evaluation, potency, and responsiveness.[5] In positive interaction situations, there is an increase in positive evaluation, as indicated by a closer position, more forward lean, more eye contact, and more direct orientation. There also seems to be an increase in potency, which is reflected in postural relaxation. Increased responsiveness in positive social relationships is indicated by more facial expressions and more active vocal mannerisms. In an ongoing relationship, individuals are constantly communicating an evaluation of the other person in either a positive or a negative way by their nonverbal responses.

Scholars who are working on the development of theory of nonverbal communication are not entirely in agreement regarding the classification of nonverbal behaviors. Thus, these behaviors will be arbitrarily grouped under four headings: (1) personal appearance, (2) vocal tones, (3) eye and facial movements, and (4) body posture and gestures.

PERSONAL APPEARANCE

There is considerable evidence that the general impression one forms of another person has significant influence on the way one responds to that person.[6] One of the most important factors in such an early impression is one's general appearance. Studies have shown that appraisals of others are made easily and with little conscious awareness. In a few minutes, perceivers form an image of another person that will guide their responses. In a study by Barker, for example, strangers who had no opportunity to interact verbally showed significant agreement with each other in their impressions of personality traits. Preferences for working together were correlated with these impressions. After several months of working with one another, 55 percent of these subjects reported the same impressions and working-partner choices.[7]

Clothing, cosmetics, and jewelry that are not parts of an institutional or professional uniform often represent a personal choice and are frequently taken as clues to the way people want others to respond to them in certain circumstances. Clothes and personal effects serve many purposes—protection, concealment, sexual attraction, group or organization affiliation, status, role, and self-expression. One study found significant correlations between clothing choices and personal behavior. Subjects scoring high in decorative dress were found to be conventional, conforming, and submissive, whereas those high on economy in dress were responsible, efficient, and precise.[8]

Clothing retailers and advertisers believe that dress is a way of expressing one's self-concept. A study by Compton of clothing choices and desired self-image tended to support this belief.[9] Further studies have shown an association between dress and perceived status with consequent differences in response behavior.[10] There is some evidence that persons are influenced by perceived differences in status clothing; in a well-known study, pedestrians were more influenced to cross "against the traffic lights" by well-dressed (high-status) persons doing so than by poorly dressed persons.[11] In the nursing profession, small items of personal appearance may influence observers' responses. One study has shown that the use of lipstick affected potential responses of males to females.[12] Another study has suggested that wearing glasses may produce more favorable judgments of intelligence and industriousness.[13]

Although the studies completed to date can only be taken to be suggestive of a relationship between personal appearance (including apparel) and predictable interpersonal response behavior, it is quite clear that ordinarily people are influenced by it in a fairly dependable way. An interesting example of this principle was demonstrated by Schauer.[14] Subjects including students, police cadets, and school teachers judged persons whose apparel *did not match* to be *less credible* than persons whose attire matched. "Matching" elements included beards, sport jackets, fringed leather shirts, "dress slacks," blue jeans, and "dress shirts." When apparel did not appear to present a clear, composite picture, observers reflected doubt and suspicion.

At present, no research provides a clear, complete index of the way dress and appearance can be taken as dependable *indexical* (cause and effect) or symbolic signs of potential interpersonal responses of nurses. However, as *iconic* signs, nurses rely on uniforms, gross differences in clothing, and general appearance as signs of status, authority, knowledge, and desired patterns of response behaviors. In a hospital or clinic, it is generally considered helpful to use some systematic code of dress to differentiate role, function, and status of all personnel.

VOCAL TONES

Actors and their audiences have long had great respect for the nuances of feeling that can be expressed by the voice alone. Most people have a similar respect, and they are often more willing to trust a person if they can hear the person's voice when a statement is made than if the same substantive information is conveyed in writing. To some extent, people are interested in judging personality patterns as they listen to another's voice. To a great degree, however, they are interested in noting emotional states of one another. Generally, one's judgment of the current emotional state of a client will be based as much on the tone of voice as on what is said. Such a judgment is very likely to have a significant effect upon one's interaction with that person.

The earliest studies of the voice alone indicated that age, sex, bodily build, intelligence, and occupation might be dependably judged from vocal differences. Efforts to find a significant relationship between vocal characteristics and major personality factors have been somewhat tenuous.[15] Only recently have more carefully selected samples of voice usage and more precise specification of personality factors produced support for the voice/personality relationship.[16] For example, introverted female speakers have been found to be low in variation of pitch, force, and rate. Introverted males were found to have breathy, muffled, high-pitched voices.

Probably of more immediate value in interpersonal communication have been studies of *stereotypes* of voice usage. That people use such stereotypes may be objectionable on moral or ethical grounds; however, the fact that they are used is an important consideration as people meet and interact with one another. Negative listener attitudes are often associated with low-volume, high-pitched voices of males and with husky, harsh, low-pitched voices of females. It is unfortunate that opportunities for employment and/or advancement are influenced by attitudes toward such vocal variations; there are recorded instances in which employers apparently have judged the potential success of applicants on such bases.[17] Other studies have shown that these attitudes are the result of cultural accidents or social prejudice, and they are subject to change if a society wants them changed.

Of even greater practical significance to a nurse is the value of the voice as a cue of the current emotional state of a patient. Early studies by Fairbanks and Pronovost demonstrated that internal states of fear, anger, and grief were expressed with different vocal rates, pauses, and pitch.[19] Later studies showed that often emotional states could be identified reliably by voice quality alone.[20] Considerable differences have been noted in the capacity (at least in ordinary circumstances) to use vocal variations in pitch and force (volume); for each individual, a general "baseline" of ordinary variation must be considered. Even so, experimental evidence clearly indicates that vocal qualities accurately convey indications of a current emotional state. Love, fear, and hate are most easily identified.

Of particular interest to persons in health care is the judgment of the credibility of a speaker. Considerable evidence has been found that judgments of credibility are linked to a speaker's vocal behavior—"firmness" (force) and avoidance of nonfluencies (*uh, er,* and so forth), as well as pleasing tones (pitch and resonance). The amount of trust you offer to a speaker will likely increase as a more "conversational" style and use of the voice are achieved.[21]

As the discussion of various nonverbal communication behaviors continues, it would be well to remind you that seldom does one of them occur alone. Vocal usage is reinforced (or confused) by facial expression, gestures, posture, and other behaviors. In any given instance, all of them should be noted collectively, and a judgment of a person's attitudes, ideas, and intentions made on the basis of an integrated response to all of them together.

The voice is often considered by nurses to be an index to the general level of energy available for clients. And awareness of this index can also be applied to oneself, to peers, and to colleagues. One might note the difference in voices of the nurse just returning to work after several days off, of the nurse after working 10 straight nights, and of the intern who has been on call for 48 very busy hours. The rested, alert person usually has a voice full of variations and inflections in tone and rapidity, whereas the fatigued person tends toward low, mumbled monotones and perhaps incomplete sentences conveyed slower than normal for that person. Awareness of this index of energy can aid in maintaining relationships with peers when one gives extra consideration for their low energy levels.

FACE AND EYES

Of all the nonverbal behaviors in interpersonal communication, very probably those involving the face and eyes are the most important in interpreting the meaning that events have for you as a nurse. Specifically, the mutual glance or meeting of the eyes and the exchange of mutual smiles set the tone for the encounter and influence the interaction behavior that follows.

The smile has been identified as the most primitive of human responses and the earliest evidence of recognition and acceptance of another person.[22] In one experimental study, approval-seeking persons gave significantly more smiles than avoidance-seeking persons.[23]

The significance of the mutual glance in interpersonal communication was given an early emphasis (1921) by a sociologist, George Simmel. He called it the purest form of reciprocity: "By the same act in which the observer seeks to know the observed, he surrenders himself to be understood."[24] The mutual glance is a way of indicating degree of willingness to be involved with another person, as well as the absence of fear, hostility, or suspicion; it is a primary display of readiness to communicate. This information is of special significance to a nurse interacting with peers and others. Too much eye contact may be misinterpreted by male peers as an invitation for a personal rather than a professional relationship, especially when accompanied by more than usual smiles. Averting the eyes is a basic way of attempting to insulate oneself from appeals, arguments, commands, threats, and affection of others. Studies by Exline have shown that persons being praised increase the frequency of their glances, while persons given negative criticism avert their eyes.[25] He also found that women use eye contact in interpersonal communication more than men, and that persons high in affiliative or affection needs tend to return glances more often.[26] Some clients seem to search a nurse's face for affection, information, and support. Other studies have shown that persons requested to talk about themselves use far more visual contact with persons who show nonverbal approval,[27] and that they use significantly less eye contact while answering embarrassing questions.[28]

There is some evidence that emotional states of a person can be identified by observing the face and eyes in live, expressive communication; however, familiarity with that person's usual behavior is helpful. Even so, identification of inner emotional states from facial expressions alone is rather undependable.[29] Still, it is quite clear that certain parts of the face tend to be used more than other parts to express various emotional states; the eyes to show surprise and the mouth to signal disgust.[30]

Mutual glances have been shown to aid in defining the nature of a desired interpersonal relationship. The two basic relationship dimensions, degree of dominance-submissiveness and degree of hostility-affection, are communicated.[31] Such use of mutual glances serves to monitor and control the interaction, guiding the participants in their responses to one another.[32]

To make a useful interpretation of other persons' mutual glances, you will need to take into account their sex, the nature of the task in which you are engaged, and their desire to maintain a friendly relationship with you. This information is very valuable to a nurse seeking to fulfill one's professional role. Research has shown that generally women spend more time looking at other women than men. Both women and men spend *less* time looking at each other if they are more concerned with maintaining a friendly relationship than if they are concerned primarily with completing a task, and they look at each others' eyes *more* if they are *competitively* oriented toward achieving a task.[33]

Gazing into another person's eyes may be perceived as a warm, affectionate gesture if the relationship is warm and affectionate; however, between strangers or new acquaintances it may be viewed as a prelude to combat! Studies of animals show that a direct gaze into their eyes signals a threat unless mitigated by friendly vocal signals and/or touch (petting and so forth). Centuries of evolution have produced a ritualization of glaring and looking away. Glaring is used by dogs and monkeys to threaten and control, and looking away is used as a signal of submission.[34] Some experiments suggest that this signal system is similarly employed by people.[35] Arousal of hostility by prolonged eye contact (e.g., staring) varies considerably from culture to culture. Prolonged eye contact is rather common among white Americans; it tends to arouse hostility among black Americans, South Americans, and Southern Europeans.[36]

The readers should be reminded once again that interpretation of eye contact and facial expression should be done in conjunction with interpretation of other nonverbal behaviors, especially vocal tones and gestures.

POSTURES, GESTURES, AND BODY LANGUAGE

The human body is quite versatile, capable of expressing a wide variety of feelings and ideas. Ray Birdwhistell, one of the early pioneers in the study of "body language," identified 60 elements of behavior that could be reacted to as different and separate from each other.[37] A problem of interpreting these behaviors is that they function as continuous variables, not as individually discrete, interpretable behaviors. In a somewhat gross way, they can be interpreted usefully; for example, Howard Rosenfeld has found that persons seeking the approval of others use more head nods and gestural activity.[38]

Posture alone can convey useful information. It will, in the first place, indicate activity being pursued that might deny or diminish an opportunity for interpersonal communication—for example, getting into an automobile, starting its motor, and so on. More specifically, posture can communicate two conditions that may influence interaction: (1) attitudes toward a person or object, and (2) an internal emotional state.[39]

In a long series of studies, Mehrabian found that posture can indicate reliably two basic attitudes: (1) attention (to a person or object) and (2) relaxation.[40] Attention was indicated primarily by leaning forward or toward the person or object, and relaxation by leaning backward with accompanying variety (less uniformity) in arm and leg positions. The attentive style is used toward people who are liked, of higher status, or currently more important; it is used by females more than by males. The relaxed style is used toward persons of lower status, toward females more than toward males, and to a person of the opposite sex more than to a person of the same sex. Other studies have suggested that persons who are dominant in a relationship tend to stand or sit erect; compliant or submissive persons tend to be less erect with head often lowered or tilted up toward the dominant person.[41]

Body posture has been found to show the intensity of an emotional state although facial expression conveys more information about the emotion (fear, joy, anger) being experienced.[42] Extreme emotions can thus be identified when people are severely disturbed; for example, those suffering deep depression tend to droop and sit listlessly looking at the floor.[43]

As nurse meets patient and they engage in interpersonal communication, general postural behavior acts as an extension of gestures, but narrower and shorter than use of space, spatial positions, and relationships (e.g., how close to one another they stand or sit).

Gestures, particularly hand and arm movement (but including other elements of body movement: head nodding, slumping, foot shifting, and so forth), perform several functions: illustrating an idea, expressing an emotional state, and signaling by using a conventional or agreed-upon sign.

Illustration of an idea or object is usually connected to verbal speech. Nonverbal illustrations are iconic, that is, they show movements or relationships (shape, distance) with hands, arms, or other parts of the body that show similarity to an object or condition. They are especially useful in describing an idea that is difficult or inconvenient to describe in words, by use of pointing, showing tempo or rhythm, or showing body movements.[44] One study has shown that people who have greater verbal facility also use more gestures.[45]

Although facial expressions generally are more dependable for inference of an emotional state, gestures and hand movements also display emotions. These movements are often diffuse, otherwise meaningless, and often idiosyncratic (peculiar to individuals).[46] Hand movements especially convey the level of excitement of a speaker—hands waving, clutching each other, straining. Anxious speakers often show such nonverbal signs that are not intended to be communicated, and attempts are often made to conceal them.

Gestures, especially hand movements, may reveal feelings and emotional states that persons don't intend to reveal.[47] Many of these feelings or attitudes are directed toward oneself.[48] Self-directed gestures may include covering the eyes, touching or covering part of the face, and other hand movements designed to groom or hide parts of one's body. Such movements are frequently indicative of shame or embarrassment.[49] One research team asked subjects to view a film and then to (1) describe their feelings *honestly* in an interview and (2) *dishonestly* in another. Observers were able to identify *twice as many* self-directed motions when the subjects gave *dishonest* reports; further, they rated the dishonest reports significantly lower in credibility.[50]

On the other hand, many people are quite aware that small, unobtrusive movements may reveal more of their emotions or feelings than they wish to reveal. To compensate, they may be fairly clever at deliberately using other movements to convey a contradictory impression; for example, artifices may be used to show confidence in order to conceal real anxiety. In such a case, gestures that can usually be taken as *indexical* (the *result* of an inner emotional state) are being faked; such gestures should be interpreted only with considerable care.

It has been noted that gestures can be used to illustrate ideas and may be an index of an inner emotional state. A third way gestures aid interpersonal communication is by signaling, that is, using a conventional symbol that has an agreed-upon meaning. Paul Ekman and Wallace Friesen, probably the foremost researchers in this area, have identified nonverbal acts that have a direct verbal counterpart as *emblems*.[51] Well-known emblems are hand-raising in an auction signaling a bid, or traffic officers' hand signals for stop or go. In addition to emblems, however, there are conventional or symbolic gestures that have no direct verbal counterpart—for example, handshakes, salutes, clasped hands (double-fist) waved above one's head. Some of these conventional signals may be iconic in nature or origin, such as giving the "sign of the cross," and may be used in ceremonial or religious settings. Some of them may be given additional meaning by the manner in which they are performed—for example, degree of pressure in a handshake, or who salutes first when salutes are conventional.

Occupational groups often develop systems of conventional or symbolic signals where conditions of noise or distance make verbal signals difficult or inappropriate—for example, crews in airline terminals or broadcasting studios. Languages for the deaf employ both iconic and symbolic signals. These languages may have a single signal for a complex idea—for example, "heavy rain is coming"—or a signal may be used for one word, such as "go." In addition, signals are used for each letter of the alphabet to spell out significant or difficult words. In these nonverbal communication systems, the vocabulary is often quite large, yet the communication is surprisingly rapid.

Nonverbal intercultural communication is ordinarily best achieved with the use of *iconic* gestures, for example, pointing or using motions that represent an action such as eating. Interpersonal communication between persons who know no common verbal language is not easy but is often surprisingly effective by use of iconic gestures.

TOUCHING

Touching another person is one of the most primitive and important means of nonverbal interpersonal communication. The most valuable use of physical contact is to establish and enjoy interpersonal relationships. This action is especially valuable from a nurse to a patient.

Touching and all forms of physical contact communicate interpersonal attitudes and inner emotional states. Touching is particularly valuable in communicating degrees of personal regard. If feelings are mutual, it can produce increased feelings of warmth and caring.

Touch often has a sexual meaning, usually conditioned in part by one's culture; certain kinds of touching between various types of persons are regarded primarily as sexual signals in some cultures. Degree of contact between two persons can imply a certain level of intimacy—by frequency of touch, duration, and how much clothing is in the way.

Touching and body contact have different significance for various age groups depending on the sex and relationship of the persons involved; such behavior is usually governed by a strong set of cultural rules. Infants cling to their mothers, and for them it is a primary means of communicating. At adolescence, contact with parents is much reduced, especially beyond the age of about 12 years; a study by Jourard found that few college students were touched anywhere beyond their hands and arms by their parents.[52] He found that 75 percent of English male students had been touched by girlfriends on the head, arms, and torso; 75 percent of females had been touched by boyfriends on head, neck, arms, and knees, and more than 50 percent on legs and torso (this study was done in 1963).

In a field study, Mary Henley found that men touched women much more frequently than women touched men, and much more than either sex touched persons of the same sex; also, in other relationships, higher-status persons did much more touching of lower-status persons, for example, physicians and patients, lawyers and clients, and teachers and students.[53]

This discussion has indicated that body contact is used to communicate nurturant attitudes and feelings toward children and dependents and to communicate attitudes toward sex in a relationship. A third use of body contact in a relationship is to express hostility and/or aggression. Aggression is a fairly normal response to attack, frustration, and a perceived threat. Human infants kick and beat with their fists; these aggressive tendencies may be either strengthened or reduced during childhood. To a large extent, the increase or reduction is a result of cultural norms: children wrestling, parents spanking, youths engaging in boxing, judo, military training, and so on. In Western culture, aggression by body contact is to some extent replaced by verbal, symbolic interaction, but not entirely by any means.

Body contact, particularly touching, is a basic biologic way of expressing interpersonal attitudes. In adult life, these forms of nonverbal communication are often replaced by use of gestures and verbal symbols. Even so, when people are ill or injured, their feelings about themselves can be improved by the warm, friendly touch of a person they respect.

USE OF FEEDBACK

To understand fully the use of nonverbal behaviors in interpersonal communication, one must remember that it is constantly changing and flowing, one fleeting movement following another with similarly fleeting cues making impressions not fully realized by the observer, but adding to the impressions and interpretations of one another's attitudes, feelings, and communicative meanings. In addition, responses are given to responses to responses, and so on, so that, as changes in nonverbal behavior are noted, they provide feedback and constant little changes in the general impressions and interpretations of one another's meanings.

In addition to the ebb and flow of body communication, verbal communication is used to check these impressions and interpretations of meaning. Verbal inquiries about attitudes and feelings may act as checks on impressions picked up from nonverbal cues. In a review of research involving both modes of communication, Kanzer concluded: "Only an intellectual bias and misunderstanding proposes that vocalized expression must somehow be higher . . . than other forms."[54] When contradictory messages are concurrently given by verbal and nonverbal communication, confusion results. When they concur, observers are more certain of the other person's attitudes and meanings. Feedback, both verbal and nonverbal, is an important adjunct to nonverbal communication.

SUMMARY

This chapter has reviewed semiology, the science of signs, as a basis for considering the essential elements of both nonverbal and verbal communication. It has noted that communicative signs may be iconic, indexical, or symbolic; this principle applies to nonverbal communication as well as to verbal communication.

This chapter has examined the use of nonverbal behaviors for communicating in four somewhat arbitrarily chosen areas: personal appearance, vocal tones, the face and eyes, and "body language" of posture and gestures. In each case, the focus was on the type of behavior employed and the kinds of messages that may be conveyed. The chapter concluded with an emphasis on the value of feedback in enhancing nonverbal communication behavior.

REFERENCES

1. This exchange and analysis are suggested by VIRGINIA SATIR: *Conjoint Family Therapy* (Palo Alto, Calif.: Science and Behavior Books, 1967), p. 79.
2. P. WATZLAWICK, J.H. BEAVIN, AND D.D. JACKSON: *Pragmatics of Human Communication* (New York: Norton, 1967), p. 104.
3. ALBERT MEHRABIAN: "Communication Without Words," *Psychology Today,* February 1968, p. 53.
4. PAUL EKMAN AND WALLACE FRIESEN: "The Repertoire of Nonverbal Behavior: Categories, Origins, Usage, and Codings," *Semiotica,* 1 (1969): 49–98.
5. ALBERT MEHRABIAN: "A Semantic Space for Nonverbal Behavior," *Journal of Consulting Psychology,* 34 (1970): 248–257.
6. See, for example, LEONARD ZUNIN AND NATALIE ZUNIN: *Contact: The First Four Minutes* (New York: Ballantine, 1973), pp. 6–10.
7. ROGER BARKER: "The Social Interrelations of Strangers and Acquaintances," *Sociometry,* 5 (1942): 169–179.
8. L. AIKEN: "The Relationship of Dress to Selected Measures of Personality in Undergraduate Women," *Journal of Social Psychology,* 59 (1963): 119–128.
9. N. COMPTON: "Personal Attributes of Color and Design Preferences in Clothing Fabrics," *Journal of Psychology,* 54 (1962): 191–195.
10. R. HOULT: "Experimental Measurement of Clothing as a Factor in Some Social Ratings of Selected American Men," *American Sociological Review,* 19 (1954): 324–328.
11. M. R. LEFKOWITZ, R. BLAKE, AND J. MOUTON: "Status Factors in Pedestrian Violation of Traffic Signals," *Journal of Abnormal and Social Psychology,* 51 (1955): 704–706.
12. W. MCKEACHIE: "Lipstick as a Determiner of First Impressions of Personality: An Experiment for the General Psychology Course," *Journal of Social Psychology,* 36 (1952): 241–244.
13. G. THORNTON: "The Effect of Wearing Glasses upon Judgments of Personality Traits of Persons Seen Briefly," *Journal of Applied Psychology,* 28 (1944): 203–207.

14. P.M. SCHAUER: "Some Effects of Variations in Personal Appearance and Apparel on Judgments of the Credibility of Potential Sources of Communication," Unpublished M.A. Thesis, The Pennsylvania State University, 1975.
15. ERNEST KRAMER: "Personality Stereotypes in Voice: A Reconsideration of the Data," *Journal of Social Psychology*, 62 (1964): 247–251.
16. J.C. WEAVER AND R.J. ANDERSON: "Voice and Personality Interrelationships," *Southern Speech Communication Journal*, 38 (1973): 262–278.
17. ROBERT HOPPER AND FREDERICK WILLIAMS: "Speech Characteristics and Employability," *Speech Monographs*, 40 (1973): 296–302.
18. HOWARD GILES, R. BOURKIS, P. TRUDGILL, AND A. LEWIS: "The Imposed Norm Hypothesis: A Validation," *Quarterly Journal of Speech*, 60 (1974): 405–410. See also W.E. LAMBERT, R.C. HODGSON, R.C. GARDNER, AND S. FILLENBAUM: "Evaluational Reactions to Spoken Languages," *Journal of Abnormal and Social Psychology*, 60 (1960): 44–51.
19. GRANT FAIRBANKS AND WILBUR PRONOVOST: "An Experimental Study of the Pitch Characteristics of the Voice During the Expression of Emotion," *Speech Monographs* 6 (1939): 87–104.
20. JAMES DAVITZ: *Communication of Emotional Meaning* (New York: McGraw-Hill, 1964), pp. 23–27.
21. W. BARNETT PEARCE AND F. CONKLIN: "Nonverbal Vocalic Communication and Perceptions of a Speaker," *Speech Monographs*, 38 (1971): 235–241.
22. K. GOLDSTEIN: "The Smiling of the Infant and the Problem of Understanding the 'Other,' " *Journal of Psychology*, 44 (1957): 175–191.
23. HOWARD ROSENFELD: "Instrumental Affiliative Functions of Facial and Gestural Expressions," *Journal of Personality and Social Psychology*, 4 (1966): 65–72.
24. GEORGE SIMMEL: "Sociology of the Senses: Visual Interaction," in R. PARK AND E. BURGESS, EDS.: *Introduction to the Science of Sociology* (Chicago: University of Chicago Press, 1921), p. 358.
25. RALPH EXLINE AND L. WINTERS: "Affective Relations and Mutual Glances in Dyads," in S. TOMKINS AND C. IZARD, EDS.: *Affect, Cognition and Personality* (New York: Springer, 1965).
26. RALPH EXLINE: "Explorations in the Process of Person Perception: Visual Interaction in Relation to Competition, Sex, and Need for Affiliation," *Journal of Personality*, 31 (1963): 1–20.
27. J. EFRAN AND A. BROUGHTON: "Effect of Expectancies for Social Approval on Visual Behavior," *Journal of Personality and Social Psychology*, 4 (1966): 103–107.
28. RALPH EXLINE, D. GRAY, AND D. SCHUETTE: "Visual Behavior in a Dyad as Affected by Interview Content and Sex of Respondent," *Journal of Personality and Social Psychology* 1 (1965): 201–209.
29. ALLEN DITTMAN: *Interpersonal Messages of Emotion* (New York: Springer, 1973), pp. 78–80.
30. PAUL EKMAN, W.V. FRIESEN, AND S.S. TOMKINS: "Facial Affect Scoring Technique: A First Validity Study," *Semiotica*, 3 (1971): 37–58, 113–114.
31. RALPH EXLINE: "Visual Interaction: The Glances of Power and Preference," in J. COLE, ED.: *Nebraska Symposium on Motivation*, 1971 (Lincoln, Neb.: University of Nebraska Press, 1972), pp. 163–206.
32. MICHAEL ARGYLE: *Social Interaction* (New York: Atherton Press, 1969).
33. EXLINE: "Explorations in the Process of Person Perception," pp. 1–20.
34. *Ibid.*

35. PHOEBE ELLSWORTH, J.M. CARLSMITH, AND A. HENSON: "The Stare as a Stimulus to Flight in Human Subjects," *Journal of Personality and Social Psychology*, 21 (1972): 203–211.

36. MARIANNE LaFRANCE AND CLARA MAYO: "Gaze Direction in Interracial Dyadic Communication," paper presented at the Eastern Psychological Association Convention, Washington, D.C., May 1973.

37. RAY BIRDWHISTELL: *Kinesics and Contexts* (Philadelphia: University of Pennsylvania Press, 1970).

38. HOWARD ROSENFELD: "Effects of an Approval-Seeking Induction on Interpersonal Proximity," *Psychological Reports*, 17 (1965): 120–122.

39. MICHAEL ARGYLE: *Bodily Communication* (New York: International Universities Press, 1974), p. 276.

40. ALBERT MEHRABIAN: "The Inference of Attitudes from the Posture, Orientation and Distance of a Communicator," *Journal of Consulting and Clinical Psychology*, 32 (1968): 296–308.

41. MICHAEL ARGYLE, V. SALTER, H. NICHOLSON, M. WILLIAMS, AND P. BURGESS: "The Communication of Inferior and Superior Attitudes by Verbal and Nonverbal Signals," *British Journal of Social and Clinical Psychology*, 9 (1970): 221–231.

42. PAUL EKMAN AND WALLACE FRIESEN: "Head and Body Cues in the Judgment of Emotion," *Perceptual and Motor Skills*, 24 (1967): 711–724.

43. G.B. ROZENBERG AND J. LANGER: "A Study of Postural-Gestural Communication," *Journal of Personality and Social Psychology*, 2 (1965): 593–597.

44. JEAN GRAHAM AND MICHAEL ARGYLE: "A Cross-Cultural Study of the Communication of Extra-Verbal Meaning by Gestures," *International Journal of Psychology*, 24 (1975): 21–31.

45. J.C. BAXTER, E.P. WINTER, AND R.E. HAMMER: "Gestural Behavior During a Brief Interview as a Function of Cognitive Variables," *Journal of Personality and Social Psychology*, 8 (1968): 303–307.

46. PAUL EKMAN AND WALLACE FRIESEN: "Nonverbal Behavior in Psychotherapy Research," *Research in Psychotherapy*, 3 (1968): 179–216.

47. MARIA RUDDEN: "A Critical and Empirical Analysis of Albert Mehrabian's Three-Dimensional Theoretical Framework for Nonverbal Communication," Ph.D. dissertation, Pennsylvania State University, 1974.

48. N. FREEDMAN AND S.P. HOFFMAN: "Kinetic Behavior in Altered Clinical States: Approach to Objective Analysis of Motor Behavior During Clinical Interviews," *Perceptual and Motor Skills*, 24 (1967): 527–539.

49. EKMAN AND FRIESEN: "The Repertoire of Nonverbal Behavior," pp. 49–98.

50. PAUL EKMAN AND WALLACE FRIESEN: "Hand Movements," *Journal of Communication*, 22 (1972): 353–374.

51. EKMAN AND FRIESEN: "The Repertoire of Nonverbal Behavior," pp. 49–52.

52. SIDNEY M. JOURARD: "An Exploratory Study of Body Accessibility," *British Journal of Social and Clinical Psychology*, 5 (1963): 221–231.

53. MARY HENLEY: "Status and Sex: Some Touching Observations," *Bulletin Psychonomic Society*, 2 (1973): 91–93.

54. F. KANZER: "Verbal Rate, Eyeblink, and Content in Structured Psychiatric Interviews," *Journal of Applied Psychology*, 61 (1960): 341–347.

6
BUILDING RELATIONSHIPS

The quality of interpersonal relationships is important to the professional work of a nurse. Both the way you relate with clients and your way of relating with coworkers can have significant outcomes. There is considerable evidence that when a person is ill or recovering from an operation or an accident, the way one thinks about oneself can make a difference in the speed of recovery and the level of physical wellness eventually achieved.[1] If a client has thoughts that are self-degrading, negative, sad, feelings of being left alone, that no one cares, the effect can be negative on the speed and strength of recovery. If the client thinks positive thoughts about self-image, physiologic (mal)functioning, surroundings, and hope for the future, one's physical condition can be enhanced. The kind of responses a client receives from a nurse can directly affect thoughts about oneself, feelings regarding self-image, and attitudes regarding one's condition. You will need to know as much as possible about building good relationships with your clients.

You will also need to know how to build good relationships with other nurses, aides, physicians, and administrators. The quality of a work relationship can affect your performance in that situation. Workers in health-care centers, hospitals, and other agencies must depend upon one another for information, assistance, and judgment. This need to work together imposes a high requirement for interpersonal trust. Without at least some degree of trust of one another, nurses, coworkers, and colleagues will have difficulty in providing the kind of health care expected of them. Development of interpersonal trust requires that relationships be developed which are durable and as comfortable as possible. To a nurse, good interpersonal relationships at work are more than a luxury; they are of primary importance. Consider, for example, the following case:

> Kathy Dalsy, a graduate with 1½ years' experience who has been working on the unit for 5 months, has been caring for Mrs. Thomas, a 52-year-old woman who recently had surgery for a colostomy. Mrs. Thomas has been recovering and has slowly begun to accept the change in body image resulting from the colostomy. Today, with a great deal of help from Kathy, she irrigated it for the first time. In the afternoon, Dr. Marshal sees Mrs. Thomas and tells her she has recovered well, and he will discharge her the next day. As an afterthought, he asks her if she has yet irrigated her colostomy, and upon hearing that she has, replies "good; then everything is set," and promptly disappears.
>
> When Kathy returns from lunch, she hears from Mrs. Thomas that she is to be discharged the next day. Somewhat shocked, she asks Mrs. Thomas how she feels about this. Mrs. Thomas replies that it will be good to be home, but she is afraid that she won't be able to care for herself, nor will her 68-year-old sister with whom she lives. Kathy tells Mrs. Thomas that she will look into the situation. She approaches Jane Ward, the head nurse, and asks her if she is aware that Mrs. Thomas is being discharged the next day. Miss Ward replies that she is and that Mrs. Thomas seems to be recovering quite nicely. Kathy then tells her of Mrs. Thomas's concerns and inability to adequately care for her colostomy. Miss Ward tells Kathy to allow her to irrigate it tomorrow and that should be adequate, replying "she will learn the rest at home." Kathy tells Miss Ward that she believes Mrs. Thomas needs a follow-up visit or two at home. Miss Ward reminds Kathy that the physician must order any follow-up visits of the community nursing service in this hospital.
>
> "Why?," Kathy asks.
>
> Miss Ward replies that although she personally doesn't agree with it, that's the way it's always been here. She reminds Kathy that it is a very conservative and traditional hospital where the physician is considered head and calls all the moves.
>
> "Well," replies Kathy, "I'll get in touch with Dr. Marshal and see what he says."
>
> "I would prefer that you didn't," replies Miss Ward, "He is busy and doesn't like people suggesting how he should follow his patients. Something like this happened about 2 months ago, and he went into a rage, and relations on the unit were tolerable at best for sometime until he cooled down."
>
> "Well, I can see the problem and can understand why we probably can't call Dr. Marshal, but what can we do about Mrs. Thomas?" asks Kathy. "Don't worry about it," replies Miss Ward, "she will be fine, you'll see."

It is easy to see that Kathy is trying to do her job in the best way she knows how. A good relationship with the patient, Mrs. Thomas, apparently has been established. To do her job well, Kathy also must maintain a good working relationship with Miss Ward, the head nurse. To the extent that such a relationship can be developed, to that degree Kathy will be able to understand Miss Ward as well as be understood by her.

As two people interact, the relationship between them tends to stabilize, "freeze," become rigid and unchangeable. To improve an existing relationship or to achieve the most satisfying potential from a developing one, one must analyze it, evaluate it, and, if need be, change it if at all possible. This chapter focuses on the process of analyzing, evaluating, and changing an interpersonal relationship.

A relationship may be analyzed in terms of its basic patterns of interaction and degree of rigidity. Both are important to your understanding if changes or improvements are to be sought. As you interact with another person, it is likely that you gain a general impression of "where you stand" with that person. You seem to be fairly close, sympathetic with each other, and seem to like each other. Generally, you cooperate, confide, and respect each other's wishes. The questions being raised are these: Can the primary behavioral *dimensions of a relationship* be defined and identified? In how many *different* ways do people relate to each other? How many of these are really *important*, significant? In a given situation, can these be observed and the *intensity* of each estimated?

ANALYZING A RELATIONSHIP

Three decades of research support the conclusion that any interpersonal relationship has three primary dimensions: (1) the degree of involvement, (2) the emotional tone or feelings, and (3) the amount of interpersonal control.[3]

INTERPERSONAL INVOLVEMENT

The degree of involvement in a relationship refers not only to the *amount* of interaction between the participants, but also to the importance each attaches to this interaction. If two people seldom see or talk to each other and, when they do, simply exchange impersonal greetings, the degree of their mutual involvement with each other is small. This is especially true if they do not notice that for days they don't see each other. For example, you work with a nurse who ordinarily works on the opposite wing of the hospital. Did that nurse attend the in-service meeting yesterday? If you can't remember, your degree of involvement in this relationship is low, even if you tend to see and talk to each other two or three times a week. Conversely, you and your father may live in different distant cities, see each other twice a year, and communicate only four or five times a year, and still have a high degree of involvement in your relationship. If each idea he presents and each sentence he speaks or writes are given careful thought and attention, then your degree of involvement is high.

The degree of involvement is closely related to the amount of personal information exchanged. To be involved with someone, you must know some things about the person that matter to you, things that are significant. If your involvement with another person is to be high, you and that person will have to reveal significant parts of yourselves to each other. There are fairly dependable research data showing that when self-disclosure is high, interpersonal involvement is heightened.[4]

Scholars who are studying the development of interpersonal relationships generally agree on three principles according to Michael Roloff in his summary of their research:

1. A relationship requires sharing of information by the persons involved.
2. As information is shared, participants make more discriminating predictions about one another's responses.
3. As more discriminating predictions are made, the relationship becomes more valuable to the participants.[5]

Essentially, four requirements must be met if a relationship is to develop: self-disclosure by both participants, positive interpersonal perceptions, sharing of information about one another's self-concepts, and predictions made and fulfilled regarding desirable responses to each other.[6]

Suppose, for example, that you (a woman) meet someone (a man) on the tennis court. You like his looks. This personal information initiates a degree of involvement on your part. You chat awhile and you like the sense of personal values implied by the conversation: He expresses regard for friends, appreciation of personal skill and achievement, and interest in conversing with you. You play tennis for an hour and receive an impression of honesty in keeping the score, determination to do one's best, and fairness in judging out-of-bounds serves. At lunch, you are impressed by his courtesy and consideration for others, cleanliness in eating habits, and friendliness in meeting your needs or wishes. During the next half hour, you hear of his hopes for graduation, ambition to be a pediatrician, frustration over required courses, and sadness over the recent loss of a grandfather. If, over the ensuing days, such self-disclosure continues and you can continue to be interested in such personal information, involvement in the relationship will increase. In addition, disclosure of the way he *feels about you* can lead to greater involvement. If he shows interest in and respect for your hopes, ambitions, values, and frustrations, your degree of involvement will be heightened, and the relationship will be of greater importance both to you and to him.

As people interact and disclose items of personal information to each other, they tend to reach little agreements on what is important and what is not. Out of this sharing comes a working consensus of mutual sympathy and consideration. There is also a tendency to close the gaps between their individual differences of opinion. In essence, *involvement* in a relationship means that participants interact in ways that are important to each other. As involvement is increased, the other two dimensions of a relationship become important: *control* and *affect* (emotional tone). In an *established* relationship, the degree of involvement is usually quite stable. The amount of interaction may vary from day to day, but such variations are expected and routine. In such a relationship, control and affect are of greatest concern.

Work relationships will have varying degrees of involvement depending largely on the roles involved. For example, your professional role with a client demands a degree of distancing and detachment. You may be involved due to roles of nurse-client, but restraint will be needed to keep the relationship one of a professional nature, that is, not becoming involved to the degree that you make poor judgments about the client's health care.

THE EMOTIONAL TONE

Behavior related to *affect*, or emotional tone, in a relationship involves expressions of warmth, acceptance, and love, as well as hostility, rejection, and hate. It is frequently characterized by such positive terms as "friendship," "emotionally close," "sweetheart," and such negative terms as "dislike," "coldness," and "distant emotionally."

In a relationship, affectionate behavior on the part of one person tends to produce affectionate responses on the part of the other; on the other hand, hostile behavior tends to produce hostility. Behavior that can be characterized as severe hostility nearly always produces resentment, dislike, and anger; over time, many people learn to hate. People may thus conclude that interpersonal affect behavior falling on their affection-hostility continuum ordinarily elicits similar responses.[7] Affection elicits affection in response; hostility elicits hostility. With clients, friendliness and warmth are contagious. Nurses can greatly influence the feelings of their clients with positive expressions of feelings.

CONTROL: DOMINANCE-SUBMISSION

Dominant behavior in a relationship tends to produce submissive responses; this, of course, is true only if interaction continues.[8] If dominant behavior by one person continues and resistance is shown by the other person, the relationship may very likely be terminated. If a power struggle continues in a relationship, this struggle may last for days, months, or even years. In some families, it may never be resolved; it may lead to the use of manipulative games or strategies that continue endlessly. Whereas the appetite for sex or comfort is limited, the appetite for power can be limitless.

Submissive behavior in a relationship tends to elicit domination by the other person.[9] If you are dominated, it is not entirely the other person's fault. Submission reinforces dominating behavior, and vice versa. Sometimes power struggles emerge between nurses or between a physician and a nurse. Such conflict should be recognized for what it is—a struggle for *power.*

THE D-A-S-H PARADIGM

These three dimensions of a relationship—involvement, emotional tone, and degree of control—can be analyzed in terms of a model, or paradigm. Drawing from the research of scholars in a variety of fields,[10] it is suggested that an established relationship can be diagrammed in terms of two areas: amount of dominance-submission and amount of affection-hostility. When these four elements are placed on an axis, this is the D-A-S-H paradigm (Fig. 6-1).

The value of the D-A-S-H paradigm as one attempts to analyze one's own interpersonal relationships is that it makes one's work easier and more efficient. It gives one primary targets for analysis. Instead of saying to oneself such things as, "We are usually friendly toward each other but I always feel uncomfortable and my feelings get hurt," one can review one's interpersonal behavior with another person *in toto.* In so doing, one can usually arrive at a satisfactory summary of the relationship in terms of the two dimensions: Am I *generally* dominant or submissive? Are we mostly affectionate or hostile (or in between)? In arriving at answers to these questions, one reviews prior interpersonal behavior and observes more carefully interaction events as they transpire from day to day. One looks for evidence of one's tentative conclusions—smiles, disagreements, squeezes of a held hand, a smile unreturned, frowns, "hard looks," and many other such behaviors that Erving Goffman calls "tie-signs"—indications that the relationship is affectionate or hostile, that one is dominating or being dominated.[11]

The D-A-S-H paradigm can be useful to you as you attempt to summarize your relationship with another person. The *essential* characteristics of any interpersonal relationship can be graphed on this model. For example, relationships between you (Y) and any other person (P) might be summarized in terms of the degree of *dominance, submission, affection,* or *hostility* shown by the distance of Y or P from the center of the D-A-S-H axis.

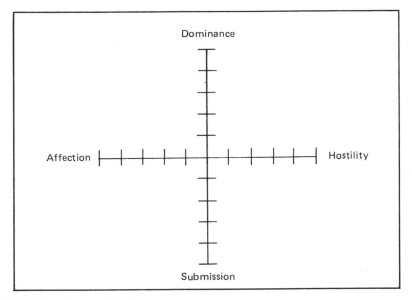

FIGURE 6-1. The D-A-S-H paradigm.

As you have been reading along, undoubtedly you have also been thinking about one of your own interpersonal relationships. Perhaps it is the one you have with your supervisor. After giving it some thought, you may conclude that your relationship with the supervisor involves considerable mutual affection but contains some dominating efforts by your supervisor to which you give small tokens of submission.

As you consider your relationship with another person, graph it as best you can on a D-A-S-H model. Reflect for a while; compare this relationship with other relationships of your own or with some you have observed on the part of other couples or groups. Make a tentative assessment and plot it on a graph. Then pay special attention to interaction events that transpire between you and the other person over a number of days. See if your tentative summary tends to be supported; if not, change it to comply with your observations.

As a nurse, you will need to analyze your relationships with your clients. Are you able to show them, to their satisfaction, warmth and caring? Can you establish relationships with them that help them to feel better about themselves? Do you have the emotional energy in reserve to express concern for their feelings, even though, and especially when, they are not feeling good about themselves and their condition or surroundings? To be able to provide the desirable degree of nurturance, you will need to be able *to express* a warm, caring attitude in these relationship.

In your work as a nurse, you will need to analyze your relationships with your coworkers—aides, head nurses, administrators, physicians, and other nurses. The primary need here will be for you to be able to reach comfortable agreements with your coworkers on the issue of dominance-submission. Can you establish relationships in which you have comfortable arrangements regarding authority—who is in charge; who can ask you to do what; who can, in an emergency, demand of you certain types of behavior without your being upset or resentful? Can you work with persons in authority who are demanding and not very warm or friendly if a client's health or life is in the balance? Are such relationships comfortable and rewarding for you? The authority issue—agreements regarding your dominance over or submission to others in your work—will be a very important part of your nursing career. You will need to analyze your own needs and abilities regarding this issue as you proceed with your career. One way to do this is to look carefully at the relationships you are developing at the present time, giving careful attention to the stages or steps you go through as a relationship develops.

STAGES OF A RELATIONSHIP

The next section considers the patterned regularities in the conversations of dominant-submissive pairs to note the rules used by interactants.

RULES IN DOMINANT-SUBMISSIVE RELATIONSHIPS[12]

Dr. Bonnie Garvin has studied physicians and nurses in their interactions with clients as a model of dominant-submissive relationships. The physicians and nurses are dominant because of their control in the hospital setting over surgery schedules, hospital resources, and everyday routines as well as their greater knowledge in the health and disease process affecting patients. The interactions were videotaped during patient's first day in the hospital. Based upon analysis of the transcripts, Dr. Garvin validated 13 rules in the relationships:

Rule 1. The dominant interactant talks first.

In all the development data episodes except one, the dominant interactant began the sequence of talk. Several forms of conversation initiation were found. Ritual greetings and summons/answer sequences started some conversations; however, in more than half of the episodes, a greeting was omitted and in its place the dominant interactant asked a question.

Rule 2. The dominant interactant selects the first topic in the first utterance.

An inquiry into the state or activity of the other or the statement of an activity to be performed was made as in the following first utterances of episodes:

1. MDS (Medical Student) 1: You goin back to bed or do you want to wait for awhile for your dad to come?
   CT (Client) 2: (I don't care)
2. MDS 4: How's the tube? Working?
   CT 6: Well it's functioning all right . . .
3. RN 5: Did they talk to you yet about your surgery?
   CT 5: No.

In each instance, the clients appropriately answer the questions posed and assume an open state of talk.

The omission of greetings and summons-answer pairs indicated several assumptions about the initiation of interaction. First, the submissive interactant was available for talk, and a greeting or summons was not necessary to establish availability. Second, the submissive interactant had already given commitment to further interaction. Third, the interactants were already in a state of open talk.

The combined use of the two rules of dominant interactant talking first and dominant interactant supplying the first topic provides for a large amount of control in the management of the interaction. The asymmetry in the opening statements affects how those statements are linked with the following statements.

Rule 3. The dominant interactant asks questions; the submissive interactant answers questions.

Approximately two thirds of the utterances were question-answer interchanges, and one third were assertion interchanges. Questions not only structured the episodes, they also served to introduce topics.

Rule 4. When in a question the dominant interactant asks about a topic X, the submissive interactant is obliged to imply topic X.

This rule was identified by Litton-Hawes[13] in relation to physicians and patients in medical interviews. She found additionally that physicians did not need to abide by this rule and could defer answering on a topic implied by the patient. This, however, did not occur in the present study.

Physicians and nurses have the right to present topics related to the client's health state, and the client has the obligation to provide the information. Topics related to the physician's health state or the nurse's health state are not appropriate topics. The appropriate topic is the basis for the next rule.

Rule 5. Topics in dominant-submissive interactions have to do with personal information regarding the submissive interactant.

Episodes are managed and topics are presented using predominantly a question/answer format. The following three rules demonstrate variations of question use in dominant-recessive interactions.

Rule 6. When the submissive interactant has answered a question, the dominant interactant can then ask the same or similar question.

This rule is illustrated in the following examples.

4. MDS 1: We <u>might</u> even be able to engin<u>eer</u> taking you home <u>Chris</u>tmas in the helicopter, would you like that?, Land at your farm?
CT 2: (Yeah.)
MDS 1: Hum?, as a special treat? . . . if you <u>don't</u> wanna just speak <u>up</u> we won't <u>do</u> it if you <u>don't</u> wanna.
CT 2: (That'd be alright.)
MDS 1: Would you <u>like</u> that?
CT 2: Yeah.

5. RN 24: Did you see? some films? today?
CT 5: Nope.
RN 24: You didn't.
CT 5: Hun uh they never did come.
RN 24: They didn't? did they instruct you on anything? about, going to surgery you know.
CT 5: One of the nurses come up and was talkin to us.

The second and third questions on the same topic serve to get more information from the patient. They also serve to question if the patient is sure of what the patient is saying. This also occurs in a more abbreviated form, but the result is the same: the patient must repeat the original answer:

6. MDS 1: I'm gonna <u>stick</u> you up in a <u>chair</u>, how's that?
CT 2: (OK)
MDS 1: Uhm?
CT 2: (OK)
MDS 1: OK?

7. (Referring to the TV monitor in patient's room)
MDS 4: What's this? uh new kind bug?
CT 6: Oh no this is televised for some reason.
MDS 4: Huh-?
CT 6: This is <u>tele</u>vised.
MDS 4: Televising you?
CT 6: Yeah.

8. RN 6: How do you feel?
CT 4: (OK)
RN 16: OK?
PT 4: Um hum.

Goffman speaks of these replies as rerun signals. The obvious function of an apparent "unhearing" or misunderstanding can be a resource for saying one thing while meaning another. Goffman states:

For to ask for a rerun can be to admit that one has not been considerate enough to listen or that one is insufficiently knowledgeable to understand the speaker's utterance or that the speaker himself may not know how to express himself clearly. . . . (p. 273)[14]

Several reasons have been suggested for this practice. It may be that repeating is habitual and is learned in the educational process or that the physician or nurse was not listening to the previous answer.[15]

Whatever the reason for the repeated question, it serves to disconfirm or not accept the first answer of the patient in and of itself. Furthermore, it requires the patient to repeat answers to the questions. Another variation in the question-answer structure follows the next rule.

Rule 7. The dominant interactant may ask a question and without waiting for a reply may ask a second question.

9. MDS 1: How often do you get these on your legs changed?
   MDS 1: Have you been getting them changed very often?
   CT 2: Yeah they've been changed.
10. RN 16: Um? do you have any questions? before I go?
    RN 16: What about the family? it's kinda good to talk with everybody in here.
    CT 5: Yeah, um, she said that I'd probly be down there for awhile you know before they put me to sleep.

Two questions in a row provide for "the rather enforced option of deciding which to answer."[18] The second question, however, often delimits the particular aspect of the topic presented in the first question to be addressed. It provides further topic direction for the submissive interactant.

Another exception to the usual two-pair parts of an adjacency pair was the frequent occurrence of a three-turn sequence. This sequence occurred with the addition of an evaluation by the dominant interactant to the usual QA sequence.

Rule 8. A dominant interactant may verbally evaluate in the next turn the answer or response of the submissive interactant.

11. RN 16: So she like she talked to you pretty much what was going on an stuff.
    CT 5: Yes ma'm.
    RN 16: OK very good.
12. Res: Can you wiggle your toes? like this.
    CT 2: I can't straighten my foot out?
    MDS 1: No you got it very straight you can't <u>bend</u> it is what you can't do, <u>Push.</u>
    MDS 1: Good now lift this back up toward your <u>head</u>, back up like that.

The dominant interactant's reply serves to evaluate—to confirm, disconfirm or revise—the answer given by the submissive interactant. This operation assumes that it is the right of the dominant interactant to evaluate the response of the submissive interactant. Goffman notes the inappropriateness of the reversal of speakers in this operation; it is not the right of the recessive interactant to verbally evaluate the response of the dominant interactant.[19] In one instance where the patient did evaluate the physician, the patient was interrupted when that evaluation was heard by the physician.

Rule 9. The dominant interactant proposes membership categories which are accepted by the submissive interactant

Specifying a membership category is an operation used to label another person. Sacks describes the membership category "baby" as belonging to two membership category devices, "family" and "stage of life."[20] In the following utterance, the physician introduces a nurse to a patient:

13. MDS 1: Do you know who that is standin at the door thats Miss G. she's the boss of ya up here.

The specification "boss" is a satisfactory reference to the membership categorization device—boss and subordinate. By categorizing the nurse as the boss, the physician has categorized the patient as submissive. The same operation occurs when the dominant person refers to the submissive as big boy or girl:

14. MDS 1: Got a little bit more skin grafting to do big boy.
15. RN 24: That's a girl.

Although the person referred to as "big boy" was 16 years old, the person referred to as "girl" was a mature woman. In this study, in no instance did the submissive interactant deny, challenge, or attempt to revise the categorization by the dominant interactant. The definition of the submissive's position was offered by the dominant interactant and accepted by the submissive interactant.

Dominant interactants can further suggest a membership category by suggesting a category-bound activity of the submissive interactant that is usually associated with a category.

16. MDS 1: Here's a playboy ((hands patient comic book)) do you wanna read? I'll putcha back . . . want the footstool? . . . (OK)
17. MS: You and I are going to be playin together everyday for awhile, OK?
18. RN 5: O?kie dokie so I'll see ya this afternoon.
    CT 5: Alrightie.

Reading comic books, playing, and adding the suffix "ie" to words are activities bound to the category of child in the categorization device "stage of life." The category-bound activity of reading a comic book was further emphasized by calling the comic book a *Playboy,* a magazine for adults. The strength of the suggestion of a category can be seen in the response of the patient in the last example. Prior to this interchange, words with the "ie" suffix were not used. The nurse used language as if a child were being addressed; the patient responded with the language of a child.

The dominant interactant frequently made statements that served to manage the pacing or timing of an episode. These statements, which Goffman calls bracket markers, helped with the cadence of activity.[21] Statements like "OK," "now then," and "well" mark the end of an episode phase or the beginning of another. These statements conform to the following rule.

Rule 10. The dominant interactant manages the timing of the episodes by using bracket markers.

The following examples illustrate the use of this rule.

19. MD 1: Uh I'd say in about another week or so.
    MD 2: Now lets look at your ears.
    CT 2: Its sore.
20. RN 16: This bothering you at all?
    CT 4: Hum ((shakes head))
    RN 16: OK can I see in your mouth again?
    RN 16: OK let me give you the nurse's call light.

Dominant interactants use bracket markers to delimit boundaries in the episode. They were employed to voice the fact that a task has terminated or is about to begin. Bracket markers are asymmetrically used in the interactions. They are a resource that the dominant interactants use to manage the timing and progression of the interaction.

Rule 11. The submissive interactant uses a more formal term of address than the dominant interactant.

The client's first name was used by the physician in all cases of address; in no instance was the physician's first name used by the client. Nurses used either the first name or last name of the client; clients did not address nurses by name.

Forms of address in this study were consistent with American forms of address. Friends or colleagues and persons of lower rank or lesser age are addressed by first names. Occupational titles are accorded people in certain statuses such as "Judge," "Doctor," or "Professor."

Because the title "nurse" is not used alone nor in conjunction with the last name, nurses were not called by name. This difference in title reflects the relative difference in status of physician and nurse. This differential status may also account for the nurses' use of both forms of address—the client's first name or the patient's last name. Further, the form of address in nurse-client dyads reflects the lesser amount of status difference between interactants as compared to the physician-client dyads. The influence of the interactants' age was also evident in the forms of address. Physicians, in general, were older than the male patients; however, the women clients were older than the nurses. Forms of address in nurse-patient interactions demonstrated more status ambiguity and flexibility than those in the physician-patient interactions.

Patterns of interruption in this study varied from the normative model presented by Sacks and coworkers (1974)[22] for conversation according to the following rule:

Rule 12. The dominant interactant may interrupt the submissive interactant's talk before a transition-relevance place occurs.

A transition-relevance place is a possible completion point. The following examples illustrate this rule.

21. CT 2: (OK) I's hopin I'd be (home by Christmas).
    MDS 1: Pardon?
    CT 2: I's hopin I'd get home.
    MDS 1: and sisters You got *eight?* brothers.
22. CT 4: No I think I'll just, I'll just get my rest.
    RN 16: I've got some beds next door if you get some time . . . you can come help me?
23. CT 6: Tell me one other thing . . . you seem to have all the answers, what gives me so much trouble with my testicles.
    MDS 5: Have I seen what?
    CT 6: You seem to have all the . . .
    MDS 5: I don't know what kind of what kind of trouble have you got in your testicles.

In two of the examples, the interruption occurred after an "unhearing." The interruption occurred when the hearing was comprehended regardless of where the submissive interactant was in the performance of the repeat. The last example also demonstrates what happens when the submissive interactant breaks the previous rule on evaluation.

The previous discussion contained rules that govern the ongoing conversational activity of dominant-submissive relationships. The last rule addresses how the conversational activity comes to a close.

A widely operative form of terminal exchange is the adjacency pair composed of conventional parts, for example, an exchange of goodbyes. This form is the institutionalized form for closing ongoing conversational activity. The speaker of the first-pair part proposes a close. The speaker of the second-pair part demonstrates by a response that the speaker understands what the first speaker is saying and is willing to go along with it. In this study, the dominant interactant produced the first-pair part, and the submissive interactant produced the second-pair part. The following rule governs the closing of episodes.

Rule 13. The dominant interactant initiates the closing of the episode.
Examples of this rule are listed.

24. RN 24: OK thank you.
    CT 5: Um hum
    ((Nurse exits))
25. MDS 5: I'll be back to see ya uh little bit later.
    CT 6: OK.
    ((Physician exits))
26. RN 16: So I'll (go out) and be back in a minute.
    CT 4: OK.
    ((Nurse exits))

In all cases when there was a typical ritual closing, it was initiated by the dominant interactant. The submissive interactants initiated no closings. If the dominant interactant did not initiate a closing, it did not occur. Frequently, in its place was the reference to some type of activity by the dominant interactant:

27. MDS 1: Its about lunch time.
    CT 2: Uh ((groan))
    ((Physician exits))
28. MDS 1: I'll talk to your parents S.
    ((Physician exits))

In these examples, there was no conversational closing. The open state of talk was interrupted when one interactant left the room. This apparent lack of a closing can be understood if the patient is assumed to remain in an open state of talk as discussed under interaction openings. In this case, a closing is not needed and is not supplied by either interactant.

SIGNIFICANCE OF THE RULES

The rules identified in this study demonstrate the procedures interactants use as resources in talk to enact their different statuses in the relationship. The dominant interactant controls the interaction timing by starting, pacing, and stopping the episodes. Control of space is demonstrated when the dominant interactant may, without asking permission, enter the submissive interactant's territory, implying the right to personal address, a state of open talk, and access to personal information about the submissive interactant.

This study makes explicit certain subtle and taken-for-granted operations so that they may be examined by health professionals. The value of this study rests on your recognition of these operations in everyday conversations. It is recommended that you as a nurse be aware of the way in which you may subtly dominate patients, neglect to give them opportunity to be heard by you, make them feel misused or abused, and, in some ways, hinder their chances for optimum recovery.

PUNCTUATION OF INTERACTION

As you attempt to summarize your relationship with another person, you may find some difficulty with what has been called the "punctuation" of ongoing interaction behavior.[23] As people interact with others, they are usually aware of little interaction events, encounters, or communication sequential units. For example, one meets someone, the person smiles, one responds, the person tells one some news, one shows what one thinks of it, one talks, then one notes one must move along to do other things; so one shows pleasure regarding this meeting and says they will meet again at some specified time. What happened first, second, third, and so on may be viewed collectively as an interaction unit or encounter.

In an ongoing series of such events or encounters, people tend to find one event overlapping with another. They may "pick up where they left off" or relate back to some midpoint item. It may be difficult, even a bit arbitrary, to decide when any particular sequence of communicative acts started—who did what first, who "responded" to whom, and so on. Even so, as people reflect back on such happenings, they usually have an impression of what behavior preceded another and what response it received. The way individuals reflectively or cognitively break up a series of ongoing recurring actions into units may be termed their *punctuation* of such an ongoing series. Although the concept of "punctuation" may seem to you to be vague or complex, it is brought up because it can have considerable significance as you attempt to analyze your relationship with another person. The way you punctuate your interaction with the person can make a difference in the way you view the relationship.

The punctuation made by one of the interacting persons may be quite different from that made by the other person in the relationship; differences in punctuation can thus produce confusion and misunderstanding. Consider a couple having marital difficulties. Suppose that the husband generally shows passive withdrawal and then re-entry into the communication situation. In explaining the couple's disagreements and frustrations, he will indicate that withdrawal is his only defense against her nagging. He will indicate that she nags, he withdraws; he goes back into the situation, she nags, he withdraws. The wife's interpretation of the interaction sequences, however, will very likely be that he withdraws and she has to nag to get him back into talking with her. Their two interpretations have been identified as follows:

1. "I withdraw because you nag."
2. "I nag because you withdraw."[24]

Seldom, however, do people recognize such a problem or talk about these things. The point to be noted is that in analyzing your relationship with another person, your own punctuation of communication events or encounters should be noted and shared as accurately as possible. It is suggested that you seek help, if needed and possible, of a trusted observer outside the relationship.

A major punctuation problem for nurses is the transition needed between clients. For example, if you have just attended a terminally ill client having severe problems and move on to a client with only minor problems, your mind may still be on the former. Your nonverbal manner may cause the second client to suspect that "something is the matter." It is often difficult to make such abrupt transitions, and sometimes candor is called for if your client senses that you are bothered and perturbed.

DEGREE OF RIGIDITY IN A RELATIONSHIP

The degree of rigidity, the established routine, is an important consideration in analyzing your relationships. It provides a basis for estimating the possibility of change and improvement, a primary issue in a relationship's value to people.

Timothy Leary and his associates, known at that time (1957) as the Kaiser Foundation Group, suggested the principle of *interpersonal behavior reflex*.[25] In his studies of interpersonal communication, Leary arrived at this conclusion: A large percentage of interpersonal behaviors simply involve a reflex—an automatic response.[26] Such behaviors are so automatic that they are often unconscious and even at variance with the individual's own perception of them; they are involuntary responses to the behavior of the other person.

As we have noted, affectionate or hostile behavior tends to evoke similar behavior. If one person in a relationship is highly affectionate toward the other, that other person ordinarily responds with at least moderate affection. In like manner, hostility generally generates hostility. On the other hand, dominant or submissive behavior tends to produce its *reciprocal*. Ordinarily, if a relationship survives over time, dominant behavior elicits passive or submissive responses. The reverse is also true: Passivity tends to reinforce and thus produce dominant behavior on the part of the other person. Of course, in the event two dominant people try to relate to each other, a power struggle usually ensues; it may last for years and may often involve manipulative games. If neither person's behavior changes, the relationship may dissolve because reciprocal responses cannot be established.

To a large extent, the effect of one person's behavior can be explained, even predicted, on the basis of these principles: Affection or hostility elicits *similar* behavior, and dominance or submissiveness elicits *reciprocal* responses. As two people interact, one person's behavior produces responses by the other; these responses in turn produce responses on the part of the first person. Responses produce responses that produce responses. As time goes on, the two persons tend to work out a "shared definition" of their relationships.[27] The "starting" behavior may be forgotten; perhaps it was never consciously perceived or analyzed; or perhaps it was misperceived because of an erroneous expectation. Nevertheless, once in motion, responses to responses tend to produce what may be called a "lockstep" effect. Once such a lockstep series has been established, change is difficult to achieve. A singular response, once given, tends to elicit a singular response from the other person, and the lockstep effect goes into full swing. On the other hand, many persons have a wider *repertoire* of responses and can appropriately react in different ways to different interpersonal behaviors. *The range of a person's response repertoire will tend to determine the degree of rigidity of one's interpersonal relationships.* As two persons interact, the degree of rigidity in their relationship to each other will be a function of the variety in the response repertoires of the two individuals.

To test the degree of rigidity in one of your own interpersonal relationships, you can "try out" new responses to the other person's behavior. Be prepared for that person's surprise—even shock, confusion, or disgust! Note the degree to which you are able to use a wider repertoire of responses; note, also, the other person's responses, especially any new ones. This procedure can give you some index of the degree of rigidity in the relationship.

BAD HABITS IN RELATIONSHIPS

For one reason or another, some persons develop habitual ways of behaving in relationships that lead to difficulty instead of pleasure and task productivity. These negative habits include manipulative behaviors and "games people play." They are not in any sense peculiar to nurses or the health-care profession, but they can seriously damage your enjoyment of your work and the degree of professional success you may achieve.

MANIPULATIVE RELATIONSHIP STYLES

Everett Shostrom analyzed the role-playing and rigid patterns in male-female relationships and explored the unconscious foundations of these patterns in people's personality.[28] He describes certain characteristic relationship styles as exploitative or manipulative. In Shostrom's analysis, six relationship patterns are identified in which the participants are not really relating to each other; instead, they are leaning on one another, avoiding each other, or competing with each other out of personal inadequacy. He sees couples at polar extremes in their capacities to express *strength* or *weakness, anger* or *love*. These dimensions equate closely with the dimensions of *emotional tone* and *control* cited in the previous section. When a couple, either consciously or unconsciously, allows their relationship to become locked or frozen in one of these ways, it becomes one of leaning rather than relating.

Note the six pairs:

1. *The Nurturing Relationship: Mother and Son.* In this relationship pattern, the *weak* man has chosen unconsciously his opposite, the *strong,* motherlike woman. Strengths and weaknesses then become reciprocally exaggerated as the pattern persists. Later in the relationship, should either or both persons' self-perception change, major perception adjustment is required.

2. *The Supporting Relationship: Daddy and Doll.* This relationship pattern is the gender reversal of the mother/son relationship because, in this case, the man displays strength and the woman weakness. As Shostrom and Kavanaugh state:

> Each is a kind of cultural distortion of masculinity and feminity. The man appears to be strong. He is suave, intelligent, cool, charming, personable, usually successful, apparently confident and in control of every situation. In the stereotype, he sits calmly with his pipe in his mouth surveying the world and his little doll is more than willing to sit on his lap and accept his help and direction. Actually, he is not as strong as he is uninvolved in the relationship. His doll is his mannequin who frames his masculinity well, who, in a sense, establishes and supports it. She is not a person to him as much as she is an expensive plaything. He does not reveal to her his weakness, since his image depends on his revelation of strength. In reality, the doll is usually a much stronger person. She controls the relationship by exaggerating her weakness and dependency. She can whine and pout and smile her way into power. The daddy and his doll actually avoid each other; they pass in the hall, they do not make contact as persons.[29]

3. *The Challenging Relationship: Bitch and Nice Guy.* Shostrom and Kavanaugh characterize this relationship as "the real prototype of the unhappy American marriage."[30] The bitch exaggerates her expression of anger, and the nice guy exaggerates his expression of love. The bitch

tends to deny her need to love and be loved as a defense against the vulnerability she feels in love, and the nice guy is out of touch with his anger or assertiveness; from his needs to be liked and accepted, he is indirect in his hostility and often needles his bitchy wife.[31]

4. *The Educating Relationship: Master and Servant.* This master/slave relationship reflects the old cultural stereotype of the strong, unyielding male and the helpless, weak, obedient woman. This relationship has little ambiguity; the male feels strong and "masculine" and the woman is dependent and devoted. This relationship differs from the daddy/doll relationship in that the master is demanding, whereas the daddy is protective, and servants are more capable than dolls.[32]

5. *The Confronting Relationship: Hawks.* Hawks are fierce competitors who both want to control and dominate the relationship.

> Hawks are fierce competitors and the energy of competition comes from their own denial of weakness or tenderness. They fight with words, they struggle for status, they strive to prove superiority. Sex is a contest, life is a chess game. They ridicule and taunt, test and prove, scream and criticize. They blame their partners for what is missing in themselves. Each day is another contest in which the competition of the preceding day is still unresolved. *When love leaves, competition arrives.*[33]

6. *The Accommodating Relationship: Doves.* Doves are the victims of our culture, which has taught people to be "nice" and polite at any cost, even at the loss of one's identity. Doves have learned to deny their true feelings, to not talk back, argue, or fight. Peace is more important than expression of true feelings. They were taught to "control" themselves, to be kind, docile, and cheerful. Artificiality, dullness, and guilt are results. Such people don't experience love, but only play a part.[34]

Although Shostrom portrays these relationships in terms of intimate long-term relationships, the same patterns can occur in physician-nurse relationships. Consider how these six pairs can manipulate each other in a hospital setting.

RELATIONSHIP "GAMES"

In his popular book *Games People Play,* the late Eric Berne analyzed relationship patterns in terms of "games."[35] The term *game,* however, is somewhat misleading. Typically, a game is thought to imply two sides that follow mutually agreeable and coordinated sets of rules. Berne's "games" tend to operate as the victimization of one party through fraudulent, manipulative means by the other party.

A typical game as analyzed by Berne is one he calls *Corner.* Berne shows that it essentially consists of a delayed refusal to follow another's ploy to produce a show of affection. In this game, a wife suggests to her husband that they go to a movie; he agrees. She makes an "unconscious" suggestion that maybe they shouldn't because the house needs painting. He has previously told her that they don't have the money to paint the house right now; therefore, this is not a "reasonable" time to relate such an expensive consideration to the price of a movie. The husband responds rudely to the house-painting remark. His wife is "offended" and says that because he is in a bad mood, she will not go to the movie with him and *suggests that he should go alone*. This is the critical artificial ploy of the game. He knows very well from past experience that he is not supposed to take this suggestion seriously. What she really wants is to be "honeyed up" a bit, told everything will be all right. Then they could go off happily to the movie together. *But he refuses* to show her this affectionate attention. He leaves, feeling relieved but looking abused; she is left feeling resentful. In this instance, the husband won this game because all he did was to do as she suggested—literally. Berne's conclusion is: "They both know this is cheating but since she said it, she is cornered." This is a cruel game played in an attempt to achieve a *show* of affection; its target is manipulation or control of another person, and its interpersonal attitude beneath the surface—no matter who wins—is not affection but *hostility*.

Why Don't You—Yes But (YDYB), another game identified by Berne, is said to be a prototype for transactional analysis. It is initiated when A (the perpetrator) adopts a docile stance toward B (the victim) by presenting some life problem in such a manner that B is induced to offer advice, that is, to adopt a managerial counterstance. A responds to this advice by saying, "Yes, but . . . ," and adding to that some information that renders B's advice irrelevant, erroneous, or gratuitous. If A's deflationary comment has been skillfully contrived and delivered, however, B will come back with an alternative solution, still believing that B has sincerely been offered the managerial position. A shoots down B again. This may go on for several "rounds," until B finally realizes that B has been defeated, as manifested perhaps by an exasperated silence or a weak acknowledgment that A "sure has a tough problem there." A has demonstrated B's inadequacy, and B confirms it by assuming a self-effacing position complementary to the competitive position to which A has already switched. Note that A's competitive position is reciprocal to B's original managerial one. In the face of B's "demonstrated" lack of talent for the managerial role, B is literally forced out of it. Needless to say, this reversal can be, and often is, deployed in a group setting, where there are several potential victims and where an even sweeter competitive victory can be fashioned by the skillful player.

Berne cites the game *If It Weren't For You (IWFY)* as the most common one played between spouses. In this game, the blame for inaction is shifted to the partner in such a way as to become both an excuse and an accusation. For example, Mary complains that her husband so restricts her social activities that she has never learned to dance. However, once the excuse of the husband's supposed restrictions are removed, she discovers that she actually has a morbid fear of dancing. Thus, Mary has been hiding her true self behind a "It's not that I'm afraid; it's that he won't let me." A common application of this game is in terms of "If it weren't for you, I'd be out having fun."

The title of the game *Now I've Got You, You Son of a Bitch (NIGYSOB)* reveals immediately that it is one involving an aggressive payoff. The perpetrator of *NIGYSOB* initiates the game by placing oneself in circumstances (often by adopting a strongly self-effacing position) that invite competitive exploitation from one's victim. The victim, if unwise or not sophisticated in these matters, sooner or later accepts the proffered agreement and initiates a program of exploitation. At some point, however, the person teased to attack becomes careless and/or the perpetrator suddenly shows increased vigilance, and the invited exploitation is thereby publicly revealed in all its nakedness. The perpetrator, with a suitable show of rage and indignation, assumes the justly deserved, aggressive *NIGYSOB* position. The victim, if the reversal has been carried off smoothly, retires to the only remaining position—withdrawn, bitter rebelliousness or guilty self-effacement. It should be noted that sometimes the victim in this reversal is not quite as "innocent" or passive as this account suggests. In some instances the victim may be playing according to a coordinate set of rules, which would make the transaction a more complicated, two-handed one—in effect, a true sadomasochistic game.

These four examples should be sufficient to illustrate the manner in which games can be used in relationships for fraudulent satisfactions at the expense of the other person. Other games described by Berne fit similar patterns; they include *Try and Collect, Frigid Woman, Schlemiel,* and *See What You Make Me Do.* Berne's work is valuable in showing how individuals may unconsciously manipulate other people.

EVALUATING AND IMPROVING RELATIONSHIPS

To assess one of your own interpersonal relationships, it is suggested that you first determine its nature. The issue then becomes: Are you happy with what you have? In the long run, only you can describe what is satisfying to you. For example, you may feel that you need to be dominated, told what to do; that without such direction, your life is too puzzling, that problems overwhelm you. The questions still remain: By what process do you arrive at such a decision? How does a person evaluate a relationship? What procedures are involved?

CALCULATING THE COST/REWARD RATIO

The concept of social exchange, or cost/reward ratios for calculating an estimated relationship potential (ERP), has previously been introduced. As you determine the cost/reward ratio of a relationship and note the degree of causal connections between your behavior and that of the other person, you have three possible alternatives. First, you may terminate the relationship if you see fit; you avoid or at least stop seeking out this person. Second, you may maintain the relationship as it is, perhaps fairly satisfied with it as it exists. Third, you may give serious thought and effort toward improving the relationship. This decision will be made on the basis of your estimates of the cost/reward ratio and the alternative relationship opportunities available to you.

IMPROVING A RELATIONSHIP

Obtaining the cooperative help of the other person in the relationship is usually about the only way possible to achieve any significant change. The lockstep of patterned responses to responses usually dooms to failure the lone effort of a single member of the relationship. Together with the other person, you may "try out" new behaviors and note the responses. Deliberate role-playing may be useful; however, be careful of adopting roles that are not true to your own personal feelings. In most cases, artificiality in interpersonal behavior can create greater problems than the original undesirable behavior.

The other person in your relationship may resent the idea that any changes are needed. You may make the mistake of trying to point out to the person the need for such changes. If such changes are discussed, the person is likely to fear exposure of one's ideas and feelings. What the person actually fears, of course, is possible damage to one's self-image as a result of such exposure. If you try to point out the behaviors that are causing difficulty, it will tend to increase the person's anxiety. Many times this is what people do who want to be helpful but who are not knowledgeable.

What can you do to be helpful? Research findings in clinical counseling settings show the value of such attitudes and abilities as accurate empathy, nonpossessive warmth, and genuineness.[36]

Accurate empathy is the ability to sense the other person's view of the world as if that view were your own. However, to demonstrate accurate empathy requires ability to *communicate* this understanding to the other person.[37] You need to be sensitive to the person's current feelings and emotions, even the fear of letting you develop a closer relationship with the individual. You do not need to *feel* the same fear or anxiety that the other one does, but you must have an *awareness* and *appreciation* of these emotions. Such empathy is communicated by the language you use and also by your vocal qualities and behavior. Your posture, gestures, and entire attitude should reflect the other person's point of view and depth of feeling. Your behavior must show awareness of shifts in the person's emotional attitudes, subtle fears, and anxieties. At all times, the message of accurate empathy is: "I am with you; I understand."

Nonpossessive warmth is a demonstration of unconditional positive regard, involving caring about the other person without imposing conditions. The attitude you communicate should be warm acceptance; there should be no expression of dislike, disapproval, or *conditional* warmth in a selective or evaluative way. You will need to show willingness to share the other person's joys and aspirations as well as anxiety and despair. It may be difficult for you to understand how you can really show warmth and affection for a person who has ways or habits you dislike; this is indeed a serious problem and becomes the heart of the matter in trying to be helpful to others. What is actually required is caring about that person's *potential,* a warm feeling about the person *as a person*—a human being. It is imperative that the other person feel you will be *for* him or her, even through failed attempts to change. The person needs to feel that you care about one in spite of your dislike of some of one's behavior.

The attitude described here may not be clear to you; indeed, in working with problems in human relations it is the most complicated concept to be faced. However, it is also the most important. Let us note it once again: *Nonpossessive warmth* involves unconditional caring about a person *as a person with valued potential* irrespective of some behaviors you do not like. Consider a female's response to a male. She must show that she cares for him even though she may not care for some of his ways. This caring is much like the loyalty and affection shown by supporters of a football team even when that team is having problems and losing games; these fans want the team to win, but they still love it when it loses—they love it for trying and for its *potential.* If you wish to help another person, you must show that person acceptance as a human being who has both human frailties and human potential.

Genuineness consists of being open and frank at all times; it involves being yourself. You must be willing not only to express your feelings, but never to deny them.[38] There must be no facade, no defensive communication, no show of emotion followed by denial of that emotion. Your responses to the other person must be sincere, never phony. It does not mean that you need to show all your feelings or emotions; but once a feeling or emotion is shown, it must not be denied—your behavior must be consistent. You need not disclose your total self, but whatever is shown must be a real aspect of yourself, not behavior growing out of defensiveness or an attempt to manipulate the other person. Glib attempts to persuade or efforts to convince the other are dangerous pitfalls.

A "professional" facade—"Now, let us take our medicine"—can be disastrous.

In view of the preceding discussion of nonpossessive warmth, it should be noted that your show of warmth must be genuine. The requirements involved in showing nonpossessive warmth make it extremely difficult to help another person if you really do not care about that person. What you think are clever strategies will likely be viewed with suspicion. You must learn to be true to yourself if you wish to be helpful to others.

SUMMARY

This chapter has suggested that a significant phase of the interpersonal communication process is developing, maintaining, and improving a warm personal relationship. In recent years, a new emphasis has been placed on seeking such a relationship with at least one other person.

To improve an existing relationship or to achieve the most satisfying potential of a new one, one must analyze it, evaluate it, and, if need be, change it.

A relationship can be analyzed in terms of its (1) basic patterns of interaction and (2) degree of rigidity. Interaction behavior has three basic dimensions: (1) degree of involvement, (2) emotional tone, and (3) amount of interpersonal control.

In an established relationship in which the degree of involvement has stabilized, the other two dimensions are of greatest concern. Such a relationship can be described in its *essential characteristics* by determining the interpersonal behavior of the two persons on two independent, bipolar dimensions: *dominance-submission* and *affection-hostility*. These two dimensions were presented as forming an axis in a D-A-S-H paradigm.

In determining each person's degree of *dominance* versus *submission* and amount of *affection* versus *hostility* in a relationship, it was noted that affectionate or hostile behavior on the part of one participant tends to elicit *similar* behavior on the part of the other. Conversely, dominant behavior tends to produce its *reciprocal*, submissive behavior, and submissiveness tends to encourage dominance. Taken together, these two principles tend to produce a "lockstep" effect of responses that produce responses. Once set in motion, such a behavior pattern is difficult to change. The possibility of change can be estimated by noting the variety of the participants' response repertoires—to what extent they tend to respond differently to different behaviors.

Evaluation of a relationship is accomplished by calculating the ratio of individual costs to personal rewards and by comparing this ratio with estimates of relationship potential for any available alternative relationships. Decisions to terminate a relationship are based primarily on the cost/reward ratio, but may also consider the potential value of available alternate relationships. A decision to attempt to improve a relationship is ordinarily based on a comparison of what exists with an ideal version of what might be.

Improving a relationship ordinarily requires a determined effort on the part of both members. Procedures for improvement include optimum use of the process of interpersonal communication, special emphasis on self-disclosure followed by feedback, and working with the other person. Cooperation of the other person may be facilitated by showing accurate empathy, nonpossessive warmth, and genuineness.

Relating to others is a basic key to a satisfying life. It can aid personal growth, confidence through self-acceptance, and beneficial cooperation through shared responsibility with others. To negotiate satisfactory conditions with one's social and physical environment, one must achieve cooperative, agreeable relationships with a number of associates. Furthermore, to achieve a deeply satisfying opinion of oneself, it is essential to achieve a warm, personal relationship with at least one other person. Satisfactory relationships are the basic goal of interpersonal communication and the true test of the process.

REFERENCES

1. For a review of relevant theory and research, see ELAINE L. LAMONICA: *The Nursing Process: A Humanistic Approach* (Reading, Mass.: Addison-Wesley Publishing Company, 1979), pp. 398–412.
2. D.A. BROOTEN, L.L. HAYMAN, AND M.D. NAYLOR: *Leadership for Change: A Guide for the Frustrated Nurse*. (New York: J.B. Lippincott Company, 1978), pp. 139–141.
3. For a review of this body of research, see KIM GIFFIN AND BOBBY R. PATTON: *Personal Communication in Human Relations* (Columbus, Ohio: Merrill, 1974), pp. 55–60; for further corroboration by a more recent study, see MYRON WISH, MORTON DEUTSCH, AND SUSAN J. KAPLAN: "Perceived Dimensions of Interpersonal Relations," *Journal of Personality and Social Psychology*, 33 (1976): 409–420.
4. W. BARNETT PEARCE AND STEWART M. SHARP: "Self-disclosing Communication," *Journal of Communication*, 23 (1973): 409–425.
5. MICHAEL D. ROLOFF: "Communication Strategies, Relationships and Relational Change," in GERALD R. MILLER: *Explorations in Interpersonal Communication* (Beverly Hills, Calif.: Sage Publications, 1976), pp. 173–194.
6. See the following four studies: I. ALTMAN AND D.A. TAYLOR: *Social Penetration: The Development of Interpersonal Relationships* (New York: Holt, Rinehart and Winston, 1973); S.W. DUCK: *Personal Relationships and Personal Constructs: A Study of Friendship Formation* (New York: Wiley, 1973); C.R. BERGER AND R.J.CALABRESE: "Some Explorations in Initial Interaction and Beyond: Toward a Developmental Theory of Interpersonal Communication," *Human Communication Research*, 1 (1975): 99–112; and G.R. MILLER AND M. STEINBERG: *Between People: A New Analysis of Interpersonal Communication* (Palo Alto, Calif.: Science Research Associates, 1975).
7. T. LEARY: *Interpersonal Diagnosis of Personality* (New York: Ronald, 1957).

8. T. LEARY: "The Theory and Measurement Methodology of Interpersonal Communication," *Psychiatry,* 18 (1955): 147–161.
9. See LEARY: "Theory and Measurement Methodology," pp. 155–161.
10. For a detailed discussion of the origins of this model, see KIM GIFFIN AND BOBBY R. PATTON: *Fundamentals of Interpersonal Communication* (New York: Harper & Row, 1976), pp. 186–189.
11. E. GOFFMAN: *Relations in Public* (New York: Basic Books, 1971), pp. 194–199.
12. BONNIE GARVIN: "A Rules-Based Study of Communication in Dominant-Recessive Relationships," a paper presented to the Third Annual Conference on Communication Languages and Gender, Lawrence, Kansas, June 1, 1980. The rules are the result of her research. We have changed Garvin's term "recessive" to "submissive."
13. ELAINE MARIE LITTON-HAWES: *A Discourse Analysis of Topic Co-Selection in Medical Interviews.* Doctoral Dissertaion, The Ohio State University, 1976.
14. ERVING GOFFMAN: "Replies and Responses," *Languages in Society,* 1976, 5, p. 273.
15. LITTON-HAWES: *op. cit.*
16. M. COULTHARD AND M. ASHBY: "Talking with the Doctor," *Journal of Communication.* 1975, 25, pp. 140–147.
17. WILLIAM LABOV: "Rules for Ritual Insults," in DAVID SUDNOW, ED: *Studies in Social Interaction* (New York: Free Press, 1972).
18. GOFFMAN: *op. cit.,* p. 287.
19. *Loc Cit.*
20. H. SACKS, E.A. SCHEGLOFF, AND G. JEFFERSON: "A Simplest Systematics for the Organization of Turn-Taking for Conversation." *Language,* 1974, 50, 690–735.
21. GOFFMAN: *op. cit.*
22. SACKS, ET AL: *op. cit.*
23. Cf. P. WATZLAWICK, J.H. BEAVIN, AND D.D. JACKSON: *Pragmatics of Human Communication* (New York: Norton, 1967), pp. 80–93.
24. *Ibid.,* p. 56.
25. For a brief summary and evaluation of the work of this group, see R.C. CARSON: *Interaction Concepts of Personality* (Chicago: Aldine, 1969), pp. 103–106.
26. T. LEARY: "Theory and Measurement Methodology," pp. 147–161.
27. E. GOFFMAN: *Behavior in Public Places* (New York: Free Press, 1963), p. 96.
28. E.L. SHOSTROM: *Man the Manipulator, the Inner Journey from Manipulation to Actualization* (New York: Arlington Pres, 1967); and E.L. SHOSTROM AND JAMES KAVANAUGH: *Between Man and Woman* (Los Angeles: Nash, 1971).
29. From EVERETT SHOSTROM AND JAMES KAVANAUGH: *Between Man and Woman* (Los Angeles: Nash, 1971), with permission.
30. *Ibid.,* p. 149.
31. *Ibid.,* pp. 149–165.
32. *Ibid.,* pp. 167–186.
33. *Ibid.,* p. 190.
34. *Ibid.,* pp. 213–234.
35. E. BERNE: *Games People Play* (New York: Grove Press, 1964).
36. C.B. TRUAX AND R.R. CARKHUFF: *Toward Effective Counseling and Psychotherapy* (Chicago: Aldine, 1969).
37. *Ibid.,* p. 46.
38. *Ibid.,* p. 58.

7
COMMUNICATING
IN GROUPS

Much of a nurse's work day is spent working with others, developing procedures for health care and executing these procedures as members of a health-care team. Whether as administrators or practitioners, nurses are involved in mutual commitment with others in a cooperative enterprise. The key to effective functioning in groups involves *two* types of activities: reaching decisions, and relating interpersonally. The *first* is a task-oriented behavior and includes identifying and analyzing a mutual problem, evaluating possible ways of solving it, and preparing for the implementation of a selected solution. The *second*, from a humanistic perspective, involves acting in a decently human way by listening to how others *feel* about *their* ideas, not just noting those ideas, and by listening to how they *feel* about *one*, not just to how they feel about *one's* ideas. The thesis of this chapter is that both task-oriented and relational behaviors are essential for efficient decision making in nursing groups.[1]

GROUP PROBLEM SOLVING AND DECISION MAKING

From the previous chapters, you have a good idea of what effective communication is, what some of the barriers are to it, and what one can do to achieve it; this chapter looks specifically at one communication process for which boards of directors, committees, task groups, and teams are organized: problem solving and decision making in groups. It is hoped you can see that, once nurses as individuals become more effective communicators and active listeners, they will have an impact for the better on their group interaction.

Problem solving and decision making most often occur in group situations because rarely does one person make all the decisions in an office or hospital, which means they are influenced by the "dynamics" or forces within the group itself, such as motivation, interpersonal relations, group structure, communication patterns, and norms.

In addition, the stages of development of the group itself can have an impact on these processes. It is important that nurses as group members learn to look at how their work gets done, how decisions are made, and how people get included (just how do people involve newly elected members of the board in their already ongoing process?), so that they can engage in these processes more effectively.

One theory of group development is that of B.W. Tuckman in "Developmental Sequence in Small Groups." He identified four stages of group development: forming, storming, norming, and performing.[2] What this theory demonstrates is that a group changes as it solves certain interpersonal issues and achieves certain tasks. This happens time after time in nursing groups, especially with new committees. It's more difficult to see all these transitions in standing committees, because by the time nurses, as new members, join such committees, they have usually moved beyond the initial stages of development and it is the new members who must try to catch up.

In the first phase, "forming" a group is primarily concerned with the issues of "Who's in charge?" and "What are we supposed to do?" and "Who are we responsible to?" Individuals tend to depend on the designated leader to provide all the structure, to set the ground rules, to establish the agenda, and to do all the "leading." As far as one's task is concerned, one must identify one's "charge"; what exactly has one been asked to do, what data does one already have to work with, what is the time frame within which one is to work, to whom is one accountable, what are the resources each member brings to the task? Too often, rather than providing for new members' dependency and orientation needs, groups just barrel along, taking up where the last meeting left off, with the frequent result that these new members do not become effective on boards and committees for a long time.

The second phase, "storming," refers to the conflict experienced in groups as the members organize to get the work of the group done and make decisions regarding who is going to be responsible for what; what are going to be the work rules and procedures (e.g., who will approach the candidates one would like to nominate to the board?); what are going to be the limits (e.g., how long will the group spend on this; how many buildings shall they look at as possible facilities?); what is going to be the reward system (how many of the members ever thought of that in the committee work?); what are going to be the criteria by which they will know they have accomplished their task? People's effectiveness as a group depends on how well they solve these interpersonal conflicts over leadership and leadership structure, power, and authority.

The third phase refers to the stage of development during which members of the group begin to experience a sense of groupness or cohesion, a feeling of catharsis at having resolved interpersonal conflict and of having "gotten their act together." They begin sharing ideas, feelings, giving feedback to each other, soliciting feedback, exploring actions related to the task (getting on with it!), and sharing information related to the task (through phone calls, formal and informal reports). They begin to feel good about their work and about being part of the group, and there is an emerging openness with regard to the task at hand. We have seen this happen on various committees on which we have served, and we have observed it in groups that we have observed. There is a sense of flow, of something clicking, and this leads to brief indulgences in playfulness where people abandon the task and just enjoy being with one another. Everyone has probably been at meetings when this has occurred—nothing was ever so funny, one never had such a good time as at that moment. Rising out of a sense of accomplishment and the joy of being able to depend on one another, it further contributes to both.

The fourth phase, "performing," is the culmination of the work as a group—people are both highly task-oriented and highly person-oriented. The group's tasks are well defined, they have a high degree of commitment to common activity, and they are able to support experimentation in solving problems. A trusting climate makes it safe to take risks.

It is hoped that this explanation of group development will make it easier for you to understand your feelings when joining a group already in progress (like a board or a standards committee or a task group) and will help you understand the various phases that a new group goes through. It has been said that part of the reason people feel dissatisfied at the "storming" stage (where researchers have discovered a real dip in what is known as the "morale curve") is that their expectations are often too high as they first get involved in a new group. When reality sets in, people often feel depressed and frustrated. But if they know that it's normal to feel that way, they can cope more easily with this stage of development and look forward to resolving these issues and moving on to the "norming" phase and becoming more productive.

One researcher, Lancoursiere, identifies a fifth phase, "mourning," which occurs with the termination of the group.[3] In nursing groups, it doesn't happen with the whole group of the board and most committees, but individuals do go through a "withdrawal" period following board or committee service, especially if they have served for a long time. Going off the board is often accompanied by a feeling of being left out in the cold, which is distinctly related to the feeling, "How can they manage without me?" The best way to handle those feelings is to get involved in something else that's meaningful as soon as possible!

Figure 7-1 identifies seven steps in the process of problem solving that lead to effective decision making.

I. *Identifying areas of mutual concern.*

First of all, when approaching work as problem-solvers, whether as board or committee members, it is important to identify areas of mutual concern. Nurses must not assume that they and other members of the board/committee/work team share a completely mutual concern about an alleged problem or situation—in spite of the fact that belonging to the health profession implies a mutuality of concern. Nurses should take the time carefully to determine the actual degree of shared concern. This stage may occur during a meeting in which they might re-clarify their statement of purpose. If they don't go through this clarifying process, not all members of the group will be committed to working on what they have determined is the problem, and this can increase interpersonal difficulty within the group and delay the problem-solving process (they would be stuck in the "storming" phase). Taking the time to verify areas of mutual concern helps build group cohesiveness (gets to the "norming" phase), at which level "data flow" (information sharing) can happen, and helps improve the interpersonal relationships within the group.

A fairly simple procedure can be followed to identify this mutual concern: each individual should be asked to indicate honestly "This is how I see . . . (the situation or need for change), and I feel . . . (very strongly, or somewhat bothered, or quite upset) about it." If this process is done in an open and supportive climate, the true degree of mutuality of concern can be determined, and fewer hidden agendas will prevail.

Sometimes it is difficult to identify specific areas of mutual concern. It's easy enough when a disaster happens (e.g., the facility burns down or the electricity goes off) for all to pull together and exert their combined energy to solve that problem. But in the absence of disaster and a "common enemy," there may be differences of opinion about where the group should spend its energy and human resources. Sometimes group members have to find complementary goals (trade-offs) or search for superordinate goals that transcend the specific objectives of the moment in order to put their conflicting ideas into perspective and allow the group to get on with its task(s). If all agree or a statement of purpose, for example, they may not have absolute agreement on all goals they might try to achieve, but they can usually come to an agreement on "the three most important" goals for the group to achieve in the next 5 years. To be able to focus on specific problems and seek to solve them is something many nurses as staff members need to know. Rather than complaining to one another about a procedure or a work-flow problem, as staff members, a

I. Identify areas of mutual concern
II. Analyze the problem
    A. Compare the existing condition with the one desired to find the gaps
        1. Define the scope of the problem
        2. Identify impelling and constraining forces
        3. Analyze problem intensity
    B. Set the group objective
    C. Obtain relevant data to achieve the objective
    D. Overcome the barriers to problem analysis
III. Generate and evaluate proposed solutions
    A. Identify possible approaches to solve the problem
    B. Evaluate the approaches according to at least three criteria:
        1. Will this approach meet the need/gap we have identified?
        2. Can it be implemented by us?
        3. Does it contain any serious disadvantages?
IV. Make a choice (decision) among the alternative approaches
V. Make a detailed plan of action for implementation
    A. Identify specific steps to be accomplished, their sequence, and "due date" (time line)
    B. Determine the required resources
    C. Agree upon individual responsibilities
    D. Provide for emergencies (plan B)
    E. Plan for evaluation at a future time
VI. Implement the plan
VII. Evaluate the plan and feedback the results to step II above for future planning and problem solving

FIGURE 7-1. Steps in problem-solving.[4]

statement of purpose can be a very helpful step toward increased effectiveness.

II. *Analyzing the problem.*

    A. *Compare the existing condition with the desired condition.*

There are four steps in problem analysis (see Fig. 7-1). The first one is to compare what exists with what is desired. For example, nurses may look at the number of clients using their services and decide that the staffing budget and facilities are inadequate. Others may state the problem differently: "We rely too much on neighboring health-care agencies." Each person's perception of the need (the gap between what is and what is desired) needs to be clarified, understood, and evaluated so as to form the best possible group perception of the problem (you see how this could not happen in a defensive climate?).

The ultimate value of this process lies in achieving the best possible insight into the nature of the problem as well as gaining optimum group member effort and cooperation in working toward the solution. Effective group action requires such a group commitment. Of course, there are times when such a process cannot be undergone, and nurses slip back to crisis management—as when a head nurse suddenly resigns and a replacement has to be found immediately. But even here, after the crisis is over, every attempt should be made to trace the steps leading up to the crisis and see how it might have been averted or anticipated by a training program. At the very least, get in the habit of developing a "Plan B" for most major undertakings.

There are three things necessary to do when analyzing problems:

1. We need to determine the scope of the problem—the size or extent of the difficulty involved. "We" means those who are in charge. This is related not only to the actual gap perceived, but to the intensity of people's feelings about it. Nurses need to ask themselves: How many people are involved in this problem? Is it just the nursing staff's problem or is it tied into other departments within the institution? What are the prevailing attitudes in the community regarding this problem? How strongly does each person feel about this problem?

2. Next, nurses need to identify the impelling and constraining forces at work in the problem. Too often, they think simplistically about their needs and perhaps tend to identify "the cause" of all their problems as "needing more nurses," for example. Diagramming the problem on a "force field" (see Fig. 7-2) should help to identify all the factors impinging on the problem and how strong each of those forces is.

Force-field analysis is a diagnostic tool adapted by Kurt Lewin from the field of physics. It is based upon the principle that any situation is the way it is at any given moment (the "status quo") because sets of counterbalancing forces are keeping it that way. The basic force-field diagram is shown in Figure 7-2.

How does it work? Take the problem identified as "not enough nurses to implement any primary nursing." What forces might be at work to produce and keep that situation the way it is? Maybe administrative support of nurses' pay structure is really minimal. Maybe there is an apathetic board. Are nurses brave enough to point it out?

And what forces are at work impelling a change in the status quo? Maybe a new nurse wants to revitalize the RN staff-recruitment program. Perhaps the new comptroller is going to establish a system of purchase orders to better control in-house spending. Perhaps the board has set as a priority objective this year the increase of salaries for nurses.

Once the forces have been identified, the relative intensity of each force must be indicated on a scale of 1 to 5, with 5 being the strongest.

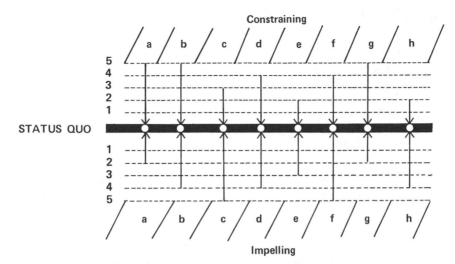

FIGURE 7-2. Basic force-field diagram. (From K. Giffin and B. Patton: *Decision-Making Group Interaction* [Harper & Row, New York, 1978], p. 131, with permission.)

That's so that when nurses attack one of the forces to change it, they'll have a realistic appraisal of its relative strength and perhaps choose initially to work on one less strong, since success is important in keeping them motivated. People who have used this method of analyzing a problem caution that once various forces have been lined up on the diagram, it is better to concentrate energies on reducing the intensity of the constraining forces than on increasing the intensity of the impelling forces, since doing the latter may just increase tension without resolving the problem. The point to be made is that if one has not analyzed the problem and isolated the various forces impinging upon it, one can spend one's energy fruitlessly solving the wrong problem and/or trying solutions that only increase the tension instead of reducing it.

3. Problem intensity also needs to be analyzed. The degree of intensity of a problem may be determined by noting the degree of dissatisfaction with the present condition. The board members' degree of commitment to solving a problem will be the direct result of their view of the intensity of the problem, that is, their own emotional investment in the situation. It seems to be true that one's degree of commitment to solving a problem is directly related to one's perception of the personal intensity of the problem for each person. And one's commitment, of course, will directly affect our board's efficiency in implementing a workable problem-solution. And, of course, the same principle applies in all committee and group work.

B. *Set group objective.*

After going through all these analytic steps, the group objective is then set. For example, the group decides to devote its energy to the need for more volunteer support and the objective is to develop a volunteer problem. Remember that it isn't enough just to say "increase the number of volunteers"; the objective must be specific, measurable, achievable, and compatible with the goals of the organization.

Objectives must be specific for three reasons:

1. The members must be able to know what type of proposal will take them to their goal.
2. The leaders must be able to tell them when, if ever, a specific problem has been solved.
3. An effectively high commitment and concerted group effort cannot be maintained forever. Within some reasonable period of time, the group will need to feel that something specific has been accomplished. (It is felt that the best time to take the measure of group accomplishments is at the annual meeting.)

C. *Obtain relevant data.*

The next step in this process is to obtain relevant data to achieve the objective. Obtaining relevant, factual information is absolutely essential in problem analysis. Information needed regarding a volunteer program would include, Has anyone else done such a thing? How do the volunteers feel right now about working with this hospital? Are their needs being met, and, if not, what unmet needs exist? What is the record-keeping system like (resource/talent file)?

When attempting to get this relevant and accurate information regarding volunteer attitudes in the community, what criteria should be used to measure this information? The group would certainly want to know if its sources of information are reliable and credible—do they really know, or are they reporting hearsay? What is their track record in this regard? Do the sources know how to conduct an attitudes survey? Can they report the results without undue distortion?

For example, suppose one of the board members conducted some kind of feedback session in which volunteers were asked, "What are all the good things about working at our hospital? What are all the bad things?" Does the group realize that sometimes people would use these sessions as "dumping" grounds, and perhaps only the disenchanted ones will show up? Furthermore, some people, when asked to list "bad things," will make them up if they hadn't thought of them before, because it seems to be expected. Those are important considerations in designing and interpreting feedback/information-gathering opportunities.

D. *Overcome barriers.*

The fourth step that must be taken during the problem analysis phase is to overcome various barriers to problem analysis. There are four such barriers, common pitfalls that help account for the difficulty many groups have in reaching agreement. There are certain assumptions frequently held by people in this culture that must be identified, evaluated, and abandoned if people are going to be able to analyze their problems effectively.

1. *Too early emphasis on possible solutions.* Before taking the time to look at all impelling and constraining forces, people latch on to one solution, relieved to be finished with that problem. But it stands to reason that the "best" solution cannot be found if only one solution is generated. In addition, it is psychologically important that each member of the group feel satisfied that one's particular insights into the forces inherent in the problem have been expressed and given adequate consideration by the group. This is necessary if members are later to give their full commitment and support to the problem solution chosen by the group.

Because board meetings are often inefficient and the tough part of the agenda, the problem-solving part, is typically put at the end of the meeting, people often, in the "interests of time," cut others off from participating in the discussion regarding the problem. By doing so, they are diminishing the chances for that problem to be solved effectively and with the full support of the group. How many times have you heard someone say, "Well okay, have it your way, but don't ask me to help!" Or maybe they don't say anything, and you simply never do understand why they don't accept responsibility for a piece of the implementation of your problem solution.

2. *Lack of specific information.* It's probably never going to be possible for groups to have all the information they need to make a perfect decision every time. Nonetheless, it is believed that often a mistaken assumption that time and/or money will be saved makes people skip the needed fact-finding missions that might have given them the significant information to make a better decision. Of course, sometimes people find it hard to admit that they don't fully understand the information they have, because to do so causes them to lose face (appear stupid), particularly in some defensive climates.

3. *The assumption that "truth will win out."* The basis for the old town hall meetings, this assumption neglects two requirements: that adequate information be obtained on all relevant aspects of a situation and that such purportedly factual information be tested for its validity. Otherwise, half-truths and untruths masquerading as truths may supplant "the truth."

4. *Confusion between disagreement and dislike.* Unfortunately, some people perceive disagreement with their ideas as dislike of themselves. Remember how one's self-concept needs to maintain itself under threat—disagreement can be perceived as threat. Perceived dislike tends to breed further dislike, and pretty soon a situation arises in which no creative group activity can take place.

III. *Generate and evaluate proposed solutions.*

Please note that the last word is plural.

The process of generation can be achieved by brainstorming, a process wherein evaluation is withheld until a large number of ideas have been generated. But before the possible solutions generated during the brainstorming process are given priorities, people need to evaluate them according to three criteria:

A. Will this proposal produce the desired changes in the current situation? Will it meet the need for change as it has been identified?

B. Can this proposal be implemented by the group? It is a workable suggestion? What is the ratio of yield (results) to effort, time, and energy required, also referred to as "cost" (money, time, other resources) to "benefit" (good outcome) analysis?

C. Does this proposal inherently contain serious disadvantages? Inherent dangers usually consist of risks that the group cannot afford to take—hiring an administrative assistant to the Director of Nursing, for example, when the hospital really doesn't have the cash reserves to pay this person should a grant not come through and/or fees go down.

Once proposed solutions have been evaluated according to those (and any other) criteria, a choice of alternatives must be made.

IV. *Need to Make a Decision.*

By comparing solutions to the above criteria, the group should be able to choose the one or two or three proposals that would be most satisfactory for the group, and it should also be able to obtain the group members' agreement and commitment for their implementation.

V. *Need to Develop a Detailed Plan of Action for Implementation.*

This stage involves:

A. Identifying specific steps to be accomplished and the sequence and "due date" for each. This is sometimes called a "time line." Examples might include: (a) set up a volunteer committee by June 1, 1983; (b) committee defines specific problem areas with volunteers by July 1, 1983; (c) committee updates the resource file by August 1, 1983; (d) committee contacts Midland Hospital regarding their hired volunteer coordinator by August 1, 1983.

B. Determining required resources—human and material. Who should chair the committee? Who should serve on it? What will it cost for an annual recognition program?

C. Agreeing upon individual responsibilities for parts of the implementation. Marie will check the resource file; Annette will make the phone calls; Marge will get in touch with the instructor; Deanna will design the awards; Terry will serve as emcee at the awards ceremony; Marianne will conduct the feedback session.

Groups do need to plan and keep in reserve a "Plan B" in case the initial solution, despite all the analysis, does not work. And they should plan for an evaluation at a future time.

VI. *Mobilize Resources And Implement Plan.*

Experience shows that few plans, even when well developed, work perfectly without mishap. Accidents occur, unforeseen barriers are encountered, and some persons become ill or find that their capabilities were overestimated. Your overall plan should provide for such unforeseen emergencies; some group members should have the responsibility of handling such problems in case they arise. In the military, it is common to have some units in reserve, "just in case." Some persons in your group should have this responsibility, should try to guess where potential needs or crises may arise, and provide contingency plans in case they are needed.

VII. *Evaluate the Outcome.*

Remember, this evaluation was built into the time-line to assure its taking place. Evaluation is one of the most effective planning tools available, and it is the one used least often in most organizations. It will tell members what worked and what didn't work, and will give them valuable data for future planning and problem-solving.

One of the authors once worked for an oil pipeline company; this organization seemed to have an established policy that identified problems, analyzed them, selected a plan of action, put it into operation, and went on to other problems. Most of these action plans worked, more or less. Only if they failed or worked poorly were they brought up again for further attention. A management consultant pointed out the potential value of systematically evaluating each "solution" after it was put into action. He suggested that the most appropriate time to plan or arrange for such evaluation was during the detailed planning of the program implementation. At this time, procedures for evaluation could be built into the overall procedure; equipment for collecting performance data could be installed while other installations or modifications were being made. In this way, total disruption and confusion would be reduced. The company adopted his suggestions and found them very useful.

We similarly recommend that your group include an evaluation of the proposed plan of action as one of the basic elements in implementing the plan. Seek information on the following items: (1) Did the predicted change actually occur; that is, did the proposal, when implemented, meet the need earlier identified by the group? (2) Did the plan, when implemented, cost no more (demand no more time, energy, or money) than predicted? (3) Were there any unforeseen risks or dangers after the plan was put into operation? Only if such questions are answered can a new policy or procedure be properly evaluated.

CONFLICT MANAGEMENT

Needless to say, many books have been written on this subject, and these few pages can merely go "once over lightly"; nonetheless, it is hoped this brief discussion will spur you on to further reading and will help you "give yourself permission" to discuss the issue with your board, committee, and supervisors. Remember, as long as a norm exists that "we don't talk about conflict," nothing constructive can be done about it.

According to experts in the field of group dynamics, reaching a "consensus" on a solution to a shared problem is a major goal of many problem-solving groups. In order to achieve consensus (as opposed to majority rule—which is often related to negative or personal power), the views of all members must be heard, given fair consideration, and be critically evaluated. Conflict, or disagreement, is a natural and essential part of this process.

If everyone agreed on everything, there would be no purpose for having discussion or, for that matter, for having problem-solving groups like task forces, committees, and boards at all. The differences that arise as a result of each person perceiving and interpreting the situation according to one's own perceptual filters are good; they generate many possible solutions and approaches to each problem. The result is that, after evaluating all ideas, the group is much more likely to find a "best" solution. A group should be committed, then, to developing a climate of trust, a climate that will foster creative inquiry, a climate in which all members will be willing to risk making suggestions for the solution to the problem.

THE NEED TO ENCOURAGE CONFLICT

Communication specialist Julia Wood says that there appear to be at least three noteworthy reasons for encouraging conflict in problem-solving discussion:[5]

1. By entertaining diverse ideas and perspectives, it is possible to gain a broadened understanding of the nature of the problem and its implications. One time, one of the authors was working with a group of directors of nursing services that was identifying all the impelling and constraining forces contributing to their perceived need for more nursing staff. The ideas were all in a similar vein—until the 14th person had the courage to say that the problem, as far as she was concerned, was with the directors—they were not looking at what nurses need and how directors could redesign jobs to be more attractive. That took real courage, and it was a whole new perspective on the problem, one with which many of the group agreed but had been too afraid to say so.

2. By encouraging the expression of different ideas, a group has potentially more alternatives from which to select a final solution. That group of directors, because of the addition of that one member's input, was able to focus on all the impelling and constraining forces at work, thereby providing a wider range of choices from which to choose.

3. The excitement that comes from conflicting ideas stimulates healthy interaction and involvement with the group's task. (That group

had a new excitement as a result of the release of energy that had been tied up in suppressing and denying possible conflict.)

By way of analogy, it is suggested that rain (conflict) is a nurturing climate needed by all living things on this planet. It is only when rain becomes a wild storm or deluge causing flooding that it becomes destructive rather than supportive of life. The same is true of conflict. It is important, we believe, for nurses to learn to manage conflict so its generation of differing alternatives and approaches is a constructive force in their organization's life; if they don't learn skills in the managing of conflict, it may intensify to the point that it destroys the organization. How many times have you heard that a group split up because of "personality clashes"? That is nothing but mismanaged conflict.

SOME WAYS OF HANDLING CONFLICT

Donald T. Simpson has identified five ways of handling conflict.
1. *Denial or Withdrawal:*
   This happens when people simply deny that a difference of opinion exists. Since conflict is inevitable whenever groups get together to exchange ideas, you can bet that in a group where denial is the technique for handling conflict, the conflict goes underground and emerges as "hidden agendas."
2. *Suppression or Smoothing Over:*
   The group norm is that "nice people don't fight." So, instead of clearing the air by getting all the aspects of the conflicting views out on the table, the group "moves to table" or "moves to adjourn," with the result that the atmosphere degenerates into "muggy and sticky." It tends to sap the group's energy and could result in apathy.
3. *Power or Dominance:*
   This method is used often, especially in groups where the majority rules. Power strategies (these are "personal" or "negative" power strategies) result in winners and losers, however, and the losers often sabotage the winners by refusing to support and implement decisions made in this manner.
4. *Compromise or Negotiation:*
   Often proposed as the way to handle conflict, this approach can result in no one's getting the best result. The compromise may be so watered down that it will never address the problem. However, when all else fails, compromise may be the only way to solve the conflict.
5. *Integration or Collaboration:*
   This approach rests on the assumption that all persons participating in the conflict have something worthwhile to contribute to the discussion. Everyone is assumed to be "partly right." The emphasis of the group is

on solving the problem at hand, rather than on taking sides. From the beginning of the process, all members expect to have to modify their original views. The goal is solving the problem, not winning a debate.

Another assumption in this approach is that the work of the whole group will be qualitatively better than the work of any one of its members. Of course, this can happen only in a climate characterized by trust, open communication, active listening, and commitment to thorough analysis of a problem area that the group has mutually agreed needs its best attention.

Our own experience in meetings involving nurses leads us to believe that most people are afraid of conflict and will avoid it at all costs and therefore can be dominated by people who use it to manipulate them. We think it's time people asked themselves "What's the worst that can happen?" We'll bet they would find out conflict isn't half as bad—when it's still at a low-intensity level—as they thought it would be. And if "the worst that can happen" is destruction of the group, perhaps now's the time to call in a consultant to help the members learn to work creatively with conflict, for the good of their organizations.

PLANNING AND RUNNING MEETINGS

Our view of leadership is that it is the potential behavior of any or all members of a group cooperatively working together to solve a mutual problem. Leadership can and should be exercised by any and all participants with the consent and approval of the other participants, whenever such behavior helps the group to achieve a mutually desired goal. Thus the central problem, as we see it, is to avoid fostering the manipulation of others and to encourage all to recognize the common need to identify mutual concerns, analyze mutually shared problems, find appropriate solutions, and put them into action. In addition, all members need to learn to recognize the behavior that contributes to these objectives and to allow it and, better, encourage it, whenever it serves the needs of the group.

Figure 7-3 provides a guide for a meeting in which you are the designated leader. To the extent possible, try to observe this format.

THERAPEUTIC GROUPS AND PSYCHIATRIC TEAMS

Many nurses will be called upon to work in special groups designated as *therapeutic groups* or as a part of a *psychiatric team*. Such assignments require special training and advanced work beyond the level of this book. They are mentioned because such groups are based on the principles of

1. Specify objectives for the meeting.
2. Build an agenda for the meeting, including all reports, discussion items, and action items, and the time allotted to each.
3. Decide who needs to come to the meeting, and give each person a copy of the agenda and any support documents needed for action and/or discussion items.
4. Make provision for appropriate space and for all supplies and resources (including people).
5. Begin and end the meetings promptly at the announced time.
6. Provide brief "group building" activities at the beginning ("coffee and conversation" time; small-group discussion) and time for summarizing and reflecting on the achievements of the meeting and planning the next meeting.
7. Continually look for ways to relate the work of the group to the purpose and goals of the organization.
8. Provide a short break for each hour or hour and a half of the meeting.
9. At the beginning of each meeting, always share the objectives and review the proposed agenda for possible revision. Try using newsprint for this purpose.
10. The size of the group affects how the group works together. If the task group is only four to six persons, then all group work can be done together. If there are more than four members, some group assignments could be done in subgroups.

FIGURE 7-3. Suggested format for planning and running meetings.

humanistic interpersonal communication emphasized throughout this book.

A number of scholars have studied mental hospital systems and, more specifically, the role and function of clinical staff members who aspire to treat psychiatric patients. Perhaps the best-known study was conducted by Caudill, who was interested in the day-to-day personal relations of physicians, ward personnel, and patients.[6] Many of his observations continue to be valid today in spite of the rapid changes in hospital care over the last 20 years. The methods used in his study were observations and interviews over a 10-month period. Data were collected from 63 consecutive administrative conferences that were held Monday through Saturday for 15 to 20 minutes. The analysis of the conferences were made using Bales' 12 interaction categories (Bales' categories are discussed in detail in Chapter 9). The results of the study showed that higher-status persons tend to participate more heavily in group discussion. Studies by Strodtbeck and Mann[7] and Mishler and Tropp[8] demonstrated similar results.

Membership and awareness of the roles of other professionals are the focus of a study by Mill.[9] He believes that team members carry out functions best if there is an awareness of individual roles and of the roles of coworkers. A study was done by direct interviews of physicians (N = 63), psychologists (N = 24), social workers (N = 30), nurses (N = 55), and attendants (N = 122) of six mental hospitals and one training school for mentally retarded persons in Virginia. Each subject was asked, "What does a (physician, psychologist, and so forth) do in a hospital like this?" Verbatim replies were rated on a five-point scale by a team of psychologists. The results of the study showed that psychologists, social workers, and attendants described their own roles better than those of others; physicians described the role of social workers better than their own role; nurses described attendants' roles better than their own role. The most adequate descriptions of professional roles were done by psychologists, social workers, attendants, nurses, and physicians, in that order. Of the professions most poorly described, physicians described the work of attendants less, psychologists described physicians and nurses less, social workers described nurses less, nurses described the physician's role less, and attendants were least acquainted with the social worker's role. This study suggests that role-definition may be a need for effective team functioning.

Schatzman and Bucher were interested in the ways psychiatric professions negotiate the tasks they perform in a state hospital setting.[10] The data were collected by field observations and interviews of five multidisciplinary teams. The membership of the teams included a psychiatrist-chief, physician, nurse, psychologist, social worker, recreational or occupational therapist, and psychiatric aide. One of the results of the study was that the more articulate professionals were in an advantageous position and were able to "demonstrate" their knowledge (and, by inference, their ability) in team meetings. There was a strong tendency to get to do what was considered important and to drop unimportant and degrading tasks. If a team member was not satisfied, one way to handle the problem was to transfer to another team. The negotiation of tasks by social workers and psychologists tended to run parallel, and the tasks of nurses and physicians were linked.

The decision-making process in a mental hospital was the focus of a study by Lefton, Dinitz, and Pasamanick.[11] They examined the process in a small psychiatric hospital in terms of the differences in real, perceived, and ideal influence patterns of 53 mental health specialists. The hospital contained 126 beds with three female and two male wards. The staff consisted of 5 senior psychiatrists (ward administrators), 15 resident psychiatrists, 18 registered nurses, and 5 each of clinical psychologists, social workers, and occupational therapists. Each person was interviewed and asked to estimate one's influence in six different decision-making areas of concern in patient care and treatment. The six areas were (1) working diagnosis, (2) medical treatment, (3) patient privileges, (4) occupational therapy, (5) special supervision, and (6) time and type of release of patients. Each staff member rated one's influence as it was and as it should have been. The systematic recordings of actual decisions at ward conferences revealed that senior and resident physicians made 96 percent of the decisions and social workers 4 percent. General discussions at the conferences were dominated by the medical staff and charge nurses. The finding of this study suggests that mental hospital personnel tend to perceive their influence and participation in the decision-making process in terms of their professional group membership. There were also discrepancies between desired and perceived decision-making influence causing dissatisfaction in the lower echelon ancillary staff members. The study also suggests that there was less dissatisfaction on the ward that had a traditional bureaucratic medical organization than on the ward using a more equalitarian "team" approach.

SUMMARY

As a nursing clinician, you will be involved in a number of committees in your health-care facility and in your community. When committees function effectively, they can facilitate coordination of efforts, make better decisions than can be reached individually, improve morale, promote creativity, and keep everyone involved and informed. Disadvantages include the amount of time invested by a number of people, slower capability to reach decisions and act, and diffused accountability. Administrative judgment is important in determining what matters should be handled individually and what is proper agenda for a committee.

This chapter has presented the various stages in typical problem-solving discussions and has presented our thinking concerning making the steps functional. An approach to conflict management in groups and a format for planning and running meetings have been suggested.

Maureen J. O'Brien has summed up efficiently the importance of such group work:

> Committee assignments can help to improve the quality of nursing being practiced within an institution. You should be willing to give your best effort to the committee for which you have been elected or assigned. If each member of the committee views his task seriously and is willing to prepare before the meetings so that he can participate intelligently, the work is made easier and the meeting is usually productive. This does not mean there is always agreement between the members; but each person is prepared to give his views or to share his research about a specific topic so that a task can be accomplished or at least some progress be made.[12]

REFERENCES

1. The basic theory for this chapter is drawn from BOBBY R. PATTON AND KIM GIFFIN: *Decision-Making Group Interaction* (New York: Harper & Row, 1978).
2. B. W. TUCKMAN: "Developmental Sequence in Small Groups," *Psychological Bulletin*, 63(1965): 384–399.
3. ROY LACOURSIERE: *The Life Cycle of Groups* (New York: Human Sciences Press, 1980).
4. Drawn from PATTON AND GIFFIN: *op. cit.*
5. JULIA T. WOOD: "Constructive Conflict in Discussion: Learning to Manage Disagreements Effectively," *The 1977 Annual Handbook for Group Facilitators* (La Jolla, Calif.: University Associates, 1977).
6. W. CAUDILL: *The Psychiatric Hospital as a Small Society* (Boston: Harvard University Press, 1958).
7. F. L. STRODTBECK AND R. D. MANN: "Sex Role Differentiation in Jury Deliberations," *Sociometry*, 19(1956): pp. 3–11.
8. E. G. MISHLER AND A. TROPP: "Status and Interaction in a Psychiatric Hospital," *Human Relations*, 9(1956): pp. 187–205.
9. DYRIL R. MILL: "Interprofessional Awareness of Roles," *Journal of Clinical Psychology*, October 1960, Vol. XVII, #4, pp. 411–413.
10. LEONARD SCHATZMAN AND RUE BUCHER: "Negotiating a Division of Labor among Professionals in a State Mental Hospital," *Psychiatry*, August 1964, Vol. 27, #3, pp. 266–277.
11. MARK LEFTON, SIMON DINITZ, AND BENJAMIN PASAMANICK: "Decision-Making in a Mental Hospital: Real, Perceived, and Ideal," *American Sociological Review*, 1959, #6, pp. 822–829.
12. MAUREEN J. O'BRIEN: *Communications and Relationships in Nursing* (St. Louis: C.V. Mosby Company, 1974), pp. 143–144.

8
COMMUNICATING IN PUBLIC

A poll shown in the popular *Book of Lists* indicated that the greatest personal fear of most Americans was having to speak in public. Virtually all people are anxious before giving a speech because they want to be well received and to have their message understood and accepted. As nursing clinicians, you are going to be called to speak to other groups of nurses and staff, to groups of clients and families, and to the general public. This chapter examines the process of speaking in public and suggests procedures for developing your skills. Important to remember is that all of the principles of humanistic communication apply; you now have typically the opportunity to preplan and enlarge your presentation to include more people.

YOUR VISION OF YOURSELF AS A PUBLIC SPEAKER

It is extremely important that you try to picture yourself using the kind of behavior that you would like to have as a speaker. Deliberately try to imagine how you will look and sound; think through the things you would like to do. If you cannot in your own mind develop an image of yourself as being a competent communicator with an audience, it is not likely that you will be able to behave in that way. Ability to achieve a vision of yourself acting in a certain way will enhance your ability to behave that way. Vision sets boundaries on your ultimate potential.[1]

It is suggested that you can help yourself to become a more competent speaker by deliberately envisioning yourself doing five things; for each of these actions, you should try to create a picture of yourself "in your mind's eye" behaving in specific and particular ways.

1. *Understanding Your Listeners:*

Imagine how you would feel and behave if you clearly understood your listeners' needs and desires. Do this carefully regarding any topic or area on which you expect to speak to them. If you don't have enough information about their hopes or interests, seek to obtain this knowledge. Imagine yourself meeting these needs and interests; develop your picture of yourself and your behavior in as much detail as you can.

2. *Knowing Yourself as a Speaker:*

How much credibility do you have? Can you imagine yourself being a dependable, knowledgeable person, talking to a group of listeners? Your most valuable characteristic as a speaker is your credibility; can you imagine yourself speaking to an audience in a way that *uses and protects* your credibility? In order to do this, you will need to be very clear in your mind regarding your *intentions* toward your listeners: do you really wish to help them understand, reach useful decisions, achieve their interests and needs? As you imagine yourself achieving these goals, do you present your ideas in a clear, well-organized fashion? Use words well? Have an attractive, expressive voice? Let your body talk freely? To the extent that you can create a vision of yourself doing these things well, to that extent you may be able to succeed in so behaving.

3. *Interacting with Your Listeners:*

You may have difficulty at first trying to picture yourself speaking to a group of listeners and at the same time interacting with them. It is suggested that you can note their facial expressions, eye contact with you, and general body movements and posture. Do they, in your imagination, show signs of interest in your ideas? Do they, at times, indicate a sense of confusion or disbelief? Do you respond to these signals in ways that clarify or increase belief? Do you verbally (really) ask them from time to time if they understand? Generally agree? Do they nod their heads? Smile in response? Show favorable reactions to your efforts? Do you hold their interest and attention? Do they show this by their responses? Remember that the limits of your imagination will set boundaries on your behavior and indirectly, to a large extent, limit the nature of their responses to you. The importance of your efforts to create, in your own mind, a detailed picture of yourself as a speaker interacting in favorable ways with your listeners cannot be emphasized too much.

4. *Helping Your Listeners Understand Your Ideas:*

You will need to work out in specific detail an image of your behavior that will be helpful in gaining your listeners' understanding of your ideas. You must first clearly identify your own specific beliefs regarding a particular topic area. Next, you must gain a clear picture of your listeners' needs and interests regarding this topic. What is it that they don't know or understand? Why are they ignorant or confused in this way? Are you clearly competent to supply needed information or insight? Can you picture yourself meeting this need? Is your image complete in specific detail, actions, and verbal behavior? Is this picture of yourself one that you think they will like and appreciate? Does it include the presentation of specific, factual, supportable information? Can you imagine your listeners' responses to your efforts? You will need to work on this problem of successfully helping your listeners to understand your ideas until, in your own mind, you have a clear image of yourself active in ways that are helpful to them.

5. *Helping Your Listeners Reach Satisfactory Decisions:*

This problem is the most difficult of the five that have been identified; it is easy to make unfounded assumptions about the desirability of decisions for others. In the first place, you will need to get very clearly in your mind your own goal in helping them make a decision. Do you respect their ability to make judgments if they have valid information on a problem? Are you simply trying to get them to do what you want? Imagine yourself with them in a persuasive situation; as you develop this picture of yourself, what is it that you feel you really want? Personal respect for yourself? Admiration for your wisdom? A decision that will serve their interests well over time? You will have to work carefully to clarify your thinking on your own goal in this kind of situation.

Second, you need to picture clearly your own assessment of the problem and its possible solutions. Do you have a clear understanding of the nature of the problem as it affects your listeners? Can you clearly see their inherent difficulties in this area? Have you clearly in mind various possible approaches to a solution, with insights and information regarding pros and cons for each possible approach? In your picture of yourself examining these elements with your listeners, do you see yourself clearly showing reasons *acceptable to your listeners* in support of the approach you believe to be best? Do you actually see them accepting these reasons? In case it is needed, do you have in mind a tentative plan of action for implementing this approach? Can you see yourself presenting it in specific details?

In creating an image of yourself helping others to reach a decision regarding a problem that concerns them, it is extremely important that you understand the thinking of your listeners and that they believe you have this understanding. People generally don't want help in making a decision unless they feel you understand their problem very well. If you can't picture your listeners showing their belief in you in this way, you will need to find out more about how they see the problem.

The most important part of picturing yourself helping others to reach decisions is to see yourself clearly as one who is *responsible to them—* a person of good will—in using psychologic principles of persuasion. It is not enough to be competent in changing attitudes of others, showing that you and they have common basic assumptions, that you believe essentially in ways that are similar to theirs, and then to be clever in planting suggestions in their thinking that will likely lead to desired behavior. It is much more important that, long after you have helped them reach a decision, they feel you have given their interests and needs satisfactory consideration. As you continue to picture yourself helping your listeners choose a solution to a problem, do you see yourself acting in a way that will bring yourself self-respect and a feeling of shared responsibility with your audience?

In each of the five ways described, it will be very valuable to you to work out in specific detail an image of yourself behaving as a responsible, authentic speaker. Following through on this suggestion will take some time; it must be done in depth and with care. However, experience with students indicates that, when well done, it is well worth the time. You are urged to do it.

The principle of responsibility as a speaker is important in two ways: this means you can start making this application today, right now. First, you can start by demanding such responsibility from other speakers any time you listen to them. You can let them know that you expect them to be open and honest with you as you listen to their ideas. In effect, you can offer them a kind of contract: you will listen as carefully and attentively as possible, giving full effort to understanding their views regardless of your present beliefs on their topic; in return, you ask that they present the entire picture as they see it, omitting nothing, either pro or con their ultimate position, nothing. This is relevant. Your expectation will be that, together, you can give the topic optimum exploration and consideration. Your critical thinking, coupled with theirs, should provide both of you the best possible result.

In the second place, you can start immediately requiring yourself to be as real as possible whenever you find others willing to listen to you express your ideas. This may be in a one-to-one interaction situation where you speak to an audience. This application of principles of humanistic communication may be made at once, today, without further delay.

Your ultimate responsibility as a speaker can be measured in these terms: It is as great as the degree of willingness of your listeners to hear and consider what you have to say. Ask yourself this question: what do you want from a speaker when you agree to give that person your attention? What do you require in terms of speakers' responsibility for what they say? We suspect that you want them to be well-informed on the topic when you agree to listen to their ideas and that you want them to tell the truth as they see it. Competency and honesty on their part, insofar as humanly possible, are very likely to be your criteria.

Your responsibility as a speaker can thus be determined: What you require of others is what you should require of yourself when others listen to you. Ultimately, this is the measure of your responsibility. Part of your responsibility is the development of public speaking skills that will enhance your capabilities as a public communicator.

DEVELOPING YOUR SPEECH

In selecting a speech subject, begin by examining your *personal resources* to discover a potential subject that will meet the needs of this audience and this occasion. Before turning to external sources, concentrate on your present and past environment, and your interests, beliefs, feelings, desires, attitudes, and experiences. Dip into your memory and search your background for those significant aspects of your life that made a vivid impression on you. Such rationalizations as "I'm not well informed" or "nothing I know anything about would interest anyone else" are absolutely false. Your insights are potentially of interest and benefit to others.

The personal nature of your communication is emphasized; you are the only person able to give this particular speech. Public speaking is a direct personal relationship of one human being with others. In contrast to writing and reading, there is no intervening agency of paper and ink. Whereas it is difficult, if not impossible, for writers to reveal very much of themselves to you, it would be possible, necessary, and desirable that they do so if they were making speeches to you. Much of an individual's communication training has probably been in writing rather than in speaking. Consequently, all persons must make adjustments in their style. You may have a somewhat impersonal tone in written communication. In spoken communication, however, not only are you allowed to talk about yourself, your activities, your thoughts and feelings, your knowledge and ignorance, your loves and hates, your attitudes and beliefs; you are *impelled* to do so by the nature of the form of communication that you are using.

Your personal resources are tied to experiences that are entirely your own. Your experience is everything inside you. It includes mental ingredients—thoughts, attitudes, memories, beliefs, opinions, and judgments. In addition to these mental components of your experience are your internal physical components: body sensations, feelings, emotions, bodily movements, and postures. Whereas external happenings stimulate your experiences, they do not cause or create these experiences. For example, an orchestra playing a particular selection of music serves as a stimulus for anyone hearing the music, but each person's actual experience of the music is unique. Just as each person's response to the music is highly individualized, so do all persons respond somewhat differently to every stimulus. The words and actions of others, the events that take place in the world, the physical objects that people encounter—each person creates one's own experience of all these things.

An experience, then, is the completely unique series of internal events that you create for yourself as you process what happens in the world outside yourself. These inner experiences become inner realities that are just as real as physical realities perceived through your senses, such as wood, metal, light, and sound. The fact that your experience and internal reality are unique provides the major impetus and challenge for communication, which, as was stated, means sharing the experiences, worlds, and realities of one another. The communicative challenge for you is to recreate your inner reality for others so they may understand and share the experience.

Thus, you cannot select an appropriate subject for your public speech by lifting ideas secondhand from some hastily read book or magazine article. Instead, you must dig deep into your experience and bring forth some of the ideas that are stored there.

Public speaking has traditionally been divided into three *general purposes:* to entertain, to inform, and to persuade. The speech to entertain is a specialized speech reserved for professionals in the entertainment field, or for experienced speakers in after-dinner situations. Although it is useful to categorize speeches according to these general purposes, recognize that rarely are the three categories totally separate from one another. You may, for example, choose to use entertaining materials freely in speeches to help your listeners understand. Or you may need to inform your listeners in order to help them reach decisions.

Identification of the type of speech that you wish to present determines the specific type of preparation required. From the general purpose, you must move to your specific purpose, which identifies explicitly what you want your audience to know, feel, believe, or do. This identification of specific purpose is similar to the central idea or thesis of a written theme. The specific purpose should guide you as you prepare your message, and it should guide your listeners as they receive and comprehend it. You cannot expect an audience to take the trouble to unravel your specific purpose. You must have it clearly in mind, and you must state it explicitly and reiterate it when necessary.

For example, suppose you have chosen as a topic, "Nursing Care for Thymectomy Patients." There are many possible specific purposes under this subject. Some informative purposes are to explain the reactions of clients; to explain a general nursing-care plan; to show the effects of preoperative assessment in certain groups of clients; to show what nursing staffs are doing to improve care; to demonstrate the proper techniques for some procedure; and to explain problems and dangers for some clients. Some possible advocacy purposes are everyone in the audience should know the proper technique of CPR; schools should do more to teach the procedures; nurses need to be more sensitive to some clients' personal needs. Unless you select a specific goal, it is unlikely that you will be able to develop a well-organized speech.

In narrowing your topic and identifying your specific purpose, do not try to cover too much. An attempt to show in 15 minutes that the federal health-care program should be reconstructed will prove most difficult to handle. Limiting yourself to one aspect of laws, such as tax incentives to hospitals for nursing staffs to experiment and innovate primary nursing, would likely be more effective. It is usually better to take a limited area and explain it fully than to give cursory or superficial treatment to a larger area. To borrow from the terminology of photography: do a close-up, not a panoramic shot.

Write out your specific purpose just as you would a telegram, trying to reduce the number of words to a minimum and being as direct and precise as possible. Be careful, however, that you don't oversimplify and overstate certainties. You will likely be showing that something is *probably* or *possibly* true, or that your research has convinced you that a given course of action should probably or possibly be taken. If, for example, after studying the relative merits of treatments of respiratory infections, you find the evidence to be inconclusive or contradictory, you should adapt your specific purpose to reflect the indecision. Instead of saying that one approach is clearly superior at this time, you may merely discuss the pros and cons.

While formulating your specific purpose, ask yourself questions such as these: Is this topic as specific and concrete as I can make it? Does it state more than I know or want to show? Does it reflect the audience's interests and needs? Does it summarize all that I want to present? (It is suggested that you formulate several specific purposes that you feel qualified to speak on and then discuss these statements with your fellow nurses.)

With your specific purpose clearly in mind, you are now ready to start exploring your topic through *research*. Your first source of material is yourself. If you have selected a subject on which you are well informed, your task may be to exclude material rather than to search for more. For most topics, however, you will want or need to supplement your present knowledge with research. For such research, you should first stop to analyze what would likely be the best sources—an interview with someone (such as one of your professors) who knows a lot about the topic; the library for books or periodicals; resource centers on your campus or in the community that are concerned with your topic; firsthand observations of an event related to your topic (a visit to a specialist, for example).

Common to all types of research is the need to take careful *notes.* Never depend on your memory if you wish to retain particulars; an "unforgettable" quotation may elude you 10 minutes later. Use note cards of uniform size (3-×-5- or 4-×-6-inch) so that you can arrange them into a variety of sequences or remove the ones you do not plan to use. Later, when you are organizing your speech, you may wish to spread the note cards on a table and group them under appropriate outline headings.

Make all notes as complete as your purpose warrants, and *be accurate*; all quotations should be exactly what the author wrote; all paraphrases should correctly represent the author. Each card should contain a complete identification of the source, so that you can properly credit your sources and so that you can go back and locate material, if necessary. Include the full name of the author(s), title, publisher, date of publication, and page number.

The *information* you gather may fall into such categories as:

1. *Significant facts and ideas.* Facts and ideas will form the central core of your speech. If a fact or idea makes a strong impact on you, make note of it. The fact may be of historical significance or may provide details of incidents or subjects.
2. *Examples, illustrations, and specific instances.* Such materials will serve to make your speech clear and concrete rather than vague and abstract.
3. *Statistical information.* Statistics are often important to demonstrate the extent of a problem or to quantify a factual situation.
4. *Quotations and testimony.* You may find that the concept that you are trying to explain has been expressed so vividly and aptly that you want to use a direct quotation. Experts and famous people may be quoted in support of your points to add credibility to your position.
5. *Jokes and anecdotes.* Jokes and humorous stories that apply directly to points you are making add interest and enjoyment to your message. Be sure they are in good taste and appropriate to the audience and the occasions.
6. *Human interest stories.* Unusual examples that involve people have a high interest level and can make abstract ideas concrete.

This phase of gathering materials should not be viewed narrowly as merely the finding of support for your ideas. It should be part of your process of learning and expanding your concepts to make you a more effective communicator. After you have researched and become saturated with your subject, you will produce an *original* speech that is different from your sources. The speech must reflect *you* in a genuine way, revealing your individuality.

As stated, your first source of ideas is yourself. To begin, ponder and list what you know about the topic. Remember where you obtained your information; that source may give you more. Regardless of how much you already know, research will help you validate your thinking and also provide additional support for your ideas. You can never be *certain* of your ideas in any absolute or dogmatic sense. Hopefully, however, your research will lend the proper qualifications and objectivity that will give your presentation the greatest impact and value to your listeners.

ORGANIZING YOUR IDEAS

Your speech outline should grow out of your specific purpose. Main points and subpoints that support your specific purpose will comprise the body of your presentation. In short speeches of a few minutes, two or three main points will likely be sufficient. Longer speeches may have more main ideas and certainly more subordinate points. In English literature classes, you may have used outlining as an analytic tool, to delineate parts of a literary work; here you are outlining as a building process. A useful first step in arriving at the best possible organization is to make a comprehensive list of the ideas that you have accumulated in your analysis and research. Work through these, finding the main thoughts and placing subordinate ideas beneath them. Then examine the list critically, adding what you think is lacking and eliminating what is extraneous. You may find, after setting up this first draft of your outline, that you need more data on some of the points. More research will thus be required. Typically, the outline will consist of three parts: the introduction, the body, and the conclusion.

PLANNING YOUR INTRODUCTION

As a general rule, the introduction to your speech should do three things: (1) gain the attention and interest of your audience, (2) establish your credentials and your reasons for speaking on this topic, and (3) give direction to your speech by revealing your topic and giving an overview of your presentation.

GAINING THE ATTENTION OF YOUR AUDIENCE

If your potential listeners don't pay any attention to you, obviously they will never understand or appreciate your main ideas. The first few moments of your presentation are particularly significant because your listeners begin to make immediate judgments about you and your message. You must gain their attention by both the delivery and the content of your message. A voice that is adjusted properly to the environment, eye contact, a relaxed yet active body, and a genuine effort to achieve rapport with your audience will be effective *physical* means to gain attention.

There are at least six ways that your *content* can attract interest.

1. *A remark that shows relationship between your topic and your audience;* for example, to nursing students, with the topic, *major requirements*, you might say:

More than half of the graduates from this school changed their specialty at least once; on an average, each change costs the student seven hours of credit.

2. *A human interest story:* Dr. Karl Menninger, the reknowned psychiatrist, once used the following human interest story in a speech on mental health:

> I remember an old story which I am sure you have heard. My dentist told it to me when I was just a little boy. If a tooth was to be extracted he would guarantee that the pain would go away if I would do exactly what he told me. Of course I said, "Well, what is it?" He said, "I will give you a hatpin, and when I tell you, stick the hatpin the full length right in your leg and you won't notice that your tooth hurts!" That principle sort of stuck with me and I wrestled with it quite a while . . .
>
> This idea that illness can be replaced or changed is one that I am asking you to concentrate on. . . .[2]

3. *A vivid illustration:* A long time ago, in 1866, Thomas Henry Huxley tried to explain "The Method of Scientific Investigation" to English working men. He did it by illustration.

> Suppose you go into a fruiterer's shop, wanting an apple—you take one up, and, on biting, you find it is sour; you look at it, and see that it is hard and green. You take another one and that too is hard, green, and sour. The shopman offers you a third; but, before biting it you examine it, and find that it is hard and green, and you immediately say that you will not have it, as it must be sour, like those that you have already tried.
>
> Nothing can be more simple than that, you think; but if you take the trouble to analyze and trace out into its logical elements what has been done by the mind, you will be greatly surprised. In the first place, you have performed the operation of induction.[3]

4. *A humorous remark:* A visiting Russian speaker recently said to an American audience:

> I have just visited Rome, Paris, London, and New York. Do you know what I saw? I saw the decline of capitalism. Do you know what I thought? A beautiful way to go.

5. *A direct reference to preceding speakers or events:* Perhaps you find yourself expected to follow a speaker who has shown exceptional wit or humor; you may find this a bit difficult. You might playfully say:

> The preceding speaker and I are a team. I want to thank him for getting my audience warmed up for me.

6. *A personal remark about yourself:* If true, you might say, "I have just made a return visit to Egypt after being away for a year; Egypt today gave me two very strong impressions," and so forth. As you capture attention, be certain that the opening is clearly appropriate for your subject and this audience.

At the start of your presentation, you and your listeners will likely believe in or stand for many similar principles. In addition, you may have had similar experiences or conditions in your background. Such similarities are often referred to as "common ground." In your introductory remarks, you may help to achieve a favorable psychologic climate for your main ideas by referring to such "common ground," thus reinforcing existing favorable attitudes of your listeners regarding you or your topic. Of course, you must be very careful that you don't make an erroneous assumption regarding your experiences.

The degree to which you will need to use any of these attention-getting techniques will in every case depend upon what is needed to divert the attention of others toward yourself. Don't use any more than is needed—such "overkill" will make you seem unbelievable; don't cry, "Wolf! Wolf!," when the threatening event is a pussycat. And, indeed, don't permanently damage the tranquility of the very people from whom you wish an unbiased hearing; if you gain their attention only by aggravating them, you may have too much of a handicap to overcome later. But, even so, you cannot demonstrate that your beliefs are credible to people who ignore your presence. First, you must get their attention.

ESTABLISHING YOUR CREDENTIALS

Audiences typically want to know why you selected this particular topic and why you are qualified to speak on it. We suggest that in your introduction you consider carefully the following factors:

1. Your listeners should perceive you as a qualified person, informed, reliable, and dynamic. Your entire life style should be seen by your listeners as honest, sincere, and genuine.
2. Your listeners should know that you are really interested in helping them understand their environment or solve their problems, even though you may see things differently than they do.
3. Your listeners should believe that you are acquainted with and understand their thinking about your topic even if they disagree with you. You must help them see that you understand their beliefs but that, for valid reasons, you have come to believe differently.
4. Your reputation should have preceded you, and it should show that you are knowledgeable about your topic, interested in your listeners, and reliable as a person.

It can be helpful to have someone introduce you to your listeners who has high credibility in *their* view. If possible, that person should review and reinforce your credibility factors listed above. Numerous research studies have shown that this procedure can influence the effect of your presentation.[4]

First impressions are extremely important. You can enhance your credibility by making yourself attractive to your listeners in physical appearance, posture, gestures, facial expressions, and vocal inflections. Researchers have found ample evidence that appearance and overt behaviors that reflect confidence, sincerity, and sociability work in your favor.[5] From audience to audience, your listeners are likely to differ on what type of appearance and behaviors make you attractive to them, and *their* tastes are important; you will have to ascertain this factor about any specific audience. Although such appearance and behaviors, especially vocal tones and gestures, are important to your credibility throughout your presentation, this factor is especially important in your introductory remarks. The first impression you make can also be your last. For example, if you initially appear to be indefinite or confused, this impression may color your listener's perception of what you say later. This advice is not to suggest that you appear to be different than you are, merely that you present yourself in the best possible light.

Most people believe in treating others fairly, at least as they have come to know fairness. Asking for a fair hearing, an unbiased evaluation of your ideas, can be a useful request in your introductory remarks. This request must be done with courtesy and sincerity; it should not be an artificial ploy. You must be prepared to be as trustworthy as you know how to be as you go on to present your ideas.

An appeal for a fair hearing cannot be effective if you provide any basis for suspicion or the appearance of subterfuge. You must give something of value to your listeners in return. We suggest that your request might be of this order:

> I would like to ask you to give my ideas a fair hearing. Please evaluate them carefully with as much objectivity as possible. And I'd like to offer something in return, to be as honest and sincere as I know how to be. I'm suggesting a little contract, a trade: your fairness in hearing me in return for my candid honesty in talking with you.

FOCUSING ON YOUR TOPIC

It is rather easy in your introduction to let your audience lose sight of the main target or thrust of your talk. Each of the things that has been suggested that you may do in your introduction is important, but as you do them you will need to help your listeners come back to a focus on the main theme of your talk.

For many years, teachers of public speaking have been suggesting to their students that at the end of their introductory remarks just before they take up the first of the major points of their speech, they should state their thesis or theme of their presentation. This should be done in a very few words, as clearly, directly, and briefly as possible. It could sound like this:

> I wish to review our present method of assigning work schedules, assess its effects, and suggest a way of improving this procedure.

As you focus your listeners' attention on your topic you will need to clarify your particular intention with this specific audience. Do you intend to help them understand a complex principle or procedure, such as cardiopulmonary resuscitation for a general audience? Do you intend to share your thinking with them on a common problem such as a dangerous condition (inadequate safety) on the job in their plant? Such a clarification of your specific intentions regarding your presentation to this particular audience should be done in the introduction right after you state the thesis or specific purpose for your presentation.

Following the clarification of your intentions is a good time to provide the preview of your major ideas. Immediately after you do this is a good time to start dealing with them one by one. The statement of specific purpose and overview lets your audience know what to listen for and provides a basis for cohesion. A speech teacher once said that the key to a speech was threefold: "Tell them what you're going to tell them; tell them; and tell them what you told them." Seldom do you have reason to keep your audience guessing about your content. This overview should merely be a brief statement of key words, phrases, or questions that constitute the main ideas to be developed in the body of your speech.

PLANNING THE BODY OF YOUR SPEECH

In informative presentations, your listeners will demand, above all, to understand what you are talking about. This need places special demands on organization.[6] Research has demonstrated the value of the use of emphasis, especially on major ideas,[7] and careful organization provides such emphasis. In addition, your listeners will need more than a clear portrayal of your main ideas; they will need to understand *how* and *why* you obtained your information. Why do you believe as you do? How was your thinking influenced? They will need to hear from you a resume of supporting material, reasons, and evidence that *demonstrate the quality of your thinking*. Relevant factual information will need to be reported in appropriate places in your presentation; working in such supporting material is a major function of organizing your speech. The same questions that you posed for others as you originally formed your main ideas will likely be in your listeners' minds.

In public speaking, a pattern or type of outline is a way of arranging your major ideas so that they make some orderly sense to your listeners. It is a means of avoiding the appearance of rambling, of having been poorly prepared, or of presenting scattered thoughts or ideas. It can help your listeners believe that you have given careful thought to your topic and that you have found a way of comprehending the major issues involved. An outline should help you avoid this vexing distraction: "Oh yes, I meant to mention one other very important consideration. . . ."

Outlines should meet three major criteria. First, they should make your major ideas stand out from supporting material—evidence, relevant testimony, examples, and so forth. Second, they should provide an orderly progression for your major ideas, a "train of thought" that your listener can follow from first considerations to logical conclusions. Third, they should accommodate your listener's present attitudes toward your topic as well as their customary way of thinking about it. For example, many educated people today think about abortion in terms of current arguments for the need of the client to decide questions involving her own physical and psychologic welfare, as well as the claim of the unborn child to an opportunity to live and survive. Very likely, any speaker today who claims to have thought carefully about this topic would not convince listeners if either of these issues is neglected.

There are two major types of patterns or outlines based upon your specific purpose:

1. Those designed to help listeners understand a sequence of events, a story, or history, a process or procedure, or a principle.
2. Those designed to help listeners solve a problem.

Each of these types will be examined in detail.

HELPING LISTENERS TO UNDERSTAND

Probably the kind of outline most familiar to everyone is the one that tells a story, a narrative of a chronologic sequence of events—the childhood experience of "once upon a time." A second type of outline designed to help the listeners understand is one that explains a process or procedure—a system of interrelated events that achieve some purpose or product. Here you may have a number of options: for example, to describe the process of group decision making, you may wish to discuss such factors as group members' consideration for one another's feelings, need for use of agenda, leadership roles, and so forth. There may be no particularly logical place to start; all major factors in the system may have equal claim on being the first item for your presentation and the choice may be rather arbitrary.

In outlines dealing with a process or procedure, there frequently is a logical starting point and patterns of events so that one cannot take place until after another one has been completed. For example, a description of the "general nursing-care plan for thymectomy patients" that we suggested earlier might be outlined as follows:[8]

I. *Planned contact with patient:*
   1. Someone near at all times, preferably in the room—either a family member to sit with patient or group nursing.
   2. Preferably the same people to care for patient day after day on each shift.
II. *Suggested equipment (in addition to suction equipment):*
   1. Large watch or clock placed where it can be seen—time is important to patient.
   2. Clipboard with large pad and pencil tied to board.
   3. Bell cord (signal light) always *at hand.*
III. *Preoperative preparation of patient:*
   1. Inhalation therapist introduced to patient *before* surgery. Postoperatively, twice daily checks (by therapists on different shifts) of patient and patients respirator.
   2. Communication code worked out with patient before surgery. Code sheet to accompany patient *everywhere* (operating room, recovery room, intensive unit, ward, and so on). A copy of the code to be attached to the patient's chart and recorded on the Kardex.
IV. *Consciousness of patient:*
   1. Remember that during the time that the patient cannot speak, the patient is very conscious and alert and can hear very well; be careful what you say.
   2. General care plan:
      a. Protect the patient's eyes; they will be light-sensitive:
         i. Avoid bright overhead lights.
         ii. Use soothing eyedrops.
         iii. Observe for changes in ability to close or open eyelids.
      b. Turn patient, at least every 2 hours during the day and every 4 hours during the night, while patient is on respirator.
         i. Check to be sure patient is comfortable after turning, for example, legs and head; do not let anything rest on the patient's chest.
         ii. Give frequent *gentle* backrubs, as back muscles will be tired and sore.
         iii. Exercise all limbs of body every 4 hours.

c. If patient is able, teach him to suction own mouth. (There will be copious amounts of mucus in mouth, nose, and throat.)
   i. Have two suction setups available—one for mouth and one for trachea.
   ii. Check with patient about need for nasal suction. Use a clean catheter moistened in saline solution or Diothane ointment and very gently suction the nasopharynx.
   iii. When suctioning the trachea use sterile catheter and gloves.
   iv. Give patient time to breathe between each insertion of tracheal suction catheter. Allow four to eight breaths (using the respirator) between each suctioning.
   v. Deflate cuff on tracheal tube every 12 hours. Tell patient what you are doing, suction, and then reinflate carefully.
   vi. Explain to patient necessity of coughing. Help by placing sterile saline down tracheostomy tube, wait a few seconds, and then suction. Patient will soon recognize coughing and can indicate when suction is needed to clear airway.
d. Keep accurate intake and output records. Patient may need to be catheterized because of loss of muscle tone.
e. Keep patient as calm and as reassured as possible. An upset patient doesn't breathe well, collects mucus, and sometimes cannot tolerate even small amounts of water in the stomach (through the gastrostomy feeding tube). Elevate head of bed 30 degrees when giving gastrostomy feedings. A frightened patient will not fall asleep.
f. If patient can write, encourage house officer to avoid using veins in the writing arm or hand for giving intravenous fluids. Patients who have a gastrostomy will not require fluids as long as those without it.
g. Avoid jarring the bed and making any loud noises, or exposing the patient to bright lights. Speak in a low, clear, soft but confident voice. Any intense environmental stimulus is a shock to the patient's nervous system.
h. Start medication with pyridostigmine bromide (Mestinon) as soon as it is reordered (usually 72 hours after surgery). Tell patient you are doing this and make sure that patient receives the drug in the proper dosage and form, and promptly at the times ordered. (This is as important as giving a diabetic patient the correct amount of insulin at the ordered times.)
i. Give mouth care every 4 hours and moisten lips with oil. Women may use lipstick.
V. *Particular Points to Remember:*
   1. Patient is alert and conscious.

2. Patient's life depends on breathing: He requires a clear airway, and a perfectly functioning respirator. And the patient knows this.
3. Patient will be afraid of not being able to breathe and not being able to communicate this fact. Do everything possible to see that patient does breathe well, and that this fear is met realistically but controlled—by your presence, skills and reassurance, and the availability of signal bell or light cord.
4. Always be honest with patient. If you can't understand what patient is trying to communicate, find someone else to interpret for you—the team leader, charge nurse, or house officer. Family members are often the ones best able to do this.
5. Always explain what you are going to do in terms the patient understands, and then do it.
6. Remember that the patient's family has learned to live with the patient and the disease. Let them use their knowledge of patient by having them participate in care; this helps them through the first critical early postoperative days.
7. Use every facility and person available at hospital to help the physician get the patient and the patient's family safely and calmly through the first few days after surgery—yourself, the head nurse, house officers, inhalation therapist, chaplain, hospital hostess, family members, and anyone else who can be useful.

COHERENT PATTERNS FOR HELPING LISTENERS SOLVE A PROBLEM

Presentations in which you advocate a specific solution to a particular problem must be designed to take your listeners over the *essential* ground you have covered in your thinking as you analyzed the problem and determined its best solution. Not every stray thought you have previously had about the problem need to given in your presentation; only the *essential* elements of your thinking need to be covered.

Each of the major points to cover in a presentation designed to help your listeners solve a problem becomes a major point in your outline:

1. Identification of the problem, a comparison of what ought to be (is desired or needed) with what exists.
2. Description of *impelling* forces (factors that are increasing the need to do something different from what is being done) and *constraining* forces (factors that keep a desired change from happening). These forces were described in Chapter 7.
3. Evaluation of alternative approaches to solving the problem; here you do not evaluate all approaches you have ever thought about,

just those that are probably uppermost in the thinking of your listeners. Comparison of various alleged alternative solutions to the problem should be made on the basis of (1) workability—to what extent do well-known alleged solutions actually meet needs (problems) similar to the one you have identified (see the first point above) and (2) disadvantages—to what extent do these various alleged solutions entail serious costs or dangers.

4. Clear delineation of your proposed plan—the one you advocate with its defense on two issues.
   a. Will it work? What evidence can be cited *to demonstrate* that your plan will actually meet the need you have identified?
   b. Are all serious disadvantages avoided? What evidence can be cited *to demonstrate* that the cost will not be severe (more than is gained by adopting your plan), or require expertise not now available, or incur serious dangers?
5. Specific action required to implement your plan; what can your listeners do now to make a start toward your goal? Sign a petition? Vote for you? Meet with you and the governing board in 2 weeks? Hand out bumper stickers? Donate funds? Meet with other supporters of your plan to discuss ways of implementing it? If at all possible, you should help your listeners know what specifically they can do to help achieve the solution you have advocated. Many inexperienced advocates fall short of this fifth step.

A fair amount of research has been done that supports the type of advocacy outline presented above. Studies of the order of presentation of the major points or elements have shown greater effectiveness for the analytic-inductive approach presented than for a headlong charge in support of your proposed plan.[9] Studies have also indicated that you should give primary emphasis and consideration to your chosen solution as you compare it with other alleged solutions to the problem.[10]

A special comment should be made about transitions between major points or elements in your outline. As you state a major point, define its terms, explain, give examples, and illustrate this idea, perhaps with visual aids; you need to be sure you have not lost your audience when you move to the next major point. They will need to see how it relates or connects with the prior major point. This process of relating or connecting one major point with another is what gives your presentation coherence. Such connection must be achieved with optimum clarity. To do this, you carefully select connecting words that show this relationship. The following are some of the ways such relationships may be shown:

1. Showing sequential progress: "Previously I have shown . . . ;" "In the second place . . . ;" "At the same time in;" "At last . . . ."

2. Drawing a conclusion: "Thus we can conclude that . . . ;" "Under these conditions. . ."
3. Summarizing a point: "We have seen . . . ;" "To summarize my support of this point . . . ;" "Briefly, I have suggested . . . ."

These are only a few of the ways that you can show that you are concluding the development of one major point and starting the exposition of another one. The major idea of such transition phrases is to help your audience follow your thinking, identify material connected with one point and then another, and, overall, to see how your major points together make a logical pattern.

PLANNING YOUR CONCLUSION

As with the introduction, special attention must be paid to your conclusion. This is your last opportunity to pull your points together and to make them remembered. A final summary is often advisable, particularly in an informational presentation. In addition, the conclusion ideally should heighten interest, add to the meaning of your speech, and leave the audience in an appropriate mood. The same techniques that were employed in your introduction to attract attention are useful here as well.

The conclusion of your presentation should serve three purposes: (1) terminate your use of your listeners' time in an appropriate manner without awkwardness; (2) help your listeners remember the essence of your thinking—the main ideas and their relationship to one another; and (3) achieve your desired outcomes, depending on the purpose of your presentation.

REVIEWING YOUR MAIN IDEAS

In your conclusion, a very brief summary reviewing your main ideas can provide additional impact for the essence of your thinking and help your listeners give final consideration to accepting your view. You may have generally led them to believe as you do, but they may not be able to explain if someone were to ask them *why* they thus believed. Such a review can help them to leave equipped with answers for others who were not present. In addition, some research evidence indicates at a later time they are more likely to maintain this belief if they can remember your reasons, that is, your main points.[11]

This basic approach is grounded on a psychologic principle called *equity theory*. A fair amount of careful thinking and empirical investigation has gone into the development of this theory.[12] Its basic tenets have been expressed most clearly by J. S. Adams.[13] In essence, *equity theory* holds that one person's response to another's behavior is generally governed by a norm of reciprocity; if one person provides another with a useful resource, the other person will tend to respond with provision of a similar resource.[14] Specifically, if one person presents to another accurate information and interpretation of it, the other person will tend to respond in kind; if one person gives fair consideration to another's ideas, the other person will tend to respond with similar behavior.

Research across cultures tends to show that in most parts of the world this equity principle holds true, at least for the majority of people.[16] It is not true to the same degree for all cultures, nor is it likely to be true for every person you meet. The personalities and response patterns of some people have been damaged by harsh or severe experiences. You may meet some persons who live in terror, view the world with severe anxiety, or respond to you with undeserved deep hostility, anger, or hatred. Even so, most of your listeners will respond to you with fair consideration of your ideas if you demonstrate to them that you are sincerely interested in their needs and views. This, then, becomes your primary objective as an authentic person seeking to help others understand their world and solve their problems: *Seek their fair consideration of your ideas.*

Your ultimate goal as a speaker should be to have your listeners *convinced by their own knowledge and reasoning* after giving fair consideration to your ideas. Presumably, their prior information plus yours will lead them to the same conclusions you have reached; if not, then you should compare their data and reasoning with yours. Maybe you have made a mistake; maybe their information is more accurate or extensive than yours; maybe their interpretation of it or their reasoning is more objective and valid.

As you compare your thinking with that of your listeners, it is important that you keep an open mind. Ask yourself and your listener these questions: What data are necessary for a complete collection of relevant information? Are we sure we know all that is necessary? Have we missed something important? Then ask these additional questions: Is there more than one way to interpret these data? Can different conclusions reasonably be derived?

If you have done your thinking well in the ways suggested, then you should be very willing to compare your ideas with those of your listeners. Your goal should not be that they *must* agree with you; rather, *you should want* to be heard fairly and have your thinking validated by others; this basic philosophy will serve you well as you seek fair consideration of your ideas by your listeners.

In the long run, it is not worth your time to try to influence people unless they understand and accept your reasoning; in such a case they will, too soon, be influenced by their own ideas. It is not to your long-range advantage to tell them what to do without their using their own reasoning power; carrying another person along this way can make intellectual cripples of you both.

You should seek to allow your listeners to consider data from their own experiences and make their interpretation of it. Then you should seek to *add* to their data and to show them how your conclusion makes sense. As you ask them to consider this new fund of data and its meaning, *your ultimate goal is that they will be convinced that your position is correct on the same basis that you, earlier, became convinced of it yourself.*

PRESENTING YOUR SPEECH

Inasmuch as the beginning speaker is usually more apprehensive about the possibility of unfavorable listener reaction than about the act of speaking, the audience is the focal point of fear. Students sometimes claim that listeners look bored and "poker-faced," seem to smirk, and in other ways noticeably indicate their disapproval. Such negative judgments usually represent students' errors in interpreting the feedback from the audience. Unless hearers are actively hostile to you or your subject, they are unlikely to show overt signs of disapproval, particularly in a speech class where active, emphatic listening skills are emphasized. As for audience criticism of your speech, it is suggested that you heed the advice of Philip Zimbardo: "Don't allow others to criticize *you* as a person; it is your *specific actions* that are open for evaluation and available for improvement—accept such constructive feedback graciously if it will help you.[15]

Focus on your desire to communicate. Immediately before the speech, we suggest that you focus on your desire to communicate. Think positively because fear of failure can become a self-fulfilling prophecy. Say to yourself: "Here's my opportunity to share my thinking. I think I can gain their attention and make them understand." If you possess keen interest in your subject and have prepared thoroughly, you know more about the subject than your audience does, and the audience will tend to respect you accordingly. Breathe deeply and regularly to relax muscle tension.

Prepare yourself by rehearsing the speech aloud, in front of a full-length mirror, if possible. Speak as though you were conversing with several of your friends. Using your outline in early rehearsals will help you to remember the content and sequencing of ideas in your speech. Don't worry about memorizing the body of your speech. Practice saying the same thing several different ways so that you won't be "thrown" by an inability to remember some exact word order. A vital part of your practice is not only to help your memory and to exercise your use of voice and action, but also to practice expressing the message in words.

Rehearsing with a tape recorder can help you to learn to vary your rate, pitch, and intensity. If you are concerned about projection, you might place the microphone far enough away from you so that you remember to raise the volume of your voice. Listen to the tape with a friend and make note of grammatical errors, mispronounced words, cliches, or disfluencies that distract.

The language of your speech should be clear, interesting, and correct. Your language should convey the ideas that you want to express. Faulty language habits can be distracting, and you should work to rid yourself of such errors if they occur in your speaking. Bad habits are difficult to break, and becoming conscious of unconscious errors is the first and most important step in making sure that you use language well in your oral communication.

We think that your attitude during practice is extremely important. Think positively about the good things that will happen to you and how good you will feel in being able to communicate your ideas to your intended audience. Remind yourself of the importance of your topic. You must make your listeners feel that what you have to say is important to them.

The practice time should make you familiar enough with your topic and the ideas that you wish to communicate so that you will not have to grope for words. At the time of presentation, you will want your listeners to feel what you feel, to understand your thinking, and to enjoy and share a memorable experience with you. You should be free to be audience-centered, rather than self-centered. Your attention can be directed toward maximizing the opportunities for interaction with the audience.

Public speaking should be for communication, not for exhibition. Unfortunately, some speakers attempt to use public speeches to "show-off": "see how much I know," "doesn't my voice sound nice?," "see how big a vocabulary I have." About the most condemnatory thing that someone can say about a speaker is, "Oh, that person has been studying public speaking." No one in the audience should be forced to pay attention to your delivery for delivery's sake.

Talking with the audience in a conversational manner should be your goal. As you gain more and more experience in public speaking, you will be more conscious of joining in conversation with members of the audience. If you truly have a message that is important to you and your listeners, the delivery will tend to take care of itself. If, however, you are poorly prepared, self-conscious, and fearful of how the audience will react, you can be certain that these factors will be communicated.

During your speech, it is suggested that you "eliminate the negative" and "accentuate the positive" in the following ways:

DO NOTs:
1. Don't focus inward; that is, avoid being overly concerned about how you feel, look, or sound.

2. Don't concentrate on how well you're doing or on whether the listeners like you personally, think you are nervous, or consider you an ineffectual speaker.
3. Don't try to camouflage nervousness by applying more pressure. For example, avoid adopting a sarcastic, belligerent, or aloof manner to mask uncertainty.

DOs:

1. Concentrate on the process of communicating your ideas to the listeners. Forget yourself and concentrate on transmitting your ideas from your mind to their minds.
2. Think positively. If you act as if you are confident, you will begin to feel more confident. If you expect your initial nervousness to subside, it is more likely to do so.
3. Look at the individual people in the audience, and talk directly to them. Consider them receptive persons who are pulling for you to do well.
4. Think about whether or not members of the audience are comprehending you. From the facial expressions and body sets of your hearers, attempt to read clues as to the reception your ideas are getting. If some persons look perplexed, perhaps you need to amplify your examples; if some listeners seem to be straining to hear, increase your volume.
5. Attempt to convert nervous energy into appropriate outlets of animated vocal and physical delivery. Without going to extremes, move around. Use the gestures that you practiced; they should be a natural outcome of what you are saying.
6. Instead of permitting tension to restrict your voice, divert the nervous energy into increased vocal emphasis and greater variety of rate, pitch, and force. Try to maintain the lively, flexible vocal and physical delivery of conversation, expanded to fit the needs of the speaking situation. The goal of this section has been not only to help you to build confidence in your speaking abilities, but to give you greater freedom for a fuller participation in public life. These are not gifts that anyone can give you. They must be sought and worked for, and when gained, held. It is entirely up to you, and it is hoped that you will choose to give it your best try.

SUMMARY

An opportunity to speak to an audience presents a real challenge. The skills and abilities to present yourself and your ideas can be developed only with practice and feedback from a caring audience. You cannot be *trained* to be a public speaker; you must learn it yourself. You can receive help from others in eliminating undesirable behavior patterns, but that is about as far as instruction can go. The verbal and vocal messages and the visual language that you use must be your own. The meanings and ideas that you are expressing cannot and will not be the same for any other speaker. You are unique, and your messages must arise from the meaning that is within you. When speakers are congruent and able to focus their energy, they will be able to communicate effectively with the audience.

It is reasonable and predictable that you will approach a speaking event and start your speech with a certain amount of nervous concern for what you are about to do. The objective is to translate this nervous energy into positive, purposeful, and animated speaking. A feeling of being prepared, a sincere desire to communicate ideas, and a direct speaking manner will all combine to use this energy to the best advantage.

REFERENCES

1. An excellent presentation of this principle has been given by KENNETH BOULDING: *The Image* (Ann Arbor: University of Michigan Press, 1956), pp. 3–18.
2. KARL MENNINGER: "Healthier Than Healthy," in WIL A. LINKUGEL, R. R. ALLEN, AND RICHARD L. JOHANNESEN: *Contemporary American Speeches*, 2nd ed. (Belmont, Calif.: Wadsworth Publishing Company, 1969), p. 58.
3. *Contemporary American Speeches*, 2nd ed., pp. 27–28.
4. See PAUL D. HOLTZMAN: "Confirmation of Ethos as a Confounding Element in Communication Research," *Speech Monographs*, 30 (1966): 464–466.
5. See W. BARNETT PEARCE AND F. CONKLIN: "Nonverbal Vocalic Communication and Perceptions of a Speaker," *Speech Monographs*, 38 (1971): 235–237; and W. BARNETT PEARCE AND BERNARD J. BROMMEL: "Vocalic Communication in Persuasion," *Quarterly Journal of Speech*, 58 (1972): 298–306.
6. D. RAGSDALE, JR.: "Effects of Selected Aspects of Brevity on Comprehensibility and Persuasiveness," unpublished doctoral dissertation, University of Illinois, 1964.
7. See R. EHRENSBERGER: "An Experimental Study of the Relative Effectiveness of Certain Forms of Emphasis in Public Speaking," *Speech Monographs*, 12 (1945): 94–111.
8. BARBARA BAIN AND JANE BAILEY: "How a Communication Tool Led to the Development of a Nursing Care Plan," *Nursing Outlook*, October, 1967, p. 49.
9. C. A. KIESLER AND S. B. KIESLER: "Role of Fore-Warning in Persuasive Communication," *Journal of Abnormal and Social Psychology*, 68 (1964): 547–549. See also A. R. COHEN: *Attitude Change and Social Influence* (New York: Basic Books, 1964), pp. 11–12.
10. See N. MILLER AND D. T. CAMPBELL: "Recency and Primary in Persuasion as a Function of the Timing of Speeches and Measurements," *Journal of Abnormal and Social Psychology*, 59 (1959): 250–253; see also N. H. ANDERSON AND A. A. BARRIOS: "Primacy Effects in Personality Impression Formation," *Journal of Abnormal and Social Psychology*, 63 (1961): 346–350.

11. See H. C. Kelmen and C. I. Hovland: "Reinstatement of the Communication in Delayed Measurement of Opinion Change," *Journal of Abnormal and Social Psychology*, 48 (1953): 330–335.
12. V. G. Foa and E. B. Foa: *Societal Structures of the Mind* (Springfield, Ill.: Charles C Thomas, 1974).
13. J. S. Adams: "Inequity in Social Exchange," in *Advances in Experimental Social Psychology* (New York: Academic Press, 1965), pp. 267–299.
14. A. W. Gouldner: "The Norm of Reciprocity: A Preliminary Statement," *American Sociological Review*, 25 (1960): 161–168.
15. Philip G. Zimbardo: *Shyness* (Reading, Mass.: Addison-Wesley, 1977), p. 159.

9
EVALUATING INTERPERSONAL COMMUNICATION

The previous eight chapters have explored the nature of humanistic communication within the nursing profession, have identified relevant variables in the interpersonal communication process, and have suggested skills to be developed in working in small groups or in presenting a public speech. Nurses must also be able to identify specific blocks to effective communication, practice techniques of active listening, identify potential areas of conflict, and practice various coping strategies.[1]

Maintenance behavior that secures satisfying interpersonal relations between people is very important; people in groups are still people with human needs, needs for individual recognition and occasionally a sign of personal warmth or regard. Only in work groups in which there is extremely high commitment to a temporary group goal can this factor be ignored. Such groups do exist: some groups in intensive-care units may be highly "mission-oriented," as in a case of open-heart surgery. For specified periods, task crews may be heavily job-oriented, as in drilling an oil well, or driving a ship through a storm; such teams at times show such task devotion that "personal feelings don't count." Even so, in most groups, the maintenance of interpersonal relations is absolutely essential if the groups are to function well. This chapter looks at ways in which these human interpersonal behaviors can be identified and assessed.

ASSESSING INTERPERSONAL NEEDS

There are a number of reasons why you as a student of interpersonal communication and nursing should be interested in the study of personality variables relating to interpersonal behavior; it is important that you become able to distinguish a *dislike* of yourself on the part of others from *disagreement* based on a different (from yours) habitual way of viewing things. Your response to others is likely to be different when you perceive them disagreeing with you because they disagree with your ideas and when you perceive their behavior as evidence of their personal *dislike*. And here is the real payoff of responding to them as persons who see things differently: Many of the ideas presented by "expedient," "tender-minded," "suspicious," "imaginative," or "apprehensive" group members may be valuable. If you listen to them conscientiously, many of their suggestions will have merit, and some of their fears will be valid. And if they, as persons, can be understood, their help and support can be valuable. It is important, of course, that they be treated in such a way that you do not seriously damage their morale, or cripple their efforts.

A number of scholars have devoted thought and research efforts to identifying those specific personality variables that directly and primarily influence interpersonal behavior. A major exploratory effort in this direction is that of William Schutz in his FIRO.[2] As noted in Chapter 2, Schutz set out to identify the "Fundamental Interpersonal Relations Orientations," those basic ways in which people characteristically orient themselves toward other people. Through analysis of a large number of research studies—parental, clinical, and small-group—Schutz found agreement on the importance of three areas: *inclusion, control,* and *affection*. His work demonstrates how measures of these three variables can be used to test a wide variety of hypotheses about interpersonal relations, leading to a better understanding of interpersonal behavior. Each of these three dimensions may be divided into two parts: (1) behavior characteristic of three interpersonal needs actively expressed by an individual toward others (that is, need to control others and to be controlled by them, and need for affection) and (2) the subjective degree to which an individual wants such behavior directed toward oneself.

Inclusion concerns the entrance into associations with others. The need of inclusion involves being able to be interested in other people to a sufficient degree and feeling that others are satisfactorily interested in oneself. Behavior aimed at gaining inclusion is seen as an attempt to attract attention and interest.[3]

Control is related to interactions involving influence and power. It includes the need to be controlled by respect for the competence of others and to control others by being respected by them. It is the need to feel adequate and reliable and also to understand the basis of legitimate control by others. Control behavior is related to decision making and is implied in such terms as "authority," "influence," " dominance," "submission," and "leader."[4]

Affection includes the need to love and be loved and to feel lovable. It is implied in the terms "positive feelings," "caring," "cool," "hate," and "emotionally involved."[5]

To have satisfactory interpersonal relationships, according to Schutz, the individual must establish in each of these three areas a balance between the amount of behavior actively expressed and the amount desired to be received from others.[6]

FIRO-B is a subjective questionnaire designed to measure the individual's expressed behavior toward others and the behavior one wants from others in the three areas of interpersonal need. It has, therefore, six scales: expressed inclusion, wanted inclusion, expressed control, wanted control, expressed affection, and wanted affection. This instrument (questionnaire) is published by Consulting Psychologists Press and may be obtained by qualified persons at nominal cost.[7]

We have used FIRO-B to help our students assess their own and each others' interpersonal needs. As we did this, our students requested some means of assessing the degree to which they were meeting each others' needs. In response to this request, we developed the *Interpersonal Perception Scale* (IPS) (Fig. 9-1), a rating scale modeled after FIRO-B and employing the same three basic dimensions. The IPS can be used to compare one's self-perceptions with the perceptions of others and can serve as a check on the degree to which an individual's interpersonal needs are recognized by the other members of one's group.

The major effect of having students use FIRO-B with the IPS in their decision-making project groups has been to call attention to the nature of the interpersonal needs of each other; this has helped them to gain insight into the importance of these needs. Usually, students then make special

---

The questions listed below refer to the group interaction experience in which you have just participated. The other members of the group will be interested in knowing how you perceive them, and you will be interested in knowing how they perceive you. Please answer the questions as carefully and honestly as possible.

Read the questions, the answer them regarding the member of the group whose name is on this sheet. Answer each item according to this scale:

Very Little	Little	Average	Much	Very Much
1	2	3	4	5

1. To what extent does this person interact with others? Circle your response: 1 2 3 4 5
2. To what extent does this person control or influence others? Circle your response: 1 2 3 4 5
3. To what extent does this person show warmth or affection toward others? Circle your response: 1 2 3 4 5

FIGURE 9-1. Interpersonal Perception Scale (IPS).

efforts to meet these needs; this consideration of the interpersonal needs of others very often has produced results that were satisfactory to the individuals involved.

ASSESSING COMMUNICATION COMPETENCIES

Ben W. Morse and Richard N. Piland conducted an extensive study assessing the communication needs and competencies of nurses in their relationships with patients, physicians, and other nurses. Specifically, an examination of the importance of nine communication skills in each of the three contexts was conducted. It was found that there were statistically significant differences across the three relationships for the importance of advising, persuading, instructing, routine information exchange, public speaking, small group communication, giving orders, listening, and management of conflict communicative behaviors. Conclusions centering on the relative openness of the nurse-patient and nurse-nurse relationships were contrasted by the closedness of the nurse-physician relationships where the situation was seen as a superior-subordinate relation.[8]

Five communication skills emerged as being of particular importance in all relationships. Those were in order of decreasing importance: listening; routine information exchange; management of conflict; small group communication; and instructing. The nurses in their sample indicated that listening was the single most important communication skill in all relationships. Although this finding was interesting, it did not speak to any qualitative or quantitative differences across relationships. Conclusions based on the other competencies, however, suggested significant differences existed among relationships.

The superior-subordinate nature of nurse-physician relationships was clearly demonstrated by the findings. For the nurse, listening to the physician was of considerable importance, while nurses report they would seldom give advice, orders, or instructions or attempt to persuade the physician. Interestingly, nurses felt routine information exchange with physicians as well as patients was important but not as valuable as exchanging information with fellow nurses. Nurses, it seems, feel compelled to listen to physicians rather than render suggestions and feel more comfortable in exchanging information with other nurses rather than with physicians. This relationship appears to be a closed system. That is, communication is essentially one-way—physician to nurse. Even in the case of routine information exchange, nurses prefer to communicate with other nurses rather than with the physician. Hence, the nurse perceives little opportunity to influence or provide the physician with feedback.

Of the three relationships, the most communicationally complex was between nurses. More skills were considered to be of primary importance for a successful nurse-nurse relationship than any other context. In fact, listening, routine information exchange, management of conflict, small group communication, and, to a lesser extent, instruction were considered exceptionally important. The inclusion of instruction was somewhat surprising. If, as the data suggested, the relationship was peer-to-peer, one would expect the advising skill to be more highly related than instruction. However, instructing was ranked more important than advising. This finding raises the possibility that nurses view other nurses as subordinates. But, since the ratings for giving orders were relatively low, that conclusion appears to be tentative. An alternative interpretation is that the nurse-nurse relationship is an exceptionally open one—one where several communication skills associated with hierarchical message changes are performed without qualitatively altering the fundamental relationship.

Similarly, an open system characterized the nurse-patient communication relationship. Primary skills included listening, management of conflict, instructing, advising, and, to a lesser degree, small-group communication and routine information exchange. These findings indicated that the nurse-patient communication context fostered participation, mutual influence, and the free flow of messages.

From a systems perspective, the study demonstrated that nurse-nurse and nurse-patient relationships were relatively open. That is, both allowed participants to influence one another via feedback and full participation. However, the nurse-physician relationship was found to be somewhat closed, characterized by a one-way flow of information and influence emanating from the physician.

Typically, proponents of the systems perspective conclude that a closed system is pathologic, that is, doomed to decay or destruction. One wonders if such a conclusion is applicable to the nurse-physician context. Indeed, future research might consider the effects on health care registered in a closed versus open nurse-physician relationship. Are physicians really in a maximal position to receive information about the health of a patient? Would health care improve if the nurse felt less inhibited in offering suggestions to the physician? Or is it preferable to allow physicians to proceed uninhibited? Would the physician's diagnosis and treatment benefit from such feedback? Would physicians be open to such feedback? These and other questions provide difficult but necessary queries to be asked of the existing health-care system.[9]

ASSESSING INTERACTIONS

Since interpersonal communication involves more than one person, the behaviors can be observed and evaluated as people interact with one another. The leader in devising methods of analyzing people's patterns of role behaviors has been Robert Freed Bales of the Center for Behavioral Sciences at Harvard University.

The basic unit of measurement for Bales is the "act," which is any verbal or nonverbal communication noted by the trained observer[5]: "In addition to speech centered around the issue being discussed, interaction includes facial expressions, gestures, bodily attitudes, emotional signs, or nonverbal acts of various kinds, either expressive and nonvocal, or more definitely directed toward other people. These expressions and gestures can be detected by the observer, given an interpretation in terms of the categories, and recorded." Twelve acts constitute the system. They are arranged in two broad areas, a *task* area and a socioemotional area, which may be equated with *maintenance* functions. The task consists of questions and answers, and the socioemotional areas are respectively "positive" and "negative."[10] Bales' system of categories is presented in Figure 9-2.

The purpose of the "Interaction Process Analysis" (IPA) system is to identify and record the nature (not the content) of each separate act in ongoing group interaction. Your first reaction to this idea may well be that it is an impossible task; this has proved to be not at all true with students after they have put forth some initial efforts. They are asked simply to try—try it out on each other, small groups of three or four working together and comparing their results with one another. Such a group observes and collects IPA data on another small group of students while they are discussing their understanding of how to use the IPA system. At

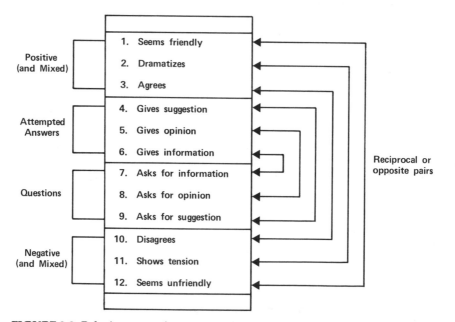

FIGURE 9-2. Bales' system of categories. (From R. F. Bales: *Interaction Process Analysis* [University of Chicago Press, Chicago, 1950], p. 59, with permission.)

a later time, the two groups reverse roles, and the previously observed group practices observing. Students are also encouraged to practice with one or two other students on popular "situation" types of television shows such as "General Hospital": there are problems galore, the range of interaction variety is great, and the actors tend to talk slowly. As students practice and compare their tabulations with one another, they are usually surprised and pleased with the results. It is suggested to them that it is not necessary to make all decisions "precisely correct" in order to generate data that are useful for raising valuable questions about ordinary interaction behavior. The objective is to provide "nearly correct" data and then to have all students think for themselves and decide whether they like what the data seem to be telling them about themselves. After this, it is up to them to decide on any personal changes they might like to make in their own behavior. We believe that such decisions require a great deal of intuitive judgment and self-questioning and that the IPA data, even if subjective and only generally accurate, may be a useful starting point.

Fragments of sentences, words, and phrases are scored as communication acts (units), when you can understand the meaning as a unit of thought in context. For example, "What?" may mean "What did you say?", or "Me?" may mean "Were you referring to me?" Such scraps of conversation as "Huh" or "Mm" may have fairly clear meaning in context. Also included are nonverbal acts, when a message is clearly implied. For example, a nod of the head may clearly signify agreement; and shaking the head may, in context, mean disagreement, or even an unfriendly reaction.

Although the 12 categories generally seem to make good sense, it is necessary and useful to provide the following category descriptions to students. Some of the descriptions are more elaborate than others because experience shows them to be more problematic. These category descriptions closely adhere to the terminology and phrases used by Bales;[11] however, for purposes of training undergraduates to use the system for self-analysis and diagnosis of their group behaviors, the following condensation from Bales' writing has been found adequate to serve the purposes. The 12 categories are briefly described as follows:

1. Seems friendly. Any act showing hospitality, being neighborly, expressing sympathy or similarity of feeling; indications of being attracted; demonstrations of affection; urging of unity, or harmony; expressing of desire for cooperation or solidarity; showing a protective or nurturing attitude; praising, rewarding, approving, or encouraging others; sustaining, or reassuring, a person having difficulty; complimenting or congratulating; exchanging, trading, or lending objects (for example, cigarettes or matches); confiding in another; expressing gratitude or appreciation; surrendering or giving in to another (for example, when

interrupted); friendly submission so that another can go ahead; confessions of ignorance; acts of apology; grinning with pleasure, smiling directly at another. This category should be used whenever an act primarily appears to convey good feeling toward another person.[12]

2. Dramatizes. Any act that emphasizes hidden meaning or emotional implications or is especially self-revealing about a person. Most frequently, these are jokes or stories with a double meaning. They may take the form of an anecdote about a particular person in which emotional feelings are expressed, or they may be symbolic actions—shrugs or bodily and facial expressions portraying great amazement, surprise, fear, or anger. More than one meaning is nearly always implicit in dramatizations as here defined; for example, a posturing, a facial expression, a remark, or all three together may imply (1) "He certainly thinks he is something!" and (2) "I don't agree." The personal tone of this dramatic bit, coupled with the overtones of partially hidden emotional feelings, is typical of acts scored in this category.[13] According to Bales, "The joke is a very common form of dramatization in group interaction. The joker expects, although perhaps not always too clearly, to produce a shock of recognition of the hidden meaning, to provoke a laugh, a sudden release or display of tension."[14] Bales goes on to suggest that the concept the joker offers is loaded and that whoever laughs admits "the hidden truth."[15] The essential quality of this category is that of some special, personal, partially hidden meaning subtly exposed in a way that is emotionally releasing even though risky; thus, one ordinary hallmark of such acts is that they seem to have two meanings, one dangerous to expose and the other somewhat amusing on the surface.[16] Behavior such as this may seem to you to be dangerous or better avoided; however, Bales makes this evaluative comment: "In terms of psychological services performed, and general importance in the group as well as individual life, these activities are not task-oriented, but they are nevertheless serious psychological business."[17]

3. Agrees. Any act that shows accord, concurrence, or assent about facts, inferences, or hypotheses: "I think you are right," "That's true," "Yes, that's it." Nonverbal agreement may involve nodding the head, showing special interest, or giving significant visible attention to what is being said. Another variation may be overtly expressing comprehension or understanding: "Oh, now I get it."

4. Gives suggestions. Any act that takes the lead in the task direction. This category includes routine control of communication and directing the attention of the group to task problems when

they have been agreed on by the group. Thus, mentioning a problem to be discussed, pointing out the relevance of a remark, calling a meeting to order, referring to agenda, and opening a new phase of activity—all of these are scored as "giving suggestions," if they are routine, agreed-on moves and if they are brought forth in a way that implies the acceptability of dissent if anyone so desires.[18] Bales gives this definition: "In general, direct attempts to guide or counsel, or prepare the other for some activity, to prevail upon him, to persuade him, exhort him, urge, enjoin, or inspire him to some action, by dependence upon authority or ascendance rather than by logical inference are called giving suggestions."[19] Such suggestions usually propose ways of modifying the problem situation, the group, certain members, or the norms.

5. Gives opinions. Any act that involves a moral obligation, offers a major belief, or value; or indicates adherence to a policy, or guiding principle. Such acts should be serious but not personal, sincere but objective. If such an act is not serious, or is insincere, you should score it in category 2, "dramatizes." Category 5, "gives opinions," includes expressions of understanding, or insight, besides those of value judgments: "I believe I see your point" or "I think we should recognize our obligation to . . ." or "I feel we are on the right track." "Gives opinions" should be distinguished from category 6, "gives information," primarily on the basis of its use of inference or value judgment.[20]

6. Gives information. Any act reporting factual (not necessarily true) or potentially verifiable (testable) observations or experiences. Bales gives this instruction: "Any statement too vague in principle to be tested is not classified as giving information, but, usually, as giving opinion."[21] Common cases of giving information are reports on problem situations confronting the group: "The legislature has not yet acted on that bill" or "We have three days left" or "I contacted the City Council and they can meet with us on Tuesday."[22]

7. Asks for information. Any act that requests a factual report. Bales' definition includes requests for a "descriptive, objective type of answer, an answer based on experience, observation, or empirical research."[23] The questions making these requests are not always direct, but sometimes indirect: "I have forgotten whom we appointed." You should include in this category only requests for simple factual answers; if an inference, an evaluation, or the expression of a feeling is requested, such should be tabulated as category 8, "asks for opinions."[24]

8. Asks for opinions. Any act that seeks an inferential interpretation, a statement involving belief or values, a value judgment, or

a report of one's understanding, or insight. It may include a request for diagnosis of a situation, or a reaction to an idea. A warning should be given here regarding such questions as "Do you know what I mean?" and "Do you see?" These are examples of attempts to elicit agreement and should be identified as persuasive effort, properly tabulated in category 4, "gives suggestions."[25] Another problem you may encounter occurs when an elected chairperson or leader serves the group in ways the group has commissioned this elected person to, and the leader is struggling to fathom, and comply with, their wishes. In such case, the chairperson might ask for an opinion in this manner: "Would you like to have a committee work on that?" If, however, the chairperson asks "What should we do about increasing our membership?" he or she is asking for suggestions regarding ways of solving a group problem, and this kind of question should be identified as belonging in category 9, "asks for suggestions."[26]

9. Asks for suggestions. Any act that requests guidance in the problem-solving process, is neutral in emotional tone, and attempts to turn the initiative over to another. Such requests sometimes indicate a feeling of confusion, or uncertainty.[27] To fit this category properly, the request should be "open-ended," without the implication of any specific answer: "What do you think we should do about that?" If, on the other hand, the question is asked in such a way that a specific answer is implied, it should be coded in category 4, "gives suggestions." An example of a veiled suggestion is "I wonder if there are any other ways of getting information from the Legislature?" This seems to imply there are other ways and suggests they be considered.[28]

10. Disagrees. Any initial act in a sequence that rejects others' statements of information, opinion, or suggestion. It is a reaction to others' action as defined by Bales: "The negative feeling conveyed is attached to the content of what the others have said, not to them as a person. And the negative feeling must not be very strong, or the act will seem unfriendly."[29] (It would, in such case, be scored in category 12, "seems unfriendly.") Statements that follow the initial rejection of another's position, such as arguments, rebuttals, and questions, are not scored as disagreement; rather, they are scored in other categories. Examples of acts scored in this category are "I don't think so" and "I don't think that's right."[30]

11. Shows tension. Any act that exhibits conflict between submission and nonconformity yet does not clearly show negative feeling toward another person.[31] Bales gives this general definition:

"Signs of anxious emotionality (that) indicate a conflict between acting and withholding action. Minor outbreaks of reactive anxiety may first be mentioned, such as appearing startled, disconcerted, alarmed, dismayed, perturbed, or concerned."[32] Other behaviors suggested by Bales are hesitation, speechlessness, trembling, flushing, gulping, and licking of the lips.[33] Of special import in this category is laughter. On the surface, laughter may seem to indicate a reduction of tension, and it may in part serve that purpose. In fact, however, it appears to be more dependable as a sign of tension rather than a sign of its reduction.[34] We are not here speaking of friendly smiles with a relaxed atmosphere of interpersonal warmth; rather, we are identifying embarrassed or tense laughter. Bales gives this explanation: "Laughter seems to be a sudden escape into motor discharge of conflicted emotional states that can no longer be contained."[35] An additional behavior to be included in this category is any embarrassed reaction to disapproval, as the appearance of being chagrined, chastised, or mortified.[36]

12. Seems unfriendly. Any act that is personally negative; it is not content-oriented, which would be classified as "disagrees" when negative, but is oriented toward another person. It includes very slight signs of negative feeling, arbitrary attempts to subjugate another, and uninvited attempts to "settle" an argument, to judge another's behavior, to override, interrupt, deflate, deprecate, disparage, or ridicule.[37] Also included are attempts to "show off," embarrass a generally accepted authority, or inordinately make a nuisance of oneself.[38] In general, Bales suggests that this category be used to identify all overt acts that seem to the observer to be in any way both negative and personal.[39]

In addition to the category descriptions and suggestions for deciding on how to use the categories for interaction analysis Bales offers four general rules to employ when an observer has difficulty in deciding where an act should be tabulated:

1. Give priority to category 2, "dramatizes," or category 11, "shows tension," whenever there is a question between either one and any other category.
2. Give priority to category 1, "seems friendly," or to category 12, "seems unfriendly," when any element of interpersonal feeling is shown.
3. Give priority to category 4, "gives suggestions," or to category 9, "asks for suggestions," over category 5, "gives opinion."

4. After an initial act of disagreement or of agreement, the scoring reverts to the appropriate impersonal categories, as the basis for the disagreement is explained.[40]

As you have been reading the category descriptions and the suggestions for scoring, you may have felt that the use of the IPA will be complex and confusing. It is a common feeling reported by students before they attempt to gain experience with it; it is also common for them to report increased confidence in their scoring ability as they follow the suggestions for practice. Students are equipped with scoring sheets, as illustrated in Figure 9-3. Familiarity with the line on the sheet where each category is located is of great help and is obtained with a little practice.

Four levels of analysis are possible. The first level of analysis involves the calculation of the percentage of total group interaction for each participant (Table 9-1).

With data from this first level of analysis, you can detect the spread of participation through your group and compare your own degree of participation with that of the others. The gross amount of participation

---

For each interactional act (a simple sentence or equivalent part of a complex sentence) put one mark in each category. For example, after some period of time your tabulation for "seems friendly" might look like this:

1. Seems friendly ⦀⦀ ⦀⦀ |||

Code number for person observed _____

1. Seems friendly	
2. Dramatizes	
3. Agrees	
4. Gives suggestions	
5. Gives opinions	
6. Gives information	
7. Ask for information	
8. Ask for opinions	
9. Asks for suggestions	
10. Disagrees	
11. Shows tension	
12. Seems unfriendly	

FIGURE 9-3. Tabulation sheet for IPA data. (From Robert Freed Bales, *Personality and Interpersonal Behavior.* Copyright © 1970 by Holt, Rinehart & Winston, Inc. Adapted and reprinted by permission of Holt, Rinehart & Winston, Inc.)

TABLE 9-1. Participants' Share of Total Observed Group Interaction

Name	Percent
Joe	10.3
Mike	7.2
Bill	42.8
Mary	28.3
Jill	11.4
Total:	100.0

from an individual member is generally a good indicator of attempts to gain status, or achieve influence over others, especially in groups in which no appointed leader is present.[41]

The second level of analysis requires the computation of the percentage of the total group interaction in each of the 12 categories; this will tell you how much your group is participating in what way. With these data you can list the estimated norms presented by Bales[42] and compare the manner of participation from your group members with these suggested norms, as illustrated in Table 9-2.

In the table, the column of estimated norms gives ranges, the high and low cutoff points. Although these points are not supported by as much evidence and experimentation as we should like to have, they may be taken as general guidelines to what may be considered high or low in each category. Whenever these boundaries are exceeded, you should give careful thought to what may be happening in your group. For example, look at the data presented in the percentage column. Here seems to be a nice, friendly group—too much so, according to data for category 12. The data for category 10 show they are not disagreeing with each other in a normal way, and the degree of tension shown by the data for category 11 tends to support our inference: they appear afraid to disagree normally. This inference, of course, is not a firm conclusion but only a lead for this group to explore further by discussing their feelings and attitudes and checking further on their ensuing behavior. An additional point for them to consider is that they appear to be giving an inordinate number of opinions and an unusually low amount of information. Are they in need of informing themselves about their problem areas? They may have intuitively sensed that they are ignorant about their problem-topic; here appears to be some solid confirmation. They should at least give this their careful consideration. From their work in analyzing data from many groups, Bales and Hare suggest that whenever the combined percentages in categories 4, 5, and 6 are less than twice the combined percentages in categories 7, 8, and 9, the group should give special attention to seeking more specific information about its problem area.[43] The normal estimated

TABLE 9-2. Percentage of Total Observed Group Participation in Each IPA Category, Compared with Estimated Norms

Category	Percent	Estimated Norms*
1. Seems friendly	3.5	2.6–4.8
2. Dramatizes	7.0	5.7–7.4
3. Agrees	18.5	8.0–13.6
4. Gives suggestions	3.8	3.0–7.0
5. Gives opinions	24.5	15.0–22.7
6. Gives information	8.3	20.7–31.2
7. Asks for information	10.3	4.0–7.2
8. Asks for opinions	12.5	2.0–3.9
9. Asks for suggestions	2.3	0.6–1.4
10. Disagrees	1.0	3.1–5.3
11. Shows tension	7.8	3.4–6.0
12. Seems unfriendly	0.5	2.4–4.4
Total:	100.0	

*Taken from R. F. Bales. *Personality and Interpersonal Behavior.* New York, Holt, Rinehart & Winston, 1970. p. 92; Bales estimated these norms by a process of inference described on pp. 482–486 of his book. Adapted and reprinted by permission of Holt, Rinehart & Winston, Inc.

ratio is 5 to 1, or 6 to 1; in the example given in the table, the ratio is less than 2 to 1, which is a fairly convincing sign of a lack of needed information for successful group problem solving. In such fashion, your group can analyze the percentage of total group participation in each category and compare it with the estimated norms given in Table 9-2.

As indicated, data collected by the Bales IPA can provide information on your group on both task-oriented (problem-solving) behavior and interpersonal (group maintenance) behavior. Data in categories 4, 5, 6, 7, 8, and 9 (giving and asking for suggestions, opinions, and information) are problem-solving, or task-oriented, behaviors. Data in the remaining categories—1, 2, 3, 10, 11, and 12 (seeming friendly or unfriendly; agreeing, or disagreeing; dramatizing and showing tension)—are primarily interpersonal in nature and relate to the maintenance of effective human relations among group members.

The third level of analysis you will wish to perform is to calculate the percentage of total group participation of each of your group members in each of the 12 categories; see Table 9-3. Comparisons between these data can give you a good idea of who is making which type of contribution and to what degree; it can also identify members who may need encouragement to participate in certain ways, as well as those who might wish to do the encouraging, especially if they are somewhat inconsiderate in their use of the total time available to the group. For example, in the group described in Table 9-4, Joe needs encouragement to participate in almost

TABLE 9-3. Percentage of Total Observed Group Participation in Each IPA Category for Each Group Member

Category	Percentage of Group Participation				
	Joe	Mike	Bill	Mary	Jill
1. Seems friendly	—	0.9	1.2	0.2	1.2
2. Dramatizes	3.4	1.3	—	—	2.3
3. Agrees	—	.4	11.4	5.5	1.2
4. Gives suggestions	—	—	2.6	1.2	—
5. Gives opinions	3.4	—	13.0	8.1	—
6. Gives information	—	—	6.2	2.1	—
7. Asks for information	—	—	7.1	3.2	—
8. Asks for opinions	—	1.2	0.1	8.0	3.2
9. Asks for suggestions	—	—	1.2	—	1.1
10. Disagrees	1.0	—	—	—	—
11. Shows tension	2.0	3.4	—	—	2.4
12. Seems unfriendly	0.5	—	—	—	—
Total:	10.3	7.2	42.8	28.3	11.4

all of the task-oriented categories (4, 6, 7, 8, and 9). Bill and Mary probably are spending a bit of the group's time talking with each other; they could well afford to encourage Joe (besides Mike and Jill) to participate more in task-oriented ways.

The fourth level of analysis is a personal one. Calculate the percentage of an individual's (your own?) total participation for each category. Looking back at Table 9-3, assume that you are Joe. In terms of total group interaction, you contributed 10.3 percent, with 3.4 percent in category 2, "dramatizes." Dividing 3.4 by 10.3, you derive 32.6 percent, that portion of your own individual participation scored in this category. In such fashion you can produce a set of data like that presented in Table 9-4.

Using the information presented in Table 9-4, you can compare your own participation with the estimated norms, the medium-range column, provided by Bales. You may recall that in Table 9-2, these normative data were used for comparison with group data; the same norms may be used for an evaluation of individual participation.[44]

According to the data in Table 9-4, Joe is extraordinarily high in interaction that dramatizes, category 2; of his own total participation, 32.6 percent was identified as fitting this category. This amount is very high compared with a normative medium-range of 5.4 to 7.4 percent.

This interpretation can give Joe a fairly good impression of the way he is seen by others for about one third of the time that he is participating. As he pursues similar interpretations of other data in Table 9-4, he may note category 5, "gives opinions": 32.6 percent (very high), interpreted as task-oriented and concerned with the work of the group. So at least one third of the time he is participating, he is seen as contributing to the

TABLE 9-4. Individual IPA Data Compared with Estimated Norms

Category of Interaction	Percent of Joe's Total	Medium Range*
1. Seems friendly	—	2.6–4.8
2. Dramatizes	32.6	5.4–7.4
3. Agrees	—	8.0–13.6
4. Gives suggestions	—	3.0–7.0
5. Gives opinions	32.6	15.0–22.7
6. Gives information	—	20.7–31.2
7. Asks for information	—	4.0–7.2
8. Asks for opinions	—	2.0–3.9
9. Asks for suggestions	—	0.6–1.4
10. Disagrees	9.7	3.1–5.3
11. Shows tension	19.4	3.4–6.0
12. Seems unfriendly	4.9	2.4–4.4

*Taken from R. F. Bales. *Personality and Interpersonal Behavior.* New York, Holt, Rinehart & Winston, 1970. p. 96. Adapted and reprinted by permission of Holt, Rinehart & Winston, Inc.

achievement of the goals of the group. As Joe thinks about these data and their interpretations, he may decide to be less of a clown and more of a problem-solving participant. He may also remember that when a tense situation arises in the group, he is seen as a person who might be able to reduce the tension by providing a good round of laughter. You should view such interpretations as suggestions rather than firm labels; these suggestions should be further evaluated by observing the reactions of other members as you continue to interact in your group; in addition, you should observe you own behavior in the light of these suggestions. In this way the approach Bales has developed and that has been illustrated here can be useful in evaluating your behavior and deciding in what ways, if any, you might wish to change.

Through observation of the words used by each person in the inter-action, the learner may achieve a growing awareness and ultimate under-standing of one's own verbal expression and that of other persons. To what extent does the nurse control the conversation or to what extent do the nurse's words elicit or permit meaningful responses from the client? (By the word "meaningful," reference is made to communication that is client-centered and, as the student grows in skill, communication that will assist the client to achieve the maximum level of health.)

Values of process recording to other phases of nurse-client interaction have been cited by Jeanette G. Nehren and Marjorie V. Batey:

> Supervision of the nurse-patient interaction may also be provided on a group basis through the student's reading and discussion of the process recording in class. This kind of supervision can be successful if the students

have a feeling of permissiveness and acceptance by their class members and the instructor. In writing a process recording, a student exposes herself, and she has to feel support and empathy before growth and insight into her own behavior and understanding of the behavior of the patients can be brought about.

One result of group sharing is illustrated by the following remark of a student, "Gee, I thought I was the only one struggling with this kind of feeling. I didn't realize the rest of you were having the same kind of problems in working with your patients." Such a realization of a common reaction can lead to the release of much tension and anxiety among the students. A climate of permissiveness in expression of feelings in group or individual counseling of student motivates students to try different approaches in talking with patients.[45]

ASSESSING LEADERSHIP BEHAVIOR

Leaders, like groups, vary in their characteristics. Different situations and circumstances require different functions to be performed if a group is to move closer to its goal. Leadership is a role that provides for vital group needs by exerting influence toward the attainment of group goals. Leadership, according to this definition, is a process. It is present no matter who the individuals taking leadership roles or what their influence.

The influence relationship is based on the motivations, perceptions, and resources relevant to the attainment of the group's goal. The multiplicity of tasks and the variety of groupings in a complex social structure have prompted a great deal of study and research in an effort to understand the nature of leadership, its proper function, and its various styles and types. An analysis of the leadership duties of the business executive, made by Barnard in 1938, suggested that two dimensions must be considered: achievement, or the performing of the group task; and efficiency, or keeping the members satisfied.[46] These two dimensions parallel the functions of task and maintenance described in the previous section.

> The leadership functions related to task accomplishment include helping set and clarify goals, focusing on information needed, drawing upon available group resources, stimulating research, maintaining orderly operating procedures, introducing suggestions when they are needed, establishing an atmosphere that permits testing, rigorously evaluating ideas, devoting oneself to the task, attending to the clock and the schedule, pulling the group together for consensus or patterns of action, and enabling the group to determine and evaluate its progress.

> The group-maintenance functions of leadership include encouraging participation by everyone in the group, keeping everyone in a friendly

mood, responding to the emotional concerns of group members when that is appropriate, promoting open communication, listening attentively to all contributions, encouraging with positive feedback, showing enthusiasm and good humor, promoting pride in the group, judging accurately the changing moods of the group, and providing productive outlets for tension.

The performance of both task and maintenance roles, then, is essential if a group is to move toward its goal. These roles are constantly being filled, adequately or inadequately, through the participation of group members. To some degree, therefore, all good group members help in fulfilling these necessary leadership roles.

One particularly interesting and important study on supervisory behavior was conducted in the psychiatric service of a large Veterans Administration Hospital.[47] The investigation focused on 25 head nurses, each of whom supervised a group of three to eight nursing assistants and one or two staff nurses. These 25 head nurses were supervised by five unit supervisors.

They filled out a questionnaire asking them to estimate the percentage of time they spent in each of three categories. These categories were:

1. Supervision of nursing assistants
2. Direct patient care (giving medicine, talking to patients, etc.)
3. Administrative duties (maintenance of supplies, preparing medicines, routine paper work, record keeping, meeting with hospital staff and other subordinates).

What percentage of time do you think you would devote to these items? The head nurses estimated that they spent 25 percent of their time supervising, 25.3 percent giving direct patient care, and 49.2 percent in administrative duties. The supervisors' estimates were 23 percent supervising, 42 percent in direct patient care, and 34.6 percent in administrative duties. Observers, however, found that the two groups spent *75 percent* of their time in administrative duties, 6.5 percent supervising, and 17.4 percent in direct patient care. These findings raise these key questions:

1. If a superior does not know how much time a subordinate manager spends on an important aspect of the job, the superior will hardly be able to tell how much time the subordinate should devote to it.
2. And if the superior has difficulty judging such objective aspects of the subordinate's job, as time use, how accurate is the superior to be in judging the overall quality of performance?
3. Finally, does the superior rate a head nurse's performance, at least to some extent, on what the superior thinks the head nurse should be doing with the time?[48]

LEADERSHIP STYLE QUESTIONNAIRE[49]

This is not a test with any right or wrong answers. It is a questionnaire designed to describe some of your attitudes about *leadership*. Below are 10 statements about situations. After each statement there are three possible attitudes or actions you might take. Place a number 3 beside the position you would *most likely* take. Place a number 2 beside the position you would next likely take, and a 1 beside the position you would *least likely* take.

For each question, you should have three answers, a "3" for your preferred attitude or action, a "2" for your second choice, and "1" for your least likely choice.

Begin when you are sure the instructions are clear!

IN LEADING A MEETING, IT IS IMPORTANT TO:

Keep focused on the agenda at hand .... 1) _____

Focus on each individual's feelings and help people express their emotional reactions to the issue .... 2) _____

Focus on differing positions people take and how they deal with each other .... 3) _____

A PRIMARY OBJECTIVE OF A LEADER IS:

Maintaining an organizational climate in which learning and accomplishment can take place .... 4) _____

The efficient operation of his organization .... 5) _____

To help members of the organization find themselves and be more aware of who they are .... 6) _____

WHEN STRONG DISAGREEMENT OCCURS BETWEEN YOU AND A GROUP MEMBER ABOUT WORK TO BE DONE, YOU WOULD:

Listen to the person and try to discover where he/she might have misunderstood the task .... 7) _____

Try to get other people to express their views as a way of involving them in the issue .... 8) _____

Support the person for raising his/her question or disagreement .... 9) _____

IN EVALUATING A GROUP MEMBER'S PERFORMANCE, THE LEADER SHOULD:

Involve the entire group in both setting goals and in evaluating one another's performance .... 10) _____

Try to make an objective assessment of each person's accomplishments and effectiveness .... 11) _____

Allow each person to be involved in determining his/her own goals and performance standards .... 12) _____

WHEN TWO GROUP MEMBERS GET INTO AN ARGUMENT IT IS BEST TO:

Help them deal with their feelings as a means of resolving the argument .... 13) _____

Encourage other members to respond to the argument and try to help resolve it .... 14) _____

Allow some time for expression of both sides, but keep
in focus the relevant subject matter and the task
at hand .... 15) _____

THE BEST WAY TO MOTIVATE SOMEONE WHO IS NOT
PERFORMING UP TO THE BEST OF HIS/HER ABILITY IS TO:
Point out to him/her the importance of the job to be
done and his/her role in it .... 16) _____
Try to get to know him/her better so you can understand
why he/she is not realizing his/her full potential .... 17) _____
Show him/her how his/her lack of motivation is adversely
affecting other people .... 18) _____

THE MOST IMPORTANT ELEMENT IN JUDGING A PERSON'S
PERFORMANCE IS:
His/her technical skills and ability .... 19) _____
How he/she gets along with his/her peers and how he/she
helps others learn and get work done .... 20) _____
His/her success in meeting the goals he/she has set for
himself/herself .... 21) _____

IN DEALING WITH MINORITY GROUP ISSUES, A LEADER SHOULD:
Deal with such issues as they threaten to disturb the
atmosphere of his/her group .... 22) _____
Be sure that all group members understand the history
of racial and ethnic minorities in this country and
the community .... 23) _____
Help each person achieve an understanding of his/her own
attitude toward people of other races and cultures .... 24) _____

A LEADER'S GOAL SHOULD BE TO:
Make sure that all of his/her members have a solid
foundation of knowledge and skills that will help them
become productive and effective people .... 25) _____
Help people to learn to work effectively in groups,
to use the resources of the group, and to understand
their relationships with one another as people .... 26) _____
Help each person become responsible for his/her own
education and effectiveness and take the first step for
realizing his/her potential as a person .... 27) _____

THE TROUBLE WITH LEADERSHIP RESPONSIBILITIES IS:
They make it very difficult to cover adequately all the
details that must be attended to .... 28) _____
They keep a leader from really getting to know his or
her group members as individuals .... 29) _____
They make it hard for a leader to keep in touch with
the climate and pulse of his or her group .... 30) _____

DO NOT TURN OVER UNTIL YOU HAVE
ANSWERED ALL QUESTIONS

*When scoring the questionnaire be sure to note that the scoring columns
on the next page *are not* in the usual sequential order.

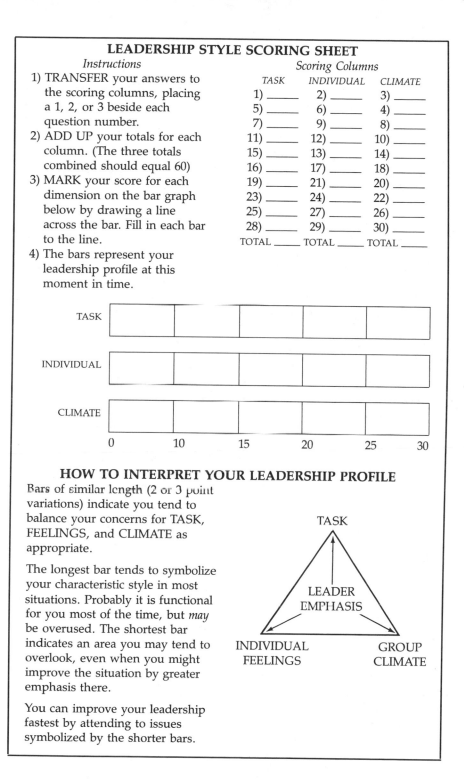

LEADERSHIP STYLE SCORING SHEET

Instructions

1) TRANSFER your answers to the scoring columns, placing a 1, 2, or 3 beside each question number.
2) ADD UP your totals for each column. (The three totals combined should equal 60)
3) MARK your score for each dimension on the bar graph below by drawing a line across the bar. Fill in each bar to the line.
4) The bars represent your leadership profile at this moment in time.

Scoring Columns

TASK	INDIVIDUAL	CLIMATE
1) ___	2) ___	3) ___
5) ___	6) ___	4) ___
7) ___	9) ___	8) ___
11) ___	12) ___	10) ___
15) ___	13) ___	14) ___
16) ___	17) ___	18) ___
19) ___	21) ___	20) ___
23) ___	24) ___	22) ___
25) ___	27) ___	26) ___
28) ___	29) ___	30) ___
TOTAL ___	TOTAL ___	TOTAL ___

TASK

INDIVIDUAL

CLIMATE

0   10   15   20   25   30

HOW TO INTERPRET YOUR LEADERSHIP PROFILE

Bars of similar length (2 or 3 point variations) indicate you tend to balance your concerns for TASK, FEELINGS, and CLIMATE as appropriate.

The longest bar tends to symbolize your characteristic style in most situations. Probably it is functional for you most of the time, but *may* be overused. The shortest bar indicates an area you may tend to overlook, even when you might improve the situation by greater emphasis there.

You can improve your leadership fastest by attending to issues symbolized by the shorter bars.

TASK

LEADER EMPHASIS

INDIVIDUAL FEELINGS

GROUP CLIMATE

SUMMARY

This chapter has discussed the value of evaluating interpersonal communication from perspectives of *needs, competencies,* and *interactions.* It has differentiated between task-oriented behaviors and problems of human relations. The Bales *Interaction Process Analysis* form presented a useful instrument for both individual and group evaluation. It has emphasized the need to discriminate accurately between disagreement and dislike if society is going to resolve its social conflicts and cooperatively solve its mutual problems.

REFERENCES

1. BEN W. MORSE AND EVELYN VAN DEN BERG: "Interpersonal Relationships in Nursing Practice: An Interdisciplinary Approach," *Communication Education* 27 (March, 1978), No. 2, p. 161.
2. W. SCHUTZ: *FIRO, A Three-Dimensional Theory of Interpersonal Behavior* (New York: Holt, Rinehart & Winston, 1958).
3. *Ibid,* pp. 18, 21–22.
4. *Ibid,* pp. 18–20, 22–23.
5. *Ibid,* pp. 20, 23–24.
6. *Ibid.,* pp. 25–33.
7. Write to Consulting Psychologists Press, Inc., 577 College Avenue, Palo Alto, Calif., 94306.
8. B. W. MORSE AND R. N. PILAND: "An Assessment of Communication Competencies Needed by Intermediate-Level Health Care Providers: A Study of Nurse-Patient, Nurse-Doctor, Nurse-Nurse Communication Relationships," International Communication Association, Philadelphia, PA, May, 1979.
9. This discussion and interpretation are cited verbatum from the Morse and Piland report, *Ibid,* pp. 11–13.
10. R. F. BALES: *Personality and Interpersonal Behavior* (New York: Holt, Rinehart & Winston, 1970).
11. *Ibid,* pp. 471–491.
12. *Ibid,* pp. 100–105.
13. *Ibid,* pp. 105–108.
14. *Ibid,* p. 108.
15. *Ibid,* p. 108.
16. *Ibid,* p. 477.
17. *Ibid,* p. 108.
18. *Ibid,* pp. 109–112.
19. *Ibid,* p. 111.
20. *Ibid.,* pp. 112–116.
21. *Ibid.,* p. 117.
22. *Ibid,* pp. 116–119.
23. *Ibid,* p. 119.
24. *Ibid,* pp. 119–120.
25. *Ibid.,* p. 121.

26. *Cf. ibid.*, p. 121.
27. *Ibid.*, p. 121.
28. *Ibid.*, pp. 121–122.
29. *Ibid.*, p. 123.
30. *Ibid.*, pp. 123–124.
31. *Ibid.*, p. 124.
32. *Ibid.*
33. *Ibid.*
34. *Ibid.*, p. 125.
35. *Ibid.*
36. *Ibid.*, pp. 124–127.
37. *Ibid.*, pp. 127–129.
38. *Ibid.*, pp. 129–132.
39. *Ibid.*, p. 127.
40. *Ibid.*, pp. 134–135.
41. *Ibid.*, p. 478.
42. See *Ibid.*, pp. 482–486.
43. R. F. BALES AND A. P. HARE: "Diagnostic use of the interaction profile, *Journal of Psychology,* 67 (1965), 239–258.
44. BALES: *Personality and Interpersonal Behavior,* pp. 96–97.
45. J. G. NEHREN AND M. V. BATEY: "The Process Recording," *Nursing Forum,* II, No. 2, 1963. p. 72.
46. C. BARNARD: *The Functions of the Executive.* (Cambridge, Mass.: Harvard University Press, 1938).
47. NEALY AND OWEN, 1970.
48. This research is explained in more detail in FRED FIEDLER AND MARTIN CHEMERS: *Leadership and Effective Management* (Glenview, Ill.: Scott, Foresman & Company, 1974), pp. 42–44.
49. Prepared by Dr. Harry Munn, North Carolina State University, and used with his permission.

10
SPECIAL COMMUNICATION PROBLEMS

Within the health-care system, a number of potential problem areas in communication have been noted. We believe that there are four categories of communication problems that deserve special attention as they relate to the health-care system: distrust and behaviors of defensiveness; perceived differences or "gaps" between different groups of people; alienation; and problems resulting from sex roles. Each problem has the potential for serious consequences and should be examined in some detail with attention to corrective measures.

DISTRUST AND DEFENSIVENESS

Probably the foremost problem in relating well to other people is distrust—and its counterpart, defensive interpersonal behavior. The basic cause of defensiveness is inherent in one's unmet interpersonal needs. People need supportive feedback from valued others to achieve a satisfactory self-image; when this need remains unmet, a general feeling of anxiety is produced. Unresolved anxiety generates defensive fear, including postural, facial, or verbal signals that warn the other person to be careful. Defensive behavior may involve small signs of a desire to withdraw: verbal hesitancies, stepping backward, turning sideways, or simply paying more attention to some other person. These defensive behaviors are real and not devious; thus, the other person perceives them directly as signs of anxiety or fear.

A more disagreeable strategy of defensiveness is the deliberate distortion of the message received. Everyone has heard exchanges such as this: (Nurse) "You ordered pentobarbital mg 500 prn hs, and this dosage seems rather large to me." (Physician) "What are you doing? Trying to practice medicine. I'm the doctor!"

A serious form of defensive strategy is direct, personal attack. A severe problem arises when the person attacked is unaware that in some way one is perceived as a threat: in such a case one will probably view the attack as pure, unprovoked aggression.[1] Recently a nurse-midwife was working as an instructor in obstetrics, taking students into a hospital for their clinical practice. One afternoon after the students had left, she returned to the delivery room to discuss a matter with one of the nursing staff. As she was leaving for the postpartum unit, the staff nurse asked her to give a birth certificate to an attending mother. In their conversation, the new mother asked her about the Lamaze method of delivery. Being an advocate of this method and having considerable experience teaching parents' classes, our friend paused to discuss the comparative advantages of this method as opposed to methods involving greater use of medications. To our friend, the conversation had been a pleasant and informative one for both her and the new mother. The next morning, however, our friend was approached by a very angry obstetrician who said, among other things, "You have no right interfering with the manner in which I care for my patients. I will tell my patients what I want them to know about their deliveries and decide what is best for them. You and your students stay away from my patients or I will have you fired." Our friend was dismayed and interpreted the obstetrician's attack as unprovoked aggression. Apparently, he had perceived her as a threat to his practice and to the perceived confidence in him by the patient. Although she believed the patient had a right to know about alternatives to obstetric care, and although this information is reasonably available to the public, she concluded she could now do nothing without jeopardizing her job. The matter remained unresolved, and this nurse refused to do any more favors for the staff nurses for a long time. In understanding the concept of distrust and related defensive interpersonal behavior, it is helpful to be aware of oneself as a variable in the relationship; the manner in which one is perceived may tend to generate defensiveness.

COMMUNICATION BEHAVIORS THAT GENERATE DEFENSIVENESS

Sometimes one finds oneself distrusting a person without quite knowing how it came about. Knowledge about communication behavior that tends to produce or increase distrust may help one forestall one's signal reactions of defensiveness. Investigation of such incidents has identified the following contributory conditions, or causes, of defensive behavior:

1. Evaluative expressions, manner of speech, tone of voice, or verbal content, perceived by the receiver (listener) as criticism or judgment, will produce defensive behavior. A single, 35-year-old woman entered an outpatient clinic to confirm her suspicions of pregnancy and to seek an abortion. The staff covertly felt she was "old enough to know better"; the woman received the care required, but left in tears, having received little support and comfort in the process.

2. Communication perceived by the recipient as an attempt to control one will produce defensiveness. When health-care staff members begin to communicate directives regarding areas not related to clients' health needs or supervisors attempt to give orders unrelated to the task, a "need to control" others is probably being expressed by the communicator.

3. Stratagems that are perceived as clever devices produce defensiveness; partially hidden motives breed suspicion. Persons seen as "playing a game," feigning emotion, withholding information, or having private access to sources of data will stimulate defensive responses. A supervisor who feigns anger to motivate subordinates may find this strategy working a time or two, but may soon find subordinates unresponsive.

4. An appearance of lack of concern for the welfare of a person will heighten one's need for defensiveness. Such "neutrality" may be necessary at times, but people strongly need to be perceived as valued persons. A clinically detached or impersonal manner (not caring) is usually feared and resented. Such a manner is frequently encountered by a nurse who has inadvertently made a medication error or a patient who has not followed directions regarding care. Interpersonal distance on such occasions may be interpreted by the recipient as, "Well, *you* goofed, turkey, and now you are on your own. I'm not about to help you."

5. An attitude of superiority arouses defensive behavior; any behavior that reinforces the recipient's feelings of inadequacy is a source of disturbance. "Well, at the University Medical Center, such a thing would never happen! That's where I got my training!" Often this attitude is expressed among nurses in this manner.

6. Dogmatism is a well-known stimulus of defensive behavior; if you know something "for certain," it is wise to determine whether or not others want to hear it from you, and whether they want your answer to be offered tentatively or with final certainty. Giving information to clients who do not perceive a need for it or

to subordinates or colleagues who already possess the information may be perceived as presuming ignorance or incompetence.[2]

When people are perceived to be attempting to manipulate one, one tends to be suspicious, and defensive behavior increases.

CONDITIONS FOR REDUCING DEFENSIVE BEHAVIOR

More than 25 years ago, Carl Rogers began to report a movement toward a nondirective approach to psychotherapy. These practices culminated in his client-centered approach. The relevant point here is his emphasis on the patient's need for personal trust in the therapist. Rogers emphasized acceptance or psychologic safety in psychotherapy groups.[3] His findings have general applications for all groups.

Rogers' approach was a forerunner of Jack Gibb's concept of supportive climate in the communication process. Starting a long-range research effort in 1953, Gibb focused his efforts on the reduction of defensive behavior in groups. This defensive behavior seemed to be caused, in part, by lack of interpersonal trust. In later work, he began to focus on trust and its development, associating trust with interpersonal acceptance.[4] According to his findings, defensive behavior is reduced by interaction that is perceived by the individual as:

1. Descriptive rather than evaluative or critical.
2. Oriented toward solving mutual problems rather than toward personal control.
3. Spontaneous rather than strategic.
4. Empathic rather than neutral.
5. Indicative of an attitude of equality instead of superiority.
6. Expressive of provisionally held viewpoints instead of dogmatic certainties.[5]

EFFECTS OF REDUCING DEFENSIVENESS

As interpersonal trust increases, interpersonal relationships change so that there are:

1. Increased acceptance of legitimate influence by others.
2. Decreased suspicion of motives of others.
3. Increased tolerance for deviant behavior of others.
4. Increased stability when one is not trusted by others.

5. Shifting of emphasis to control over the interaction process rather than control over individuals.
6. Further increase of interpersonal trust.[6]

Changes in personality characteristics are not easy to produce; changes in behavior that seem to indicate changes in personality structure may be only temporary. Even so, studies tend to indicate that, as defensive behavior decreases and interpersonal trust increases, two important personality changes can occur: (1) People tend to achieve heightened feelings of personal adequacy (improved self-image), and (2) they achieve easier acceptance of their temporary feelings of internal conflict (less anxiety). Reducing defensive behavior and increasing interpersonal trust appear to be extremely valuable goals in terms of effective interpersonal communication.

GAPS BETWEEN GROUPS

A major problem today is that of overcoming communication barriers between different groups and groupings of people. Gaps need to be bridged between members of different reference groups and different subcultures.

BARRIERS BETWEEN MEMBERS
OF DIFFERENT REFERENCE GROUPS

In order to be socially adequate, one must achieve personal beliefs, attitudes, and convictions that help one to function well with those people who surround one. Conflicts over norms of behavior and belief usually prove to be threatening. If personal standards and norms conflict seriously with those of people in the immediate environment, the experience is likely to be painful because one's very basis of existence is at stake.

When individuals identify with a group, such as the people in their community, they almost inevitably adopt and defend the standards and behavior of that group. A group with which individuals identify is sometimes called a "reference group." This process of identification introduces a certain degree of narrowness or distortion into the perceptual field; limiting and distorting perception of "foreigners" (persons not in the reference group) then becomes a major source of breakdown in communication.

Because each person accepts one's own perceptions as "reality," the customs and attitudes of one's own reference group are judged to be superior when they are different from those of other groups. Other people and other groups are then judged according to these standards. Americans commonly place a high value on complex, mechanical and electric health-care equipment, such as cardiac monitors, defibrillators, and artificial kidney machines; as a result, many Americans consider the health care provided in the United States superior to that of the Chinese. If you say, "Well, it is!" then you have illustrated the point at issue—you have made a judgment based on a standard derived from your American reference group.

Two nurses may be colleagues on the same nursing staff; one may have graduated from a private university, and the other may have graduated from a tuition-free city college having special programs for socially or culturally disadvantaged individuals. Both may be Registered Nurses; even so, bridging the gap in the clinical setting may not be at all easy, particularly since it is compounded by these nurses having also to relate to clients presenting similar communication gaps.

How can such gaps ever be bridged? In a way, every individual bridges a similar gap whenever one tries to contact and "get to know" any other single individual. One starts by accepting and even adopting a few behaviors of others that help one to satisfy some personal need. As one accepts or adopts behaviors, one later modifies one's attitudes, beliefs, and value systems. For example, the acceptance of the rhythm method of contraception by American Catholic women tends to be facilitated by attitudes, beliefs, and values arising from tenets of the Catholic religion. However, health workers and missionaries in India attempting to persuade Indian women to use the rhythm method found their efforts rejected; differing social and religious beliefs caused the methods to be viewed as a great menace.

The process of acceptance of the ways, attitudes, and beliefs of others is speeded up if the other person has some acceptable source of status, or if the behavior satisfies some immediate and important personal need.[7] New ways of doing things that otherwise fit one's customary pattern of behavior are eventually accepted and adopted. Once the change is made, one quickly finds additional reasons why it is a good idea; one thus reduces the cognitive dissonance imposed by the new behavior.[8]

The primary tool for bridging gaps between reference groups is, of course, getting the group to look at each other without perceptual distortion. *The real barrier is the prior notion that just because a person is a member of another group, one's behavior and one's beliefs will be inferior.* People who fail to conform to a group's standards tend to be viewed as ignorant or perhaps evil. Such prejudgment—judgment without taking an objective, open-minded, inquisitive look to see first and decide later—is properly called prejudice. No people of any nation, religion, or group have been entirely free of this problem. Even nurses who ordinarily are severe critics of their own educational system have difficulty giving objective consideration to the suggestions of those who are not a part of the system. Objectivity, however, is the true basis of tolerance and makes possible the bridging of gaps between members of different reference groups.

GAPS BETWEEN DIFFERENT CULTURES
AND SUBCULTURES

Communities that pride themselves on tolerance and the absence of prejudice almost always have only a few members of a minority group in their midst. Minority groups become threatening to majority groups only when they are large or powerful. When a group feels threatened, its members tend to accentuate or idealize their own characteristics. This has two negative effects on their perceptual processes: (1) Their perceptions tend to be focused on the object of threat so that it is difficult to see broadly and clearly, and (2) they tend to be much more rigidly defensive of their existing perceptions. As a general principle, the psychologic effects of intergroup threat or conflict are felt at the lower socioeconomic levels, especially if persons at these lower levels are the victims of domination or aggression within their own group. For example, the most violent reactions to school integration occurred among the "poor white" economic classes.

The point of greatest potential for bridging intercultural gaps is at the interface between cultures, that is, the personal, face-to-face interaction between official and unofficial representatives of these cultures. Foreign travelers are generally better educated and more broadly experienced, and feel less personally threatened by representatives of the other culture. At this interface, a common language capability is helpful but not crucial. For example, caring for patients who are foreign travelers in this country can be accomplished by responding to nonverbal cues. The human reactions to pain, fear, and grief have a similarity that transcends language. Needs for action in a health crisis tends to make individuals from different cultures important to each other, and a certain pleasure is often experienced in the process.

What is severely needed by intercultural representatives at this interface is objectivity of perception. Intercultural conflict is always carried on by individuals who think of others as *members of the other* group rather than as individual human beings. Intergroup conflict at the cultural interface can be diminished by increasing the capability of members to differentiate one another as individuals.[9]

Increased interaction between such representatives is helpful; it fosters the capability of these persons to see each other as individuals rather than as blacks or whites, Israeli or Egyptian, Russian or American. A very interesting procedure has been shown to be an effective means of promoting better relationships between representatives of different groups. Instead of talking about intergroup or intercultural problems and differences, people are asked to talk about pleasant childhood memories. Members of both groups talk about their experiences in smelling and tasting enjoyable foods, playing games, and participating in athletic events. After a while, they feel as if they have had similar experiences and somewhat similar childhoods, and are, first of all, all members of the human race. Shared experiences make possible a common feeling; furthermore, shared experiences provide a more personal, human view of a member of another group or culture.

The objective view of one another, a view focused on the other person as an individual human being rather than as a specimen of a strange cultural type, is the basis for effective interpersonal communication between representatives of different cultures. Such effective communication behavior is highly useful in reducing intergroup conflict for the following reasons: (1) It maximizes human capability for tolerance of differences and acceptance of new or different folkways and attitudes, and (2) it minimizes the degree of fear and feelings of threat imposed by the other group, race, or culture.

ALIENATION

Comments on current social problems frequently use the term *alienation*. Because many persons in health-care fields appear to have negative attitudes toward other persons in their immediate social environment, the problem deserves special consideration. In common parlance, "alienated" usually refers to persons who are estranged or withdrawn from other persons whom they would ordinarily be expected to respect or admire. A teenager who has turned away from parents—that is, who has ceased to talk with them in the way they expect or desire—may sometimes be called "alienated."

Alienation does not mean simple disagreement with another person, *as long as interaction continues*. When one ceases overt communication with another person or persons and withdraws from interaction, then social alienation has occurred. Alienation of a person from another can be partial; one can be convinced that one will be denied the opportunity for communication on certain topics or at certain times or under limited conditions. As long as one is allowed to communicate on most topics most of the time, the degree of alienation is only slight. The severity of alienation increases as a person perceives an increase in the number of times one's communication is denied.

Alienation can occur between a person and one or more other people. Complete alienation from one other person may not matter much; complete or nearly complete alienation from many others can make life miserable. William James once said, "No more fiendish punishment could be devised, even were such a thing physically possible, than that one should be turned loose in society and remain absolutely unnoticed by all members thereof." Social alienation can be analyzed in terms of communication theory; that is, it constitutes a refusal to use a communication channel generally thought to be available and useful. An important question for the student of communication among nurses is thus posed: What kinds of communication behavior tend to produce alienation? Tangential questions are as follows: Is it possible that alienated nurses are responding realistically to communication events in an intelligent way? Or are they mistakenly withdrawing from social interaction that would be useful to them? Have colleagues or supervisors or other important persons unknowingly or thoughtlessly caused such withdrawal?

COMMUNICATION BEHAVIORS RELATED TO SOCIAL ALIENATION

An understanding of the ways in which basic principles of interpersonal communication may be ignored can lead to a better understanding of alienation. Such insights can provide the basis for changes in your communication behavior that may lead to a reduction of your feeling of alienation. Your own insights and your changes in the use of interpersonal communication techniques may or may not change the behavior of those persons from whom you feel alienated, but such additional insight can at least help you to understand yourself and others better.

The first principle of interpersonal communication that appears to be related to social alienation is this: *People communicate on two levels.* The first level is *message sending;* the second level is *providing information about the message.* When the message itself is in conflict with, or contradictory to, the communication about the message, a natural response is confusion and at least a partial attempt at withdrawal from further interaction. If parents say, "We really do love you, John," *but say it in a way that shows distrust, suspicion, anger, or hostility,* social alienation is a reasonable result (from John's point of view).

The second principle that appears to be related to alienation is that *one cannot refuse to communicate in an interpersonal situation.* A refusal to interact with another person is a communication in and of itself. When another person simply refuses to talk to you (perhaps for a reason thought to be excellent by that person), the message given you is conclusive: The person does not wish to talk with you. Such a conclusion provides an excellent reason for withdrawal from later interaction unless it is absolutely necessary.

The third related principle is that *nonverbal communication ultimately establishes the nature of an interpersonal relationship.* People often receive verbal messages from another person telling them how that person perceives their interpersonal relationship with the person: "I like to be with you," "I enjoy talking with you." Sometimes people believe what they hear; however, *if the other person's nonverbal behavior is in conflict with the verbal message, they usually recall the old adage that "actions speak louder than words."* In the final analysis, a person's perception of one's relationship with another is determined by the latter's nonverbal communication. In many interviews, students have said, "My parents said they loved me, but they didn't act like it." Such behavior appears to be reasonable justification for diminishing interaction.

The fourth related principle is that *the degree to which two persons similarly perceive their relationships will heavily influence the interpretation of communication between the two.* Different perceptions of their relationship can lead to serious and even violent disagreement between them regarding what one has "really said" to the other. There is the classic situation in which the Registered Nurse, contrary to directives, does not administer a medication and consequently the client improves. Upon learning this, the physician immediately becomes angry with and begins to berate the nurse. The nurse angrily argues that she actually did the appropriate thing. But the physician insists: "Well, you may have done the right thing, but you were wrong because you did not consult me." In actual fact, the real conflict was over the nurse's right to take such initiative without consulting the physician: this concerned their perceptions of the nature of their interpersonal/professional relationship. They argued about the action while actually disagreeing about their professional roles, failing completely to resolve the confusion between their two perceptions of their interpersonal relationship.

ALIENATION BY COMMUNICATION DENIAL

The initiation of any communication act carries with it an implied request: "Please validate me." This plea can be in the form of a request for recognition of one's ideas as worthwhile. Even in such a case, however, there is an obvious implication regarding *the value of oneself personally.* There are three ways a person can respond to the implicit request for validation of person: (1) agreement—a person or the person's idea; (2) disagreement—accept the person but the idea is responded to as more or less not valid; and (3) denial of the existence of the question. This denial (i.e., an attempt to refuse to give any response at all) not only denies the existence of the implicit request "please validate me," but by implication denies the existence of the other person on a functional, interpersonal, or communication level.

Little Johnny, age 5, comes home from kindergarten and says, "I have a girl friend." His mother says, "Eat your soup, Johnny." This constitutes a denial of Johnny's capability of discussing girl friends (at that time)—perhaps an event of no great consequence. Ten years later John says, "Dad, Joe Smith is taking his folks' car to the school picnic Saturday." Dad says, "Finish your homework, John." This is an example of a denial of John's right to talk about using the family car, that is, denial of

INTERPERSONAL COMMUNICATION IN NURSING

John's existence on this communication level. Two such instances in 10 years are inconsequential; two instances per day for 10 years are another matter. Also, denial of communication on one isolated topic may not pose a severe threat to an individual's self-validation. Remember, however, that the question of his validity is implied with every statement John ever makes, and that in any interpersonal situation the other person cannot refuse to respond to it: A refusal becomes at least a temporary or partial denial of John's self-identify. On a different, but similar level, communication denial is experienced when a head nurse makes a recommendation about equipment repair for her unit of the hospital and receives no response from the supervisor. There is a similar denial of the head nurse's self-identity and professional identity.

The impact of such denial depends on the value a person places on the other person or persons, perhaps on the value one places on one's relationship with them. Consistent and continued denial of a child by the parents can cause severe damage. For nurses, this denial process may be one of the causes of uniquely low job satisfaction and uncommonly high job turnover among this professional group.[10]

In commenting on our society, Martin Buber writes as follows:

> At all its levels, persons confirm one another in a practical way, to some extent or other, in their personal qualities and capabilities, and the society may be termed human in the measure to which its members confirm one another.[11]

The implied request, "Validate me," may be put by an individual, a group, a subculture, or even a nation: the responses—agreement, disagreement, or denial of existence—may be made by another individual, a group, a subculture, or a nation.

There are two major ways in which an individual can respond to the denial described: (1) One can refuse to accept it as a denial, or (2) one can accept the idea that one does not exist on that communication level. Communication behaviors exhibiting a refusal to accept such a denial include (1) repetition of the request, (2) escalation of the vocal tone or manner of the request, and (3) overt verbal communication about the denial.

Repetition of the request simply involves continuation of any verbal communication with its attendant implied request, "Please validate me." Escalation can involve changes in vocal tone or intensity, threatening posture, violent gestures, or, on a larger scale, demonstrations, riots, and the like. Overt communication about the denial would likely be something like this: "Dad, why don't you talk with me about my using the family car on the picnic?" For a head nurse to the supervisor: "I have reported the defective equipment to you on three occasions; why haven't you discussed it with me?" It should be noted that such overt communication is rarely initiated by the person in the weaker, "one-down" position who feels threatened, and, of course, such denial of one's existence (on any level) by a valued other will produce a feeling of threat.[12]

Acceptance of the implication of denial of oneself is more common than many people believe: many persons accept the idea that they are unworthy of talking to "better" people—people with more influence, more education, more experience, or just more self-assurance. For example, patients in hospitals frequently express the idea that they "hate to bother the busy nurses" when specific care is needed, so they don't ask for assistance. The acceptance of this implication is frequently a constituent of the process of social alienation.[13]

THE "DOUBLE BIND"

A particularly interesting problem arises when communication denial occurs and at the same time the denied person cannot withdraw from the situation because of the value one places on the relationships with that specific other person or group. Bateson and his associates coined the term "double bind" to identify a communication situation in which the following elements occur:

1. For certain important reasons a person cannot withdraw from the scene, for example, for one's own moral reasons, one must continue to try to talk things over with one's parents, spouse, colleague, physician, client, or supervisor.
2. Messages are sent by the other person on the verbal and nonverbal levels that are internally contradictory; that is, the subject is validated by a verbal message and invalidated by nonverbal behavior—those cues as to how one is to interpret the verbal message.
3. One's attempts at overt communication about the contradiction are denied; that is, one is not allowed to initiate discussion about the internal contradiction posed between the verbal message that validates one and the nonverbal communication that invalidates one.[14]

An attempt to justify the refusal to communicate about this contradiction, that is, denial of opportunity to engage in overt communication about it, is frequently based on rather unreasonable grounds. Moral ground rules may be invoked: "It is not right (moral) for you to question the physician in this way." Such morality is seldom expressed in overt verbal communication; rather, the cold stare or the angry expression usually carries the message of infraction of moral boundaries. In other cases, an ethic is invoked: for example, in health-care circles, it is sometimes claimed to be unethical to "deal in values." Thus, a request for overt communication about the contradiction may be construed as an attack or manipulation of the other person's status, belief system, or right to determine care of one's own body. Once again refusal of overt communication about the contradiction will likely be indicated by a cold stare or nervous fidget rather than by forthright verbal communication. If for one's own reasons or if for reasons of physical incapacity a person cannot "leave the field" and is also denied the opportunity to initiate overt communication with the other person, one is confronted with an undecidable problem. If one also feels that it is morally wrong to question the physician about confusing messages, one truly is in a double bind. If one acts on the apparent implication of the verbal message ("You are a worthwhile person" or "You have a good idea"), one will run the risk of antagonizing the physician by ignoring the negative implications. On the other hand, if one accepts the apparent implication of the physician's vocal tone and general manner, one will infer that the physician thinks one's idea is worthless, thus, again, one will run the risk of antagonizing the physician by acting as if the physician did not "properly" respect or care about the person. The point is, one is in trouble; one is "damned if one does and damned if one doesn't."

There is no way out of this dilemma; the doorways out—leaving the field, that is, quitting, or getting a transfer, or initiating overt communication—have been closed. In such a case the individual usually does one of three things: (1) One scans the interpersonal horizon (i.e., the physician's behavior) for some message or clue that one must have missed or overlooked; (2) one ignores all or most communication from the physician; that is, one interprets all or most of the physician's communication as confusing and of slight value or meaning; (3) one may overreact, jumping inside one's skin when the physician says, "How are things going tonight?" Such is the way in which the double bind can produce an unhappy relationship between two more or less well-meaning people who, according to the notions of many individuals, should mean much to each other because of interrelated task and professional goals.

When the double bind is of long duration, it will produce habitual suspicion regarding the general nature of human relationships. This suspicion leads to a self-perpetuating pattern of mistrust of communication. It can lead to alienation, not only toward others, but eventually toward oneself.[15]

There may be times when one cannot or should not respond to the overtures of another person. At times one may be tired or mentally exhausted, or may have nothing to say that has not already been said over and over. At other times, for one's own survival or peace of mind, one may deem it necessary to ignore the presence of another person. Even so, in such a case one should be aware of what is happening: if one is with other persons, and they believe one is aware of their presence, to ignore them is to deny their implicit requests for validation as persons. Furthermore, to remain silent in response to an overt request to talk with one is prima facie evidence that, for oneself, they do not functionally exist at this time.

ALIENATION BY ANGER

Research has shown that nurses frequently encounter alienation processes in daily clinical practice. In a survey of 330 RNs currently employed in hospitals, Grant[16] found that three fourths of the subjects received angry messages during the 5 days prior to completing the questionnaire, and about one third of these received three or more such messages. The angry messages were received from patients, visitors, and other hospital employees, but the major portion (40 percent) came from other members of the nursing department and from physicians (20 percent). The data show that receiving angry messages causes serious concern for the RNs. Of the many issues identified as stimulating angry messages, criticism of task performance was identified as a common topic (40 percent). The most relevant finding, however, was that the nurses tend to feel neutral to cold and distant toward the angry person rather than warm and close. By definition, this feeling of neutrality or coldness is alienation operationalized.[17] This feeling of neutrality was associated with increased turnover rates in the agencies in which the RN subjects were employed. This study tends to support the conclusion that receiving angry messages and coping with alienating processes represent a portion of avoidable job turnover of RNs.

DEALING WITH ANGER

Nurses can attempt to change their communicative behavior by increasing capabilities of coping with anger of others, and communicating their own anger in a mode that tends to *maintain* good relationships.

Certain specific suggestions can be made about how anger can be communicated in a maintenance mode, that is, a manner that involves elements of *attending, describing,* and *identifying.* These suggestions are designed to increase the probability of achieving an interpersonally gratifying closure to the anger cycle and decreasing the probability of alienation.

Research shows that the recipient of an angry message tends to perceive the angry person as unattractive; the recipient tends to withdraw.[19] However, *attending* to the angry person is important. Thus, if you receive an angry message, with courage you can show the angry person that you are listening. Nonverbal verification of your attending may include facing your speaker and maintaining eye contact. Alienation tends to develop in an interaction in which communication denial occurs. Not attending or communication denial serves only to lead to alienation. Here, it seems, lies a major difficulty in handling angry feelings. As the recipient of any angry message, you must try to overcome the tendency to withdraw from an unattractive person. You must consider the possible value of maintaining the relationship with the angry person. If the cost of interacting is judged to be sufficiently rewarding, then you will tend to become involved and attend to the messages.

Dealing with anger tends to be costly because of the prolonged psychologic imbalance involved. If one's present state of tiredness, hunger, level of coping, or incidence of more pressing issues tends to preclude a maintenance approach, then you may best avoid becoming involved *at this time.* And this can be accomplished *without communication denial.* A statement of how one feels, and a request to discuss the problem at a later time would still tend to validate the angry person. Since anger is communicable like measles, that is, tends to evoke an angry response, you need to be aware that you will be in a provocative interaction and will need to manage your own feelings. These, then, are the suggestions offered in regard to the attending element of communicating anger. One can now turn to the next element, that of describing.

If the angry person *describes* one's feelings of anger rather than just showing a heightened emotional state, there will be a tendency to achieve closure to the anger cycle and a decreased probability of alienation on the part of the recipient of the angry messages.[20] First, if one describes one's anger, one tends to feel less angry. Second, although initial responses tend to be very angry, if use of the maintenance mode is continued, the intensity of anger tends to decrease and solution-oriented responses tend to increase. Third, interpersonal involvement tends to increase with the use of maintenance mode of expressing anger. Conversely, if the destructive mode is used, which includes the use of personal diatribe and reference to past rather than "here and now events," the intensity of anger of the recipient tends to increase gradually—the "slow burn" effect. This serves to negate probabilities of achieving closure of the anger cycle. In summary, two specific suggestions can be made relative to the describing element: Describe the feelings of anger when you are angry, or positively respond to the other person's descriptions of how the anger feels when one is angry and you are on the receiving end. If the angry person is aware of one's own anger, then there may be a greater tendency for the maintenance mode of expressing anger to be used. If the recipient of the angry expressions recognizes the other's anger and states, "You are really angry!," then this further serves to validate the angry person and tends to decrease alienation. If the recipient is able to restate descriptions of the other's anger, the angry person can perceive oneself as being understood and experience the relief from tension associated with feeling no one understands. *If the recipient of the angry expressions can respond to the other's descriptions of how the anger feels in such a manner that avoid discipline* ("Don't use such ugly language!"), *denial* ("You shouldn't feel that way."), *moral-*

izing ("It's a sin to get so angry."), *punishing* ("God will get you for that!"), and *patronizing* ("Careful, dear, you will just get one of your blood pressure headaches if you get so upset."), *the anger cycle will tend to be completed more quickly* than when these negative approaches are used. Recognition of the anger and positive responses to descriptions of the angry feelings are the two suggestions offered relative to the describing element of expressing anger. The final element is that of identifying.

Identification of the source of anger involves specifically indicating the cause of the angry person's arousal. If the source of arousal can be clearly communicated, the angry person can be helped to cope with the perceived threat, frustration, or whatever causes the anger. Research has shown that if the cause of the anger is clearly stated, the degree of responses that tend to *maintain* relationships are found to increase.[21] Therefore, it is suggested that, in communicating with an angry person, one might assist the person to *identify* the specific cause or stimulus of anger by (1) asking questions, the answers to which would tend to reveal the cause, and (2) positively responding to the person's comments that tend to clarify this issue, thereby increasing the tendency for such comments to occur. If the source of anger arousal is an error in task performance on the part of the recipient, it becomes important that the recipient admit one's own honest mistakes without apology. This act aids in validation of the angry person's perceptions and evaluation of "reality." In addition, to *express how one feels about one's own errors* would be appropriate, such as, "I feel bad that this had happened," or "This was not what was intended." As signs of decreasing tension begin to appear in the angry person's behavior, attempts may be initiated to identify possible solutions to the cause of anger; the problem-solving process may now begin. However, the *recipient* of the angry expressions may now be angry; this may be particularly true in the event of angry criticism of something the recipient has, is, or has done. In this case, it will be necessary for this person to proceed through the anger cycle, communicating anger in the maintenance mode (of course!) until this cycle has achieved closure.

In many nursing teams in which one member has personal power over others, there seem to be certain cautions to be considered before applying the suggestions offered above. In the superior-subordinate relationship, it would seem reasonable for the *superior* to employ the suggestions, because the results would tend to have positive outcomes. However, if the *subordinate* clearly expressed one's feelings and identified the source or cause of anger, the hazard to one's continued membership, that is, job status or even employment status itself, may prove too venturesome and risky for some. It is possible the superior may react defensively, and punitively use power to the subordinate's disadvantage. Therefore, while the maintenance mode of expressing anger is believed helpful interpersonally, it would seem wise for one in a subordinate position to consider the risks involved. However, the other alternative—withdrawal—may also have disadvantages.

In summary, handling anger of others in the *maintenance* mode involves four basic actions on the part of the recipient:

1. Stop—whatever you are doing.
2. Look—directly at the angry person.
3. Listen—for description of feelings and source identification.
4. Respond—by (a) acknowledging and accepting the anger; (b) asking about the specific cause of anger; (c) admitting errors without apology; and (d) moving to problem solving whenever appropriate.

In addition, there are four basic responses that one should *avoid* in dealing with an angry person:

1. Disciplining the person.
2. Appealing to logic.
3. Denying the person's anger.
4. Attacking the angry person.

There are few things more difficult than to try to overcome the effects of the misuse of the interpersonal communication principles outlined; interaction with persons who have been alienated from their social environment is never easy. Of course, the primary requirement is that someone must want to make the effort. It is also helpful to provide the alienated person with insight into the process that has contributed to the alienation; sometimes this insight plus that person's own attempts to reach out and establish new contacts with people around one tend to reduce the problem. Most certainly, covert denial of communication must be avoided if interaction with alienated persons is to be achieved.

SEX ROLE PROBLEMS

One professional colleague with whom the nurse, usually a woman, needs to maintain positive and open interpersonal communication is the physician, usually a man. In this society generally, communication between men and women is becoming increasingly complex with the changing roles of women and the corresponding role change required of men. Social and cultural fixed expectations of the traditional male role of husband-breadwinner-superior and female role of wife-homemaker-subordinate are being continually challenged as women, and men as well, define more rewarding and actualizing roles that give fuller expressions of an individual's potential.[22] Kanter identifies the many ways by which women and men have difficulty communicating in the corporate setting of business and industry.[23] Sex-role stereotypes impose a unique and unexpected influence on the superior-subordinate and peer-colleague relationships. Stereotyped expectations of nurses and physicians impose still another influence that compounds this already complex relationship between men and women in the corporate-like setting of health agencies. Historically, there is considerable evidence that the relationship between the physician and nurse has been difficult at best. Ashley documents extensively the obstructionism, discrimination, exploitation, and suppression of nursing and nurses by medicine and physicians since the mid-1700s.[24]

There is an abundance of contemporary evidence that all is not well at the present time between physicians and nurses. Testimony before the National Commission on Nursing cites physicians' treatment of nurses as a major factor contributing to the nursing shortage currently occurring in all parts of the United States.[25] Wolf states the following in relation to nurse turnover rates:

> Poor physician-nurse relationships are also a primary concern to many nurses. They resent physicians' lack of professional respect for them and interest in what nursing has to offer in patient care.[26]

Simmons and Rosenthal also cite relationships with physicians to be a major factor in the successful adaptation of a nurse to the expanded role of the nurse practitioner.[27] These are a few of the authors who have cited physician-nurse relationships as a problem, and as the nursing shortage grows, more emphasis can be expected to be placed on this cause of alienation of nurses.

In discussions with nurses, two types of communications that seem to be of concern to nurses and to be heavily influenced by sex-role stereotyping have been identified. One is sexual harassment, and the other is verbal abuse.

SEXUAL HARASSMENT

"I work in a doctor's office, and this is the nicest, best job I have ever had. But that doctor has his hands all over me the minute we are alone. I don't know what to do. I guess I will just have to quit."

"As an ICU nurse, I can't turn my back to some of the doctors—they pinch my backside. I have to hold the chart in front of my breasts to prevent them from touching me there. It's really very distracting."

"I will be married in about a month. Some of the doctors found out about it and have asked me all sorts of very personal questions. I am shocked at the things they have the nerve to say to me. I don't even like being at work. I feel so angry and embarrassed. What right have they to say these things to me?''

"As head nurse, there are certain doctors who hug me and pat my bottom, almost without thinking, it seems. It's as if they are doing it so I will take good care of their patients. As a professional person, I resent that. I give nursing care according to clients' needs. No one has to bargain with me to get me to do it. I think these doctors go around hugging all the head nurses, and I am just one of the 'girls.'''

According to the Equal Employment Opportunity Commission (EEOC) guidelines, these complaints are forms of sexual harassment, verbal or physical. Sexual harassment is becoming an issue because it is a violation of individual rights according to recent interpretations of Title VII of the Civil Rights Act. It is an issue for the employing health agency and for the individual nurse; both need to know how to cope with and prevent sexual harassment. More recent interpretations of this law hold the employer responsible for sexual harassment of employees by third parties, that is, clients, customers, and others, such as the supervising physicians, who are related to the agency by contracts. Attorney Dan Norwood, a specialist in labor relations law, states this is one of the strongest laws on the books.

"Sexual harassment" is a concept new to the language and doesn't appear in dictionaries. It has been defined legally, but the interface between laws and social customs now begins. Men and women over the centuries have learned to relate to one another in a personal or social context. As great numbers of women have entered the work environment, society now has become aware of the need to clarify and redefine relationships. Relating in "personal" contexts differs from relating in "occupational" or "professional" contexts. Mistakes have been and are being made by both men and women. People are alienated and dehumanized. New laws have been established to protect individual rights. Now, there is a need to resocialize both men and women so that customs can be changed and new patterns of interpersonal relating can be acquired. There is a need to study this communication process and take steps to avoid and prevent it.

Five elements in sexual harassment are brought into play in a dehumanizing and alienating manner by the harasser to insure that the harassee will not feel at ease, but will be aware of the role of an available and subordinate sex object. MacKinnon identifies three of the five elements of sexual harassment: (1) *unwanted sexual advances,* physical or verbal; (2) *rejection* by the victim; and (3) *retaliation* by the harasser.[28] We would add the following: (4) *power* of the harasser by virtue of the job description; and (5) *employment* of the victim can be jeopardized. These elements usually work together like this: Some reference, verbal or nonverbal, is made to the victim's sexual nature, such as appearance, habits, or needs. The victim responds negatively, expressing dislike, moving away, or refusing the overtures of the harasser. The harasser tends to threaten or actually retaliate so that in some way the victim is aware of and/or experiences the harasser's threat. The harasser tends to have power over the victim's job or, if a coworker or subordinate, possess some job-related resource necessary to the victim's job performance. The employment of the victim becomes at risk, either through lowered evaluation of job performance, reduced hours, being placed on a lower-paying job, disciplinary layoff, demotion, and the like. Ultimately, the victim tends to be distracted from task performance, quality of work decreases, and loss of employment becomes probable if not initially chosen by the harassee as an early means of escape. In a personal or social context, the victim can simply walk away. In the occupational or professional context, the interaction of personal and professional needs and values produces a particularly distressing dilemma. Employment is needed to meet living expenses and obligations, and such values as dedication, loyalty, accountability, and responsibility tend to deter one's immediate resignation.

Since the typical sexual harassment situation involves a man harassing a woman, for the purposes of this chapter, the harasser will be considered the man and the victim the woman. We are aware that women sometimes harass men and that a small percentage of the harassment cases are homosexual in nature. Our major concern is female nurses, and most of the harassers of nurses tend to be nonsupervisory physicians or superiors. The typical harassee tends to be relatively powerless in the hospital organizational hierarchy, that is, staff nurses, team leaders or charge nurses, and head nurses. In the survey cited above, nurses identified physicians as being the harasser in 50 percent of the cases, and some other superior in 20 percent, and peers in 10 percent. Subordinates accounted for another 10 percent, and the remainder included clients and others. The most frequently reported form of unwanted sexual advances were found to include "being touched in a familiar manner" and talking about "personal topics." Usually, retaliatory threats were not involved; those receiving threats report very few being carried out. Apparently it's just "stuff" a nurse has to put up with—unwanted, unnecessary invasion of private lives and personal space.[29]

The effect of sexual harassment for nurses is found to be similar to that experienced by other women.[30] More than 60 percent of the nurses surveyed experienced sexual harassment in the preceding year, and more than half of the harassees experienced some negative result. Being distracted from nursing tasks seems to be the most serious. Some nurses indicated that the clients' best interests and safety were in jeopardy. More than one fourth became so emotionally upset they could not perform their jobs in the usual way. Eight percent were jeopardized legally by being so distracted that good judgment in making decisions was impaired; mistakes that ordinarily would not have been made just "happened." About 7 percent had trouble in their personal relationships with their spouse, sex partner, or lover. Physical illness was the result for about 3 percent of the respondents, but no one reported quitting because of sexual harassment. Typically, few nurses report sexual harassment incidents to a superior at work. The greater the nurses' concern, the greater the tendency to NOT report. Younger nurses tend to believe they cope well with sexual harassment, whereas older nurses report not being so confident. About 15 percent report feeling very ineffective in coping with a harasser and feeling very distressed. Thus, sexual harassment tends to lower the quality and quantity of productivity in nursing, that is, the nursing care, just as has been reported in business, government, and industry generally.[31]

The personal impact of sexual harassment on women takes its toll in several ways. First, one's confidence as an employee is undermined. The typical pattern used by the harasser is to praise a woman's work and evaluate job performance very highly. When the woman has refused his sexual advances, his evaluation of her job performance becomes very negative. This is particularly destructive; which message must the woman truly believe, the very positive or the very negative one? Even discounting the negative message after rejection, there are the nagging questions: Were the positive evaluations true or were these a sham also? How well am I really doing my job? Where is reality? Which "map" is the "territory"? Since the harasser is often the supervisor, this question often goes unanswered.

Second, women experience feelings of alienation and dehumanization. There is a discord of feelings: humiliation, degradation, shame, fear, embarrassment, repulsion, and anger. One feels helpless, powerless, and isolated, as if no one else has ever had this problem. Third, feelings of guilt predominate for many who believe they must have done something "wrong" to elicit such behavior from a man. Fourth, there can be physical illness caused by increased tension, ambivalence, and stress. Errors in tasks occur, and days are taken off for ill health. Finally, the woman experiences financial crisis if dismissed, disruption of career development, and job dissatisfaction. The overall effects are not unlike those of rape; this is a dehumanizing, alienating, symbolic rape.

The people involved in this classic scenario are generally considered rather nice, socially acceptable, regular folk. Often the men involved are responsible, reasonably successful, and respected members of their community. The women involved tend to have fine reputations, too. This is probably why people just don't discuss sexual harassment. According to MacKennon, however, sexual harassment prevails at all levels of society.[32] The man who becomes a harasser seems to be of two types. Either he is "Mr. Nice Guy" who impulsively acts out his fantasy and has to expend considerable effort mending his social relations fences afterwards, or he is a social failure in his relationships with women in his personal life, and discovers he can use the power of his job to coerce a woman subordinate into relating to him in a personal way.

The heart of this matter of sexual harassment seems to be twofold. First, it is necessary to look at the beliefs that people in the communities have about human relationships and human values. What a person believes tends to be congruent with behaviors. Second, since the element of power, control, or dominance is an element of sexual harassment, one must consider the role of power in relationships.

A little list of "do's and don'ts" that need to be considered in a sexual harassment training program is offered here. First, one needs to include a review of the supervisor's role. For the supervisor, it will serve as a good reminder of the responsibilities to *all* of his subordinates; for the naive woman, it will serve as a guide for establishing her expectations of a good supervisor. It should make all aware of the areas in which the supervisor has legitimate control. Men supervisors need to be helped to treat women as all other employees, to expect the same work performance of all, and to use the same criteria for evaluation for all. Women need help understanding that they can control their own personal lives and that they can refuse to accept control of non-job-related segments of their lives. They have choice.

Second, both men and women need to recognize their own sexual needs. They may be giving off signals unconsciously—have their "motor running." One needs to be fair with oneself. One needs to decide how one wants to behave in relation to goals and expectations on the job, and then be that way consistently.

Third, all need to do their work well, without depending on "connections" or favors on or off the job. If one decides to develop a special relationship with another employee on the job, then one must be aware of the risks involved and the implications for working relationships.

Fourth, help participants learn to identify potential sexual harassment situations and avoid trouble. Both men and women need to identify potential harassers. Secure people do not have to push themselves. Co-workers need to speak up in defense of victims and confront harassers. Code of conduct and maybe even dress guidelines can be worked out by employees within an agency to help in this area. Certainly, all are to be encouraged to avoid touching another except on socially accepted areas of the body, that is, the hands, elbow, or shoulder, and then primarily to gain a person's attention. Hall defines one's personal space as being about $1^{1}/_{2}$ to 4 feet about one's body.[33] It seems to be a good idea to follow that guideline and give everyone their personal space.

VERBAL ABUSE

"All of us (nurses) were so glad to see the doctor take her (another nurse) in the supervisor's office to bawl her out—the patients couldn't hear him from there. It wasn't her fault, and she didn't deserve such a blast. She looked absolutely crushed and all slumped over when they came out of the office. She was so upset she didn't come to work the next day."

"I work for a surgeon in his office. I was talking on the phone to one of his patients—I know she could hear him—and he just stood there shouting all sorts of obscenities at me. He wanted me to do six things at once, and, well, it was just absurd. I couldn't believe he could act so irrationally."

"The doctors have so much hostility toward us. Even the nice ones are capable of verbally attacking. It's so unexpected. It's really scary."

The above are just a few of the many testimonies that nurses have reported, examples of verbal abuse, a noisy, prolonged ranting that usually attends a berating. It is punitive and intended to be humiliating to the recipient. In the physician-nurse relationship, such abuse represents a gross misuse of power and status on the part of the physician, and demonstrates a need for understanding of interpersonal power struggles on the part of nurses. Two assumptions seem to be made by each participant. The male physician assumes he has a right to behave in this manner, and the female nurse assumes she must expect and endure this tirade. Also striking is the similarity in patterns of communication between this "abused nurse syndrome" and the battered wife syndrome as described by Martin.[34] This section develops this analogy and discusses remedies, suggested by Martin for the battered wife, that may also be useful in combating nurse abuse.

First, there is a similarity in the psychologic basis of the battering husband and the abusing physician. According to Martin, the intrapersonal dynamics that arouse the battering husband's behavior are a strong dependency need that has shifted from the mother to the wife. The battering husband experiences the inner conflict of being hostile to the wife, yet dependent upon her emotionally. Thus, the husband has a need to hold the wife in rigid control as long as his dependency needs are satisfied in the relationship.[35] In the physician-nurse relationship, the physician is dependent upon the nurse to provide information, skills, and services. His professional practice and reputation are at risk in this relationship if the nurse does not function. Like the battering husband, then, the abusing physician may be hostile and seek to control the nurse, apparently to be assured that his professional dependency needs will be met.

Second, the underlying personality and life experiences of the battering husband and the abusing physician also seem analogous. Martin describes the battering husband as a psychopath who is aggressive, dangerous, and deeply immature. He has learned that violence is the way to respond to stress in his personal life or to threats to his identity. Typically, Martin states, the middle-class male is most likely to be a battering husband who quickly regains control and seeks to re-establish the relationship. The battering husband typically has been a battered child, and 90 percent have been in the military and/or police force. In short, they have received training in aggressive behavior and they HAVE BECOME IM-MUNE TO THE PAIN OF OTHERS.[36] Physicians tend to be similar to battering husbands in that they also tend to be socially immature and aggressive. If not learned earlier, this behavior can be learned by the middle-class man as he progresses through medical school and internships in which stress and threats to identity are common experiences. A frequent complaint of families, clients, ministers, and nurses today is the great insensitivity physicians have to others' distress. The emphasis in medical schools on biologic pathology, and the exclusion of the humanities from the curriculum probably contribute to this pattern.

What, then, tends to trigger the attacks? Martin found no apparent trigger is necessary. It is simply a violent, irrational outburst on the part of the battering husband. The wife never threatens the husband; in fact, the husband may begin beating his wife as she sleeps. The outbursts seem to be attempts to force deference in the wife's behavior. Asian wives of American soldiers have an unusually high incidence of battering; these women are known for their deferent ways. Apparently, subservient behavior by these wives "calls out" battering behavior by the husbands. Yet, Martin found that if wives do not assume themselves inferior, the husbands feel they have to beat the wives down to size.[37] Erich Fromm states that the more powerless a person is, the more likely one is to compensate for one's weakness by sadism. One may even risk one's life for a moment of absolute power. Thus, the other person must be made helpless and weak.[38]

In the physician-nurse relationship, nurses are perceiving themselves as equal to physicians; perhaps the abusing physician feels a need to "beat the nurse down to size." Physicians do have sufficient reason to feel threatened in their professional roles. The practice of medicine is becoming continually more complex as third-party payments, government restrictions, and regulations increase. Physicians are meeting rejection and distrust more often than previously by a more knowledgeable public that is becoming less impressed by the quality of care received in relation to the cost of that care. Currently, there is an oversupply of physicians in our country. This has economic implications for the physicians as they view the expansion of nursing practice into areas of health care previously considered their territory. For example, in the 1981 American Medical Association Convention, there was considerable discussion of how to prevent nurses from performing the physical examination of clients . . . a health assessment practice now considered necessary to provide an adequate data base for developing nursing-care plans.[39] Thus, the physician may very well be experiencing feelings of powerlessness, and the compensatory mechanism of sadism may suddenly surface under the pressures and risks of contemporary medical practice. Physicians may thus be disposed to become nurse abusers.

At the heart of the matter is the male-female role perception. According to Martin, as long as the husband perceives his wife as chattel, he will believe he has a right to make all decisions and to mete out punishment.[40] The battering relationship will continue until he sees his wife as a person in her own right. Thus, the only solution for the battered wife, according to Martin, is to assert herself; as long as she continues to show deference, the expectation is that she will continue to be battered.[41] Perhaps this solution is also applicable for female nurses in the physician-nurse relationship.

The key to change is the woman's perception of having options. Martin states that as long as the woman remains isolated, trapped by fear, and perceives this problem as being her own, she will tend to stay in the battering relationship. When the wife can perceive that others share her problem, that it is a common problem imposed on the wife by artificial and ill-applied expectations of society and that she has a right to a better life, then will she be able to change.

The perception of the nurse is similar. As a professional person, the nurse feels she has limited options, feels isolated, and is frightened. Society generally expects one professional to act respectful to other professions. It is a shock to see a physician rant and rave. And the nurse is not only made aware of her subordinate role as a child-woman, but also is made aware that the physician has political power enough to have her fired if she retaliates in kind.

The primary theme in all correctives offered by Martin and others seems to us to be that nurses need to support one another. The most common complaint from nurses is that their head nurses or supervisors too often do not believe and do not back up the staff nurses caught in a power play or a manipulative pattern of behavior. Wagner reviews strategies of dismissal as a corrective to avoid personal abuse, and they appear to be appropriate for avoiding verbal abuse, too.[43]

There seem to be degrees of hate and hostility in relationships between men and women as individuals and collectively. While extremes of femicide and rape are blatant and overt examples of male hostility toward women, it is the covert and subtle expression of hostility, sexist values, and attitudes that keeps professional women, nurses, subordinated to men. This represents a relatively new area of interpersonal communication problems that are known to alienate nurses. The degree to which professional men, physicians, tend to so alienate professional women, nurses, to that degree there will tend to be closed communication between them, to the detriment of their clients.

SUMMARY

Of the many potential barriers to interpersonal communication in the nursing profession, at least four are important enough to deserve special consideration. This chapter discussed (1) interpersonal distrust and its consequence—defensive communication behavior, (2) prejudicial gaps between groups and between cultures, (3) social alienation, and (4) sex-role problems. It also suggested that cultural prejudice and gaps between groups and between cultures are natural but not necessary. Certain ways of overcoming prejudice are available to those who wish to reduce this barrier. Such an achievement is rarely easy; in any case, it takes determination and strong resolve.

This chapter has described the way individuals are sometimes influenced to withdraw from interaction with others. The process has been discussed in terms of social alienation, and it was suggested that such withdrawal can be the result of prior communication experiences, particularly continued communication denial and abuse based on sex role assumptions. Appropriate changes in one's communication behavior are more easily achieved if one has good insight into the need for such changes. This chapter attempted to provide the basis for such insight.

REFERENCES

1. P. WATZLAWICK, J. H. BEAVIN, AND D. D. JACKSON: *Pragmatics of Human Communication* (New York: Norton, 1967), pp. 80–93.
2. J. R. GIBB: "Defensive Communication," *Journal of Communication*, 11, No. 3 (September, 1961): 141–148.
3. C. R. ROGERS: *Client-Centered Therapy.* (Boston, Mass.: Houghton Mifflin Co., 1951), pp. 515–520.
4. J. R. GIBB: "Climate for Trust Formation," in L. P. BRADFORD ET AL, EDS.: *T-Group Theory and Laboratory Method* (New York: Wiley, 1964), pp. 279–309.
5. GIBB: "Defensive Communication," p. 148.
6. K. GIFFIN: "Interpersonal Trust in Small-Group Communication," *Quarterly Journal of Speech*, 53, No. 4 (December, 1967): 224–234.
7. R. LITTON: *The Cultural Background of Personality* (New York: Appleton, 1945), pp. 39–74.
8. S. FELDMAN: *Cognitive Consistency* (New York: Academic, 1966), pp. 45–57.
9. B. KUTNER, C. WILKINS, AND P. YARROW: "Verbal Attitudes and Overt Behavior Involving Racial Prejudice," *Journal of Abnormal and Social Psychology*, 47 (1952): 649–652.
10. J. P. LYSAUGHT: *From Abstract to Action: Report of National Commission of the Study of Nursing and Nursing Education* (New York: McGraw-Hill Book Company, 1973); T. R. TIRNEY AND N. WRIGHT: "Minimizing the Turnover Problem: A Behavioral Approach," *Supervisor Nurse*, 8 (August, 1973): 47, 50, 53–57; and G. P. FOURNET, M. K. DESTEFANA, AND M. W. PRYER: "Job Satisfaction: Issues and Problems," *Personal Psychology*, 19 (No. 2, Summer, 1966): 165–183.
11. M. BUBER: "Distance and Relation," *Psychiatry*, 20 (1975): 97–104.
12. WATZLAWICK ET AL: *Pragmatics of Human Communication*, pp. 86–90.
13. R. D. LAING: *The Self and Others: Further Studies in Sanity and Madness* (London: Tavistock, 1961), pp. 135–136.
14. G. BATESON, ET AL: "Toward a Theory of Schizophrenia," *Behavioral Science*, 1 (#4, October, 1956), pp. 251–264.

15. D. JACKSON: "Psychoanalytic Education in Communication Processes," *Science and Psychoanalysis*, 5 (1962): 129–145.
16. B. W. GRANT AND K. GIFFIN: *A Survey of Expressions of Anger and Job Turnover Among Registered Nurses*. (Lawrence, Kan.: Communication Research Center, University of Kansas, R/44/1978).
17. GIFFIN: "Social Alienation . . ." *Quarterly Journal of Speech*, pp. 347–357.
18. GRANT AND GIFFIN: "A Survey of Anger . . .", 1978; B. W. GRANT: "Anger, Cohesiveness, and Productivity in Small Task Groups" (unpublished doctoral dissertation, University of Kansas, 1978), *Dissertation Abstracts*, 1979, *39* (January) 3916A (University Microfilms International No. 7824799); B. W. DULDT: "The Effect of Training in Coping with Alienating Co-workers on Job Turnover and Attitudes: A Pilot Study Report" (Memphis, Tenn.: Memphis State University, Department of Nursing, 1981, an unpublished report); B. W. DULDT: "Anger: Are Nurses Different than Non-nurses?" (Memphis, Tenn.: Memphis State University, 1981, an unpublished report), HOEKELMAN: "Relationships," 1975; STEIN: "The Game," 1969; BONNIE W. DULDT: "Anger: An Occupational Hazard for Nurses," *Nursing Outlook*, 29, No. 9 (September, 1981): 510–518; BONNIE W. DULDT: "Anger: An Alienating Communication Hazard for Nurses," *Nursing Outlook*, 29, No. 11 (November, 1981): 640–644; "Commentary," *Nursing Outlook*, 30, No. 2 (February, 1981): 84–85; BONNIE W. DULDT: "Helping Nurses to Cope with the Anger-Dismay Syndrome," *Nursing Outlook*, 30, No. 3 (March, 1982): 168–174.
19. GRANT AND GIFFIN: "A Survey of Anger," 1978.
20. GRANT: "Anger, Cohesiveness and Productivity . . .", 1977; K. GIFFIN AND B. W. GRANT: "Communication of Anger" (Lawrence, Kan.: The Communication Research Center, University of Kansas, 1977) KU/CRC/77/10/P/42.
21. *Ibid.*
22. B. R. PATTON AND B. RITTER: *Living Together . . . Male/Female Communication*. The Interpersonal Communication Series of 8 volumes edited by B. R. Patton and K. Giffin (Columbus, Ohio: Charles E. Merrill Publishing Company, 1976).
23. M. B. KANTER: *Men and Women of the Corporation* (New York: Basic Books, 1977).
24. J. A. ASHLEY: *Hospitals, Paternalism and the Role of the Nurse* (New York: Teachers College Press, Columbia University, 1976).
25. *Summary of the Public Hearings, National Commission on Nursing*, Marjorie Beyers, R.N., Ph.D., Director (Chicago: The Hospital Research and Education Trust, July, 1981). This is an independent commission sponsored by the American Hospital Association, Hospital Research and Educational Trust, and the American Hospital Supply Corporation.
26. G. A. WOLF: "Nurse Turnover: Some Causes and Solutions," *Nursing Outlook*, 29 (April, 1981): 235.
27. R. S. SIMMONS AND J. ROSENTHAL: "The Woman's Movement and the Nurse Practitioner's Sense of Role," *Nursing Outlook*, 29 (June, 1981), p. 373.
28. MACKINNON: *Sexual Harassment*, p. 33.
29. BONNIE WEAVER DULDT: "Sexual Harassment: An Alienating Communication Hazard for Nurses (Report of a Survey)." Paper presented at the Tennessee Nurses' Association Conference on Research, "Spring Gathering '81," Nashville, Tenn., April, 1981; BONNIE W. DULDT: "Sexual Harassment in Nursing:

Another Alienating Communication Hazard," *Nursing Outlook* 30, No. 6 (June, 1982): 336–343.

30. *Ibid.*
31. *Ibid.*
32. MacKinnon: *Sexual Harassment.*
33. E. T. Hall: *The Hidden Dimension* (Garden City, New York: Doubleday, 1969).
34. D. Martin: *Battered Wives* (New York: Pocket Books, 1977).
35. *Ibid.*, p. 47.
36. *Ibid.*, pp. 49–54.
37. *Ibid.*, p. 69.
38. A Reif: "Erich Fromm on Human Aggression," *Psychology Today* (April, 1975): 22.
39. "Threatened Professions," *Health Planning and Manpower Report*, 10 (Convention Report, 1981), pp. 5, 6.
40. Martin: *Battered Wives*, pp. 73–87.
41. *Ibid.*, pp. 149–174.
42. *Ibid.*, pp. 160–162.
43. J. Wagner: "Strategies of Dismissal: Ways and Means of Avoiding Personal Abuse," *Human Relations*, 33, no. 9 (September, 1980): 603–622.

11
INTERVIEWING: PULLING IT ALL TOGETHER

The interpersonal communication that occurs between a nurse and a client is the very core of nursing. This book has emphasized the communing, the humanizing factor of interpersonal communication, and its importance in nurse-client relationships. The interpersonal communication with one's peers and colleagues is of equal significance throughout one's career in nursing. A very pragmatic and utilitarian label can be applied to all of this: interviewing. It is proposed that interviewing can be the means of implementing humanizing interpersonal communication and can be the epitome of humanistic nursing communication. This is where nurses can get it all together and make special things happen between people.

Interviewing is defined by the dictionary as a face-to-face meeting arranged for a formal discussion of some matter or issue.[1] The word interview is derived from the Latin words "entre," meaning "mutually" and "each other," and from "videre," meaning "to see."[2] Communication scholars Downs, Berg, and Linkugel state, interviewing

> is basically a specialized pattern of verbal interaction. It is specialized in that there is a specific purpose for initiating the interaction and there are specific content areas to be explored. The interview differs from ordinary conversation in that we expect more control to be exercised in the interaction, that extraneous matter be excluded, and that the interviewer-interviewee role relationship be maintained.[3]

Typically, the interview involves only two people, a dyad. Additional people increase the complexity of the relationships among the participants; thus, three or more people often are labeled a.group or a conference. This discussion of interviews will center on dyads, that is, the nurse and one other person.

There are many varieties of interviews. A few include counseling, appraisal, selection, discipline, and persuasive interviews.[4] In applying the nursing process, the health-history interview is the major tool nurses use to gather data about the client. The health-history interview data, with physical assessment data, provide the major data base upon which the nursing-care plan is developed. This is the initial meeting of two people, of the nurse and client, often strangers to one another. All the issues discussed previously in regard to interpersonal perceptions and orientations, environmental factors, and verbal and nonverbal messages come into play. All of the factors discussed in previous chapters regarding building relationships, communicating in groups and in public, and evaluating interpersonal communication can be applied to this interviewing process as implemented in nursing practice. Even the special problems that were considered are applicable too.

Nurses often function as employees in health facilities such as hospitals; as such, the nurse often participates in significant interviews within the organization of that agency. As an applicant for a position on the nursing staff, the nurse participates in the initial appraisal interview. Later, there are evaluation interviews in which the nurse may be either the superior or the subordinate. Certainly, there are daily interviews with peers and colleagues as one goes about the nursing process of assessment, analysis, implementation, and evaluation of nursing care for clients. Here, too, all of the issues and factors discussed previously about interpersonal communication are applicable.

Throughout all interviews, the nurse who chooses to communicate in a humanistic manner will be continually aware of the existential state of all human beings. This state involves being concerned about the process of being one's own self and of becoming one's ideal self, of having choice, and of being free, yet being responsible. It involves loneliness, pain, struggle, tragedy, dread, and uncertainty. It involves a search for meaning in one's own life and a sense of purpose for one's existence. Ultimately, it involves facing despair and death. All humans share this existential state. The nurse who chooses to communicate in a humanistic manner will be aware of the characteristics of humans that are uniquely relevant to nursing. These include living, communicating, negativing, inventing, ordering, dreaming, choosing, and self-reflecting.[5] Being aware of these aspects of human beings will make a special difference in the attitudes and patterns of interactions occurring in the interview process—the humanizing difference!

SEQUENCE OF THE INTERVIEW PROCESS

An interview can be divided into six sequential segments: introducing, focusing, contracting, communing, recording, and closing. This section briefly describes each segment.

INTRODUCING. Participants of any interview need to adhere to common social behaviors upon meeting. The ritualistic greetings, such as "Hello, how are you?", are important in validating the individual as a person worthy of respect and recognition. If the nurse has not met the client previously, then formal introductions are appropriate. The person in the role of interviewer usually assumes responsibility for selecting the site for the interview, for the comfort of the interviewee, and for providing an environment fostering privacy and lack of interruption. This introductory period often includes a bit of social "chit-chat" regarding noncontroversial topics. People can usually agree about the weather, but it is usually wise to avoid religion and politics as topics. If, for some reason, one finds that the interview will be late in starting, it is very considerate for the interviewer to greet the interviewee as soon as possible and briefly explain the delay, making whatever other arrangements are necessary because of the delay.

FOCUSING. Focusing involves identifying the purpose of the interview. Generally, the focus of the nurse is on the client as a whole. The purpose of the interview is to gather data about the client's health problem. As both individuals verbally and nonverbally interact to obtain information about the client's state of health, the client tends to focus on the immediate health problem. By focusing on the client as a total being, covert health problems may be identified by the nurse. In focusing on the client, the nurse then needs to limit comments that focus on one's own self. Counting the number of times one comments about oneself can be a simple index to the degree to which the focus remains on the client. The client needs to feel he or she has the total attention of the nurse.

CONTRACTING. Contracting is developing mutual agreements about the interview process generally. Specific agreements that often are made routinely involve roles, rules, costs, and decision making. The nurse may state the roles briefly: "I will help you if I can." "You tell me all you can about your health concerns and I will take note of the information." This requires self-disclosure on the part of the client, a behavior that requires trust of the nurse. How will this information be used? Who else will see it? The nurse needs to make some statement about these issues. Limitations for the interview, series of visits to the health agency, or other rules need to be agreed upon by both participants. Certainly, cost of the care to be received needs to be discussed early; this may be the responsibility of the nurse, or it may be taken care of by personnel in the business office of the agency. The client needs to know who is going to make the decisions. In a humanizing context, the client is encouraged to make final decisions regarding whether or not the health care or advice will be accepted partially or totally. The client needs to be made aware of this also. The client is to be viewed by the nurse as a holistic individual who has the power to cope and to make choices, who is an irreplaceable equal who is to be accepted with positive regard, empathy, and caring.

COMMUNING. Communing is the heart of the interviewing process. It involves intimate dialogue in that the nurse seeks to understand the client's "inner" and "outer" world. Often, communication techniques, such as restatement, rephrasing, and verifying, need to be used to assure accurate and complete information. Words chosen need to be those most probably understood by the client; too much mysterious medical terminology can be frightening. It is best to ask only one question at a time; asking two or three at once may tend to result in inaccurate or incomplete information.

As a rule, there is a format that is followed in interviewing, and this is true of the health-history interview used in nursing practice. While each nursing staff may have a specific format, the following one is typical of most:

1. Biographic information.
2. Immediate health problem.
3. Description of current illness.
4. Personal, social, work history.
5. Previous health problems.
6. Review of bodily systems.
7. Summary.

The physical assessment may be included in the review of systems, or it may be conducted a few minutes after the health history has been taken. One can expect to structure the health-history interview to a considerable degree around a format similar to this one.

RECORDING. Recording involves making a formal record of the interview. There are examples in the literature as well as in most clients' charts.[6] During the interview, the nurse needs to make brief notations of the client's health history and plan to write the history more fully as soon as possible after the interview. The notes need to be minimized during the interview so that the nurse may maintain eye contact with the client and demonstrate other nonverbal behaviors that indicate the client has the full attention and authentic concern of the nurse.

CLOSING. The end of the interview is usually signaled by the interviewer. The nurse might note that the allotted time has expired or that there are sufficient data to now develop a plan of care. The client may be given one last opportunity to add something. For example, the nurse may ask, "Is there anything else you would like to tell me or that you think I need to know?" In closing, it may be necessary to arrange for one or more subsequent interviews. When both the nurse and client are satisfied that all business is completed, then both tend to move once again to social rituals. A few minutes of social "chit-chat" immediately precede parting. Thus the interview ends. If the nurse has demonstrated behaviors that convey empathy and respect for innate human characteristics, then there is a high probability the client will feel a special bond of intimacy with "my" nurse.

SITUATIONS IN WHICH THE NURSE INTERVIEWS CLIENTS

The typical use of interviewing occurs when the nurse admits a client to a hospital or clinic and completes a health assessment. This includes collecting data through the physical assessment and the health-history interview. These data are then used as the basis of the client's nursing-care plan. To varying degrees, the physical assessment and the interviewing are repeated as needed in order to evaluate concurrently care given and/or to explore potential new health problems. Thus, each contact the nurse has with a client is essentially an interview for appraisal and for problem solving.

Some rather delicate situations truly test a nurse's interviewing skills. One is conducting an interview with a child. This situation becomes more complex because of the need to include one or both parents or responsible adults. The growth factor adds another dimension to the data needed in order to evaluate the developmental patterns of the child. The way one establishes rapport with a child differs considerably from the rapport-establishment process with an adult. Emotional responses are more spontaneous and overt than responses of an adult. If trust does not exist, a child does not try to feign trust as an adult might. Once a child distrusts an adult, a nurse, the relationship is seldom easily repaired with mere words, as might happen between adults. The nonverbal cues are particularly meaningful messages for the child, and a child senses the nurse's sincerity or insincerity. Nurses who have younger siblings or have had experience babysitting are at a definite advantage.

Other rather difficult situations involve sexuality. A nurse is often the first person to interview, collect evidence for police, and assess the injuries of rape victims. Nurses apparently have been aggressive in establishing rape crisis centers in many communities, and they have a good reputation for helping rape victims cope with the police, lawyers, and all. Clients who have venereal diseases need to be interviewed carefully in order to identify and locate all sexual contacts. These contacts need to be tested and perhaps treated for the venereal disease too. Naturally, people are reticent to reveal such personal information and jeopardize important, perhaps illicit, relationships. In public-health agencies, nurses often are assigned to conduct these interviews. And finally, the woman who seeks an abortion is also interviewed, often by a nurse, to adequately inform and prepare this client for the procedure. Special consideration is necessary for the legal and religious aspects relating to the fetus, as well as concern for the client and her needs and rights. These are all very difficult interviews and require considerable interviewing skill to reach the troubled and tramatized person within.

In all of these situations, nurses need to be particularly skillful in conveying empathy for the client. The awareness of the client as an existential being is primary to success in these more complex situations. Consideration of the client's feelings by the nurse is probably a major factor in generating trust and self-disclosure on the part of the client. The nurse needs a sense of "being with" rather than "looking at" the client.

Special Problems in Interviewing Clients

There are several problems of which the novice nurse interviewer may well be forewarned. One is the use of the interview format. One needs to become accustomed to one format and be able to use it easily. As one moves to another agency or begins to deal with a clinical specialty, however, there is often a need to change the format or to increase the depth of data collected in specified areas. Generally, if one becomes accustomed to one format, another can be mastered with a little practice and patience.

It is often difficult for nurses to find a place to interview clients in privacy and without interruption. A few, but not many, agencies provide private offices for nurses. Frequently, the client must be interviewed at the bedside or in full view of others in a clinic waiting room. Too often, only a thin curtain separates the nurse and client from others, so all that is said can be overheard by others. Only upon the insistence of nurses themselves can this situation be corrected.

Age often presents a unique problem in the nurse-client relationship. Older clients may comment on the youthfulness of the nurse, suggesting the nurse could be a child or grandchild. It may be difficult to disclose private information and to expect knowledgeable and skillful care from one so young. The older client may even seek to control the young nurse and establish a parent-child relationship. Clients the same age as the young nurse may find self-disclosure easier on the one hand, but may also attempt to influence the nurse by asking for special privileges, extra food, drugs, and the like. Both of these clients may tend to arouse feelings of self-consciousness and defensiveness on the part of the nurse. Depending on the relationship, the nurse may simply generalize the issue and proceed as usual: "Yes, a lot of the nurses here are quite young." Another approach is to confront and present reality: "I may seem like your (grandchild, sister, etc.), but I am not, am I? I am your nurse." Still another approach would be to focus on the client: "Tell me about your (child, grandchild, etc.). Do you miss 'em?" Certainly the nurse needs to be aware of one's own feelings and biases in dealing with this issue. Unfortunately, nurses age as fast as everyone else, and soon enough one is told how trustworthy one is because of one's mature appearance; some "mature" nurses really don't like to hear this either.

Certainly cultural, ethnic, and language differences between nurse and client produce difficulties. One Laotian family was told their child had cancer. They did not realize "cancer" in this case meant a terminal illness. Only when the mother sadly said she didn't think her son was improving very much did the nurse realize the misunderstanding. A teenaged mother was told to start feeding her baby cereal. After a short time the baby became ill. There were numerous trips to the emergency room for treatment of the baby's diarrhea and intestinal bleeding. The cause was a mystery until the nurse asked the mother to itemize what she had been feeding the baby—cornflakes and bran flakes! That's what "cereal" meant to her. The baby improved significantly as soon as the mother learned how to cook oatmeal.

One difficult problem is the client who rambles. Many people are not required by their life experiences to structure their communication toward a specific topic or period of time. They feel no obligation to use time carefully. Older people often ramble in their conversation, reminiscing, younger people ramble about their dreams and expectations. Still others continually talk about how bad or sad life is. In such situations, the nurse needs to be gently assertive and move on to the next topic. Somehow, in one's own unique way, this needs to be accomplished without communicating disrespect or disregard to the client.

A nurse may be so pressured by demands of the job that there is a tendency to skip details in order to "save time." The result tends to be superficiality in interviewing and an inadequate and perhaps inaccurate data base for development of the nursing-care plan. The "time saved" may lead to lost time for the client in terms of extra time required to regain one's health, and the costs of misguided care can be an unnecessary expense for the client. Nurses need to periodically review the nurse-client ratio existing in the clinical area in which they practice. Some hospital administrators have gradually increased the number of clients assigned to a nursing unit so that "cost effectiveness" is achieved. In some agencies, a nurse is routinely expected to be responsible for 75 to 100 patients on a busy medical-surgical area with only a few aides to assist. Certainly, this is an extreme case. The nurse is ultimately responsible for deciding what is a safe, workable nurse-client ratio and for being aggressive about implementing it. If nurses do not speak out, the public eventually will, through lawsuits against individual nurses or through legislation of safe ratios. If one feels pressed for time, look for correctives elsewhere, not at the health-history interview time.

Finally, some nurses feel the pressure to "do something" immediately about information obtained in a health-history interview. This is particularly true when clients ask for specific advice, such as what laxative to take or what foods have high salt content. If these questions are answered directly, important interview time will be used so that data-gathering time may be limited. In answering such questions, the nurse is really operating without an adequate data base. A nursing intervention needs to follow data collection and data analysis. Such questions can be noted, and the nurse might say, "I will be glad to help you in this area, but let's go on for now." The nurse may also ask for additional information: "Tell me more about why you believe you need a laxative," and "What is happening that makes you think a laxative is needed?" Responses to such questions may reveal data significant to the client's care.

Although a nurse can encounter many other problems while interviewing, these seem to be common ones, and nurses can prepare themselves to deal with them.

SITUATIONS IN WHICH THE NURSE IS INTERVIEWED

Interviewing plays a significant role in the development of one's nursing career. Those situations that are particularly significant are the initial appraisal interview when applying for a job, evaluation interviews for progression and promotion, and interviews as a witness in a court of law.

In these interviews, one hopes to be treated with equality and accepted as a holistic, irreplaceable individual with special power, that is, special knowledge and skills of a nurse. Unfortunately, this does not always happen. One needs to learn to recognize and expect dehumanizing treatment so that one is not caught off guard. Some interviewers are monologic, directive, and degrading. One's feelings may be disregarded, and the very purpose of the interview may be judgmental in nature. The nurse may experience feelings of isolation, helplessness, and powerlessness. Consequently, one needs to be prepared to choose; one may meet such situations with communicative behaviors conveying humanizing attitudes, or one may choose to respond in a dehumanizing manner. The wider one's range of communication skills, the more respect one will tend to receive. To be humanistic does not necessarily mean to be a pacifist; it means to be thoughtful and to care about human values and needs, including oneself.

When one applies for a position on a nursing staff, one can expect to be interviewed by persons who will be one's immediate superiors and perhaps one or more administrators within the nursing service organization. The nurse is primarily in the role of an interviewee, and one can expect to give information regarding educational and licensure qualifications as well as experience in nursing practice. It is wise to maintain a confidential professional dossier at a placement center, a service that is often available through one's college or university. A vita usually includes the following information:

Name.
Address, home and business.
Telephone, home and business.
Social security number.
Marital status and dependents (optional).
Date of birth.
Military service.
Health (limitations if any).
Education.
  Formal.
  Informal (workshops, seminars, etc.).
Professional experience.
Research.
Publications.
Papers presented at professional meetings.
Consultations.
Workshops or seminars presented.
Professional licensure (list states).
Professional affiliations and distinctions.
References (list names, addresses, and phone numbers.)
Miscellaneous.

One may request a letter from an employer or other appropriate individuals, having the letters sent directly to the placement center to be included in the dossier. This practice allows one to request only one letter of an employer rather than requesting a new letter for each new position. This dossier can be made available to potential employers, and it facilitates the application process considerably.

While one expects to give information about one's self, one can also expect to receive information about the agency generally; the interview need not be monologic or one-way. The size of the agency, the number of clients served, the services offered, the number and composition of the nursing and medical staff, and the philosophy and objectives of the agency are all vital facts to know. One can also expect to receive information about benefits received by professional nursing staff, such as salary, sick leave, health insurance, vacation, and educational and advancement opportunities. There should be available written job descriptions with criteria for advancement and promotion specified.

The nurse applicant also needs certain information to evaluate the status of nursing and nurses at this agency. One might take careful note of how equitably professional nurses' benefits compare with those of comparable professional staff, particularly in regard to parking space, food services, office or personal space, and manner of keeping personal records. For example, who has free parking spaces and who has to pay? Is the nurses' dining area segregated from others in some manner? Do head nurses have shared office space or only a locked drawer at the nurses' station? How does the office of the director of nursing services compare with that of comparable administrative personnel? Do nurses punch time clocks and line up in front of a business office window to receive their pay checks while other professionals merely sign in and receive hand-delivered paychecks? Nurse applicants need to evaluate the employer as critically as an employer evaluates the nurse applicant. If one chooses to make certain demands about benefits or courtesies, then the time to make these is prior to accepting the position. This initial appraisal interview needs to reveal significant information to be considered by both parties.

Being interviewed by lawyers while serving as an expert witness in a court of law requires special preparation by the nurse. According to Dan Norwood, attorney, a good expert witness needs to be aware of several factors.[7]

First, one needs to be sure to obtain as much information as possible about the case before deciding to give an expert opinion. This requires careful interviewing skills on the part of the nurse. While one has a professional obligation and a duty as a citizen to serve, it is appropriate for a person to decide not to serve. However, one does not always have choice; lawyers can subpoena the nurse, and thus one is required by order of the court to testify. In the event this occurs, the nurse may need protection. One's job may be endangered if one must testify against the best interests of one's employer. There may even be need for protection from bodily harm. And one may be sued by someone associated with the case who may be disadvantaged in some way by the nurse's expert testimony. In order to provide protection for oneself, the nurse may be well advised to seek legal counsel of one's own.

Second, one can expect the opposing lawyer to seek to discredit one's expertise. Prior to the trial, the expert witness can expect to be interviewed extensively by the opposing lawyer; this is called taking a deposition. The nurse needs to prepare as well for this interview as for the one later on the witness stand. The deposition is taken under oath and is transcribed by a court reporter, just as the interview on the witness stand. In the deposition, the topics covered tend to be much broader in scope than the examination in court—a fishing expedition. The opposing lawyer will seek to find inconsistencies between the testimonies. And discrepancies found can be used to discredit the nurse as an expert; the nurse can thus be impeached as a witness.

If the nurse as an expert witness uses any other authority, such as an author of a nursing textbook, as a basis of judgment, it is important that one become knowledgeable of the entire text and of all the theories and opinions of that author. If upon examination, the nurse admits to disagreeing with the author on one point, then this also destroys the credibility of the author the nurse has chosen, and ultimately that of the nurse as an expert witness, too.

Another way of discrediting the nurse as an expert witness is to suggest a hypothetical situation and ask the nurse to give an opinion. If one does not ask for all critical factors in the hypothetical situation, the nurse may inadvertently contradict previous statements. For example, if the opposing lawyer describes a situation in which a patient is in the hospital for serious heart surgery and asks the nurse how often the patient needs to be checked by a nurse, the nurse witness needs to determine all the facts before answering carefully. One needs to ask at what point, before or after surgery, is the checking to be done by the nurse? One might also ask how long after surgery the checking is to occur, if that is the case, and whether or not complications are present. The nurse as expert witness needs to have complete information before offering an opinion on a hypothetical question.

Third, the nurse as expert witness needs to listen carefully to the questions asked and give only the information requested. If one has a tendency to "show off" one's expertise in such a situation, there is a possibility that one can inadvertently give conflicting testimony and discredit oneself.

It is important that the nurse realize the interviewing process by a lawyer in a court of law is dialogic or two-way. The expert witness can ask questions of the lawyers to clarify their questions and remarks. It is important that as an expert witness, the nurse interview the lawyers, too, and become aware of all the information relevant to the case.

Finally, it is imperative that the nurse not discuss the case or one's own testimony with anyone prior to the trial. The case may be so damaged by such discussions that the rights of the parties involved may be infringed upon and limited. Expert witnesses need to be particularly careful about maintaining silence around news reporters. While it is an honor to be recognized as an expert in nursing, this honor brings with it added responsibility and accountability for confidentiality.

Special Problems Nurses Encounter
in Career-Related Interviews

Several aspects of interviewing can have an adverse effect upon one's career progression if one is not prepared to anticipate and cope with these. One problem is that most interviews related to practice do not have a format, at least one that is shared with the interviewee. The agendas of interviews and conferences related to care of clients are focused on applying the nursing process; the agenda develops according to the clients' needs or problems. Nurses usually expect this.

However, for evaluation, retention, and progression interviews, formats are not known to the interviewee. As an employee, one can expect to have one's performance compared with written criteria. Often, individualized objectives are identified jointly by superior and subordinate. It is reasonable to expect corrective criticism of one's performance at the time it is needed and to see that event have an influence upon one's quarterly or semiannual evaluation. This does not always happen. Some supervisors seem to have no criteria, do not use participative management or management by objectives styles of leadership, and tend to "gunnysack" all criticisms until the evaluation conference or "dumping ceremony." This is degrading treatment of any employee, shows disregard for the individual nurse, and is careless leadership behavior. One needs to report such unfair treatment as a grievance.

Unfortunately, in many health agencies, there is no administrative means for nursing staff to report grievances or recommendations with the same ease with which a nurse reports medication errors, malfunctioning equipment, or people falling out of bed. The nurse who alone submits grievances or recommendations for improvements needs to realize this act places one in the position of being a "whistle blower."[8] Employees who blow the whistle on employer practices have been found to have short tenures. Employers quickly rid themselves of these individuals who can be labeled troublemakers or dissenters. It is far better for two or more nurses to submit grievances or recommendations that may be viewed as controversial. Collectively, there is more power and influence so that these unpleasant messages cannot easily be disregarded by employers.

EXIT INTERVIEWS. Exit interviews are frequently, but not always, conducted by a member of nursing service administration or a member of the personnel director's staff with nursing staff members who resign. Administrators need to know whether or not some current management or utilization of human resources practices has created a work environment sufficiently alienating to precipitate a nurse's decision to leave. Often there is an interview format that serves as a guide to the interviewer, and the nurse is often asked to respond to a special exit questionnaire that may cover a wide range of topics, often including communication.

While it is easy to be complimentary about good experiences, many nurses feel hesitant to be truthful about dehumanizing experiences since a letter of reference is often needed to obtain one's next position in nursing. It is easy to indicate that everything is fine and no change is needed and to quickly take leave of a truly bad situation. That's the easy way out. What is needed, however, is an authentic disclosure of feelings and facts about any alienating and dehumanizing aspects of the nurses's role in that institution. This is necessary for change to happen. This risky business of self-disclosure takes courage, and responsible administrators need to know what is wrong. Comments of one nurse can be discounted, but if the majority of nurses who resign report similar experiences, the issues cannot be ignored. Exit interviews can be a very effective way of having an influence and making a difference. Indeed, nurses might request the initiation of exit interviews if these are currently not being used.

HUMANIZING VERSUS DEHUMANIZING

The way one communicates makes a difference—a humanizing difference! If one wishes to incorporate humanistic values in one's career and wishes to practice humanizing interpersonal communication, then one seeks to become a humanistic nurse and to practice humanistic nursing. It is proposed that this involves three major factors. First, one needs to become increasingly sensitive to the existential state of human beings. Second, one needs to be able to demonstrate communication behaviors that convey attitudes which humanize rather than dehumanize; one needs to view people as valuable and powerful human beings rather than as things to be used. Third, one needs to develop patterns of interaction that, when applied skillfully and wisely, interact strongly with one's attitudes to have a significant and positive impact on relationships, on the way people feel about themselves and one another. All three of these factors need to interact to help the nurse know how to help oneself, one's clients, and one's peers. These three factors also need to interact to help the nurse protect oneself and others, and to cope effectively with dehumanizing situations.

REFERENCES

1. WILLIAM MORRIS, ED: *American Heritage Dictionary of the English Language* (Boston: Houghton-Mifflin Company, 1969), p. 686.
2. *Ibid.*
3. CAL W. DOWNS, DAVID BERG, AND WIL A. LINKUGEL: *The Organizational Communicator* (New York: Harper & Row, 1977), p. 49.
4. *Ibid.*, p. 50. For further reference, see CAL W. DOWNS, G. PAUL SMEYAK, AND EARNEST MARTIN: *Professional Interviewing* (New York: Harper & Row, 1980).

5. See Chapter 1, pp. 7–9.
6. ARLYNE SAPERSTEIN AND MARGARET A. FRAZIER: *Introduction to Nursing Practice* (Philadelphia: F. A. Davis Company, 1960), pp. 280–288; LOIS MALASANOS, VIOLET BARKAUSKAS, MURIEL MOSS, AND KATHERYN STOLTNBERG-ALLEN: *Health Assessment* (St. Louis: C. V. Mosby Company, 1981), pp. 35–57.
7. DAN NORWOOD, Attorney-at-Law, Memphis, Tenn.: Private interview, March, 1982.
8. LEA P. STEWART: "Whistle Blowing": Implications for Organizational Communication," *Journal of Communication,* 30 (1980): 90–101.

12
THE FUTURE
OF HUMANISTIC
NURSING

One of the mysteries that has intrigued human beings for centuries is the future. What is going to happen? The well-known futurist Alvin Toffler has made some predictions of particular relevance to nursing. A few years ago, Alvin Toffler was the keynote speaker at the National League for Nursing convention in Atlanta.[1] He made some fascinating statements, and presented a challenge to nursing.

Alvin Toffler stated that there has been more change in health care in the last 5 years than in the last 50. Some areas of change include (1) development of self-help groups; (2) the awareness of the environment and its impact on people's health status; (3) the shift of emphasis toward prevention rather than cure; (4) the changing perception of the physician's role as exemplified in such movies as "Hospital" and "Coma"; and (5) healthcare decisions being made by laymen, not professionals alone. It might be noted that most of these predictions have already been experienced by many practitioners of nursing. He described the systems of society as changing so fast that they are in a state of terminal crisis—systems of services, energy, family, communication, economy, and health care. The rate of change is reflected *to* nursing *from* society. There is less time for professionals to develop relationships with clients in hospitals, clinics, and physicians' offices. Professional personnel turnover rates are high. Consequently, relationships tend to be temporary and transient. People are pressured to make more decisions, faster, and with less validated information than in the past. As he ended his speech, titled "Nursing Encounters of a Future Time," Toffler challenged the nurses to take control of change and influence *now* health care in the year 2000. "Nursing education," he said, "is the lever for the future—*use* it!" Apparently, Toffler is not pessimistic about the future because he also stated the changes being experienced can lead to richer systems, a healthier society, and a better chance of surviving. People simply are not ready now to cope with change. They need new ways of solving complex problems, new political systems, and new knowledge and specialists in the health-care system. For individuals, the primary cure, he believes, is learning. "The people who think ahead, these people will decide (the future)." This is the most unique ability among all living beings, to be sensitive and responsive to change. Nurses, both in their professional role and as human beings, have the power to influence the direction of change in health care and nursing care over the next two highly turbulent decades. Nurses cannot risk leaving their future to luck, chance, or fate. They need to take up the challenge of meeting health-care needs and deliberately focus their learning, consider alternatives, and choose deliberately the way they believe health care and nursing should become. Then nurses can work toward closing the gap between what exists today and their goals for the future.

But if learning is the cure to survival and the key to a richer nursing-care and health-care system, then *what* must nurses learn? One key to learning is improved communication, particularly in that it is the key to humanizing relationships between people. Failed communications and dehumanization are identified by Leventhal[2] as major problems of health care in particular. For correction, Leventhal believes major organizational changes are not necessary in the health-care system. He states the problems can be solved by individuals developing the ability to communicate interpersonally with others in a humanistic manner. The individual practitioner and the way in which one communicates need to change.

In this book, interpersonal communication skills have been presented. Through use of these skills, the nurse can develop an awareness of one's own interpersonal influence. We believe this can be accomplished to such an extent that the nurse can *deliberately* choose to intervene in a client's (or others') situation so that predictable and positive results can be obtained.

ASSUMPTIONS

Based on discussions presented throughout this text, the following statements are presented as assumptions of humanistic nursing communication.

1. Human beings exist in a "here-and-now" existential context from which there is no escape.
2. Human beings function as a unique, whole system responding openly to the environment.

3. Survival is based on one's ability to communicate with others in order to share feelings and facts about the environment and coping.
4. The environment is a "booming, buzzing" world of strange sensations, which must be sorted out to determine which are most important; this sorting is achieved through communication with people.
5. The need to communicate is an innate imperative for human beings.
6. Owing to innate fallacies, human beings use and misuse all capabilities, especially the ability to communicate. (An example is speaking to a person as if the person were a thing.)
7. Human beings are continually concerned with certain existentialist elements such as being, becoming, choice, freedom, responsibility, solitude, loneliness, pain, struggle, tragedy, meaning, dread, uncertainty, despair, and death.
8. The way in which one communicates determines what one becomes.
9. All elements of existential beings and the communication imperative are salient issues to be dealt with in critical life situations.
10. The purpose of nursing is to intervene to support, maintain, and augment the client's state of health.
11. Nursing is primarily concerned with communing, caring, and coaching clients in critical life situations. (The term coaching here is used to indicate the planning, teaching, and encouragement of clients to maintain recommended health-care regimens. Critical life situations are those in which perceived threats to one's health state are salient.)
12. Interpersonal communication is an innate element of the nursing process (assessment, planning, implementation, and evaluation) and occurs between nurses and clients, nurses and peers, and nurses and professional colleagues.
13. The nurse shares with the client all characteristics of being human.
14. Humanizing patterns of communicating can be learned.
15. Evaluation of one's own communication skills is subjective; each individual must make one's own social decisions and choices about communication behaviors and choose to change, depending on one's ability to use feedback.
16. Growth and change arise from within the individual and to a considerable degree depend on one's choice.
17. Satisfaction and success in one's life and work or one's state of being are derived from one's feeling human.
18. Owing to the bureaucracy and complexity of the present health-care delivery systems, there is a tendency for clients and profes-

sionals to be treated in a dehumanizing manner and to relate to one another in a dehumanizing manner.

These, then, are assumptions upon which concepts of humanistic nursing can be based.

DEFINITIONS AND CONCEPTS ABOUT INTERPERSONAL COMMUNICATIONS IN HUMANISTIC NURSING

Interpersonal communication is defined as a "dynamic process involving continued adaptation and adjustments between two or more human beings engaged in face-to-face interactions during which each person is continually aware of the other(s)." Conceptually, the manner in which communication can occur is viewed as being on a continuum. This continuum extends from humanizing to dehumanizing ways of communicating.

Humanizing	-	Dehumanizing

To communicate in a humanizing manner generally means to be aware of the eight characteristics of a human being as defined in Chapter 1. To dehumanize is to ignore these characteristics. The polarized sets are:

Humanizing Elements	Dehumanizing Elements
Dialogic	Monologic
Individual	Categories
Holistic	Parts
Choice	Directive
Equality	Degradation
Positive regard	Disregard
Acceptance	Judgment
Empathy	Tolerance
Authenticity	Role-playing
Caring	Careless
Irreplaceability	Expendability
Intimacy	Isolation
Coping	Helplessness
Power	Powerless

1. *Dialogue versus Monologue.* Dialogic communication requires the nurse and client to genuinely listen to one another to say something new about one's own unique, here-and-now life situation.

Communication in dialogue is a humanizing, two-way interaction in which each person participates by sharing with another information about oneself as well as being open and responding to similar information shared by the other. Each is aware of the other's presence—of "being there" and "being with." It is an encounter that involves the interpersonal concepts of trust, self-disclosure, feedback, assertiveness and confronting. The nurse is involved on two levels: (1) as a unique human being and a warm, genuine person; and (2) as a responsible, accountable professional person making one's special knowledge and skills available to the client. The client is also involved on two levels: (1) as a unique human being and person experiencing some degree of experiential distress and struggling to cope in a critical life situation; and (2) as a client needing and, intentionally or unintentionally, seeking the special knowledge and skills provided by the nurse.

The polar opposite is monologue or a one-way interaction in which the nurse informs, directs, and instructs the client with minimal consideration of the client as an individual. A monologue encounter tends to involve distrust, lack of self-disclosure and feedback, submissiveness, and lack of confrontation. Personal involvement is minimal. The nurse is perceived as a closed, cold, role-playing individual; this tends to reduce for the client the general availability of the nurse's special knowledge and skills. The client tends to be viewed by the nurse as a problem or a disease entity requiring the nurse's professional attention. In the more technical clinical settings, the client is ignored as the nurse cares for the equipment attached to the client.

2. *Individuals versus Categories.* Individuality requires the nurse to be aware of the client as a unique, irreplaceable human being.

Individuality is the recognition of another as a person and choosing to enter into a meaningful interpersonal relationship. Treating a person as an individual involves the deliberate use of humanizing communication attitudes and patterns of communication. The nurse remembers seemingly minor details of care or preferences in routines—details that, when attended to without prompting, assure the client's self-perception as a person. In this way, the nurse validates the client as someone special.

The opposite is to categorize the client as one of a set, to whom nursing care, treatments, or procedures are applied with minimal variation in routine.

3. *Whole versus Part.* The element of holism requires the nurse to perceive the client as a complex totality of coherent characteristics (or systems) functioning together as one undiminished entity constituting the full of a person.

Holistic is a way of perceiving the client on two levels "all at once," as a total system of the whole and as a part that is a subsystem of the total. In providing care, the nurse necessarily focuses professional attention on a particular part(s) or subsystem(s) that is maladaptative. Simultaneously, the nurse also focuses both professional and personal attention on the organized set of parts or subsystems comprising the total human being, that is, a holistic view of one seeking to maintain a harmonious relationship with the environment.

The opposite of "holistic" is fragmentation of the person by focusing only on the malfunctioning part. For example, an intensive-care nurse may concentrate so intently on the tasks and procedures of caring for the client's body that one may experience some degree of surprise when the very ill client speaks, turns over, or initiates some independent action.

4. *Choice versus Directive.* Choice requires the nurse and the client to have freedom to consider alternatives and make decisions about issues encountered in the existential here and now.

Choice is a privilege and a responsibility for all human beings and is a key concept in existential philosophy. To be able to choose allows a human being to be more than merely a "reactor" to stimuli, but to be "actor," producing novelty and change in human behavior. Having thus initiated change, the human being is then accountable for the outcomes and consequences of decisions. In humanistic nursing, both the nurse and client as persons have choice in regard to whether or not to communicate, with whom, regarding what, and in what manner. The nurse as a knowledgeable professional has choice regarding decisions about care offered and provided for the client. The client has choice, to the extent of capabilities, regarding whether or not to accept the care offered and provided. And the nurse needs to validate that the client has knowledge of alternatives and consequences of choices and to respect and honor the client's choices.

The opposite of choice is directive. The nurse may dehumanize the client by issuing orders and expecting compliance, often without questioning the appropriateness or validity of the order. Some professional colleagues and perhaps the total health-care system may dehumanize the nurse and client by issuing directives and policies that limit unnecessarily professional and personal choices of the nurse and the options of health care for the client.

5. *Equality versus Degradation.* Equality requires the nurse to approach the client with an awareness that both are human beings sharing all characteristics of existential human and living in an inescapable "here and now."

Equality involves being aware that, beneath all of the roles, status symbols, positions, and classifications people use in presenting themselves to one another, all are united in being human. People share the struggles of essence or being that involve ambiguity, anxiety, pain, joy, grief, and loneliness. The nurse is privileged to "be there" in critical life situations that involve very human struggles with inescapable "here and now" threats to health, well-being, and life itself. Equality means to perceive oneself as one person, a nurse, standing beside another person, a client, looking together at a health-related problem, concern, or burden owned by the client, but shared; together nurse and client seek ways to solve the problem, alleviate the concern, or lift the burden . . . and endure the ambiguity.

The opposite of equality is degradation, a dehumanizing process of depriving another of due rank, honor, and status. Degradation means to perceive oneself as a nurse, standing before a client, and to perceive the client as a problem, concern, or burden—not as another person. The nurse seems to be above having such a problem. Thus, the nurse keeps a safe distance, physically as well as interpersonally, as if to avoid being contaminated by the client.

> 6. *Positive Regard versus Disregard.* Positive regard requires the nurse to label the client as potentially being capable of positive growth, of being able to cope, so that the client will tend to live up to this label.

Positive regard involves establishing an interpersonal climate that assumes the client does not like one's situation or problem. It also assumes the client is capable of choosing to improve one's life situation. The client is seen as having potential for growth and learning not only in relation to health care and maintenance practices, but also in relation to personal maturity. In such a climate, help can be extended to the client, and the client may move more readily into open communication patterns that include trust, self-disclosure, and feedback. According to Rogers and Truax,

> It involves as much feeling of acceptance for the client's expression of painful, hostile, defensive, or abnormal feelings as for his expression of good, positive, mature feelings. . . It is non-possessive caring for the client as a separate person. The client is thus freely allowed to have his own feelings and his own experiencing.[6]

Disregard is the dehumanizing opposite of positive regard. To communicate to a client with disregard is to assume the client prefers one's situation or problem and is incapable of improving. To provide more than minimal or routine help is believed relatively pointless; the client is seen as incapable of using the help. The client is socialized into a submissive, uncomplaining, manipulative "client role" with limited acceptance of expressions of feelings and needs in a closed communication system.

      7. *Acceptance versus Judgment.* Acceptance requires the nurse to establish a climate of psychologic safety and support so that the client perceives the nurse as a trustworthy listener.

Acceptance involves nurses receiving clients as they are, not for *what* they are, but for their potential.[7] It includes making favorable responses to clients' expressions of feelings, personal meanings, and attempts to change and cope. Clients need to feel free to risk revealing the positive as well as the awkward, unsuccessful, and negative side of themselves, knowing the nurse will acknowledge, agree, and welcome these things without denial, manipulation, or defensiveness. Acceptance is a restful state of being approved, believed, and acknowledged in one's own life situation. The effect of interpersonal acceptance is, for the nurse, recognizing the client as a unique self and, for the client, a releasing of the individual to self-disclose and trust.

Judgment is the dehumanizing opposite of acceptance and requires both the client and nurse to meet certain criteria in order to receive. For the client, one may need to be on Social Security or Medicare in order to qualify for certain types of nursing care. Or the nurse may need to behave in a certain manner in order to be worthy of receiving a particular privilege. Since one is continually aware of the other's role of judge, one is prone to compare what is received with that of others to determine one's own ranking in the regimented scheme of things. It makes a difference what or who one is. The threat of rejection is continual.

      8. *Empathy versus Tolerance.* Empathy requires the nurse to actively listen for significant cues communicated by the client in order to sense the client's view of the world, to anticipate feelings and reactions, and ultimately to assess needs.

Empathy is the nurse's ability to communicate understanding of the client and to demonstrate a sensitivity of one's current feelings, needs, and fears. This ability is achieved through selection of language, voice qualities, posture, gesture, and attitude. The nurse does not experience the client's feelings, but has an awareness, an anticipation, and an appreciation of the expression of feelings. The nurse is able to make relationships between the client's current health status, the progress of the client's response to therapy, and the impact of the nurse's own subsequent behavioral acts upon the client. As the recipient of empathy, the client is able to cope more easily with one's life situation and perceive the nurse as communicating, "I am with you." The client is subjectively aware of the nurse's "presence."

It is particularly discouraging and disappointing to expect empathy and to receive only tolerance. Here the nurse endures, bears, or puts up with the client. There is a lack of sensitivity to the client's feelings, needs, or fears. When the latter are expressed, the nurse may deny the importance or relevance of each. The nurse also tends to receive tolerance rather than empathy from superiors and colleagues in the health-care system. This feeling is particularly true in regard to discussions involving personnel policies, salary increases, and similar issues related to job satisfaction.

9. *Authenticity versus Role Playing.* Authenticity requires the nurse to be one's own self, openly and honestly a human being, nothing more or less, in interpersonal relations with others.

Authenticity is a personal recognition and acceptance of oneself as a human being, caught up in all the struggles, dilemmas, and contradictions characteristic of being human. It is recognition and study of one's own struggles with choice; of dilemmas with knowing perfection and being trapped in an animalistic-materialistic, time-space-bound world; and of inevitable contradictions of values, feelings, and behaviors. Authenticity excludes pretense and facades; rather, it involves honesty in personal feedback to self and others, as well as an openness and spontaneity of expressing feelings. Authenticity includes a commitment to communicating deliberately with responsibility and accountability interpersonally as a person having unique and singular capabilities, limitations, feelings, values, and perceptions.

The opposite of authenticity is role playing. Here the individual, whether client or nurse, is perceived interpersonally as if an empty shell of a person or as if hiding behind a facade. The client plays the "sick" role, seemingly for secondary gain. The nurse may act "professional" seemingly to protect oneself from becoming involved. One tends to wonder where the "real" person's values, feelings, and intentions truly lie.

10. *Caring versus Carelessness.* Caring requires the nurse and client to help one another struggle and strive, cope, and achieve in the human existential state through confirmation of being and understanding of feelings.

Caring is having a positive regard for another person so that one can accept the other as each grows, unfolds, and blooms in one's own unique way. It includes validating one another in worth of self, desires, beliefs, perceptions and feelings through a process of trust, self-disclosure, and feedback. Caring is not feminine in the sense of classic sex-role stereotypes of lover-wife-mother behavior. It excludes the classic male sex-role stereotype of unemotional stoicism, dominance, and competitiveness. Rather, it is one person caring for another, regardless of sex, because one has a stake in the other's fate. One gives of oneself or becomes involved to give out of one's strengths. One gives time, energy, attention, and thought to another's existence in order to promote and sustain that existence. In humanistic nursing, the nurse gives of personal and professional strengths and resources to help the client struggle and strive to survive illness (or to die, to let go), to heal, and hopefully, to achieve wellness of body and of spirit. And this caring is reciprocal. The nurse is able to study each existential relationship with clients, to mature in personal and professional resources, and to be validated in those communication and nursing skills and behaviors that prove most effective in achieving meaningful interpersonal relationships with clients and others. Each caring experience gives promise of another caring in the future for both nurse and client.

The dehumanizing opposite of caring is carelessness. There is, for the client and nurse alike, a tendency to be ignored and disregarded. For the client, it means carelessness in nursing care. Details of care are left undone; call lights are unanswered; medications are given erroneously if at all. It means losing personal items of clothing, dentures, or eyeglasses. And it means receiving salt on the low-salt diet tray. For the nurse, it means not being informed of a change in one's duty hours, not being relieved by another nurse for lunch or bathroom breaks, and having the guards refuse to provide escort service to one's car when leaving the hospital late at night. It just seems no one notices; people seem to care less about one another.

11. *Irreplaceable versus Expendable.* Irreplaceability requires the nurse to recognize one's own life as well as those of the clients and others as having intrinsic value.

Irreplaceable means human life cannot be replaced or substituted as one might replace a ballpoint pen. Each client is to be supported, maintained, and enhanced through respect and enhancement of self-concept, body image, and reality presentation. One's self-concept is the spirit and center of the human being. One's image of oneself, of one's body, and of one's life situation is heavily influenced by interpersonal relationships.[8] It is important that the nurse recognize one's own being as having intrinsic worth and value. The nurse needs to care for one's own self-concept, body image, and life situation. It is important to treat oneself in a humanistic manner by recognizing one's feelings and needs, learning to express positive as well as negative feelings, and meeting one's needs. It is recognizing one's own worth and irreplaceability to limit one's personal and professional commitments, responsibilities, and obligations to that degree at which one can function with optimal ease. To the degree this is accomplished, to that degree the nurse will tend to operationalize humanistic nursing.

To assume the human being is expendable is the ultimate in dehumanization. Clients come to be viewed by nurses as machinery on an assembly line in a factory. For a client to die would be the equivalent of relief from a taxing routine of trying to get the machine fixed. The death may hardly be noticed at the charge nurse's change-of-shift report. And the empty bed is quickly filled with another client. There begins for the nurse to be a quality of sameness about the clients. Little progress seems to be made, and the need of making any real effort to value human beings seems pointless. This is particularly true when the clients tend to be socially unattractive, such as the retarded, the mentally ill, the senile, and the chronically ill and disabled—the very people who need the extra dose of all humanizing elements identified here.

> 12. *Intimacy versus Isolation.* Intimacy requires the nurse to be receptive of clients' need for disclosure of personal feelings, perceptions, and experiences, especially those disclosures having relevance to health.

Intimacy is listening to another's self-disclosures and caring about the meaning and implications for the other's well-being.[9] It involves establishing an interpersonal climate of trust so that the risk of self-disclosure is minimized. In nursing, there is a social "permission" to disclose so that the health care might be based on all relevant information. Clients often disclose to nurses things never before revealed to others. The nurse needs to be committed to receiving clients' disclosures with respect in order to promote the client's interpersonal growth and to support the client's coping and adaptative processes. In nursing, intimacy also includes touching as one administers nursing care. Hall[10] (cited in Chapter 3) identifies intimate space as being up to 18 inches from one's body. He describes this interaction space as appropriate for lovemaking, comforting, protecting, struggling, and fighting. In the process of "laying on of the hands," nurses need to recognize the potentially powerful impact of invading clients' intimate space, and nurses need to use this to support the clients' well-being.

The dehumanizing opposite of intimacy is interpersonal isolation, which seems to be too often the experience of clients needing care and of nurses wanting to give safe, quality nursing care. The client finds oneself isolated from familiar faces and places while experiencing strange sensations and behaviors of one's body. While many people, nurses and others, may come near to perform certain tasks, too often it seems that no one, even the nurse, is able or willing to provide adequate information or answers to questions posed. And all quickly withdraw to other tasks, busily rushing down separate trails, hopefully coordinated in some unknown way—the so-called "team" approach. Very few of these people use one's name, and those who do often merely use it to check the identification bracelet; one becomes a bed or room number or a diagnosis. If one displays the normal symptoms of isolation, the nurses soon stop using the bed or room number and begin using labels such as "difficult," "problem," or "fussy." Because contact and responsibility are fragmented in the team or functional organization of nursing staffs, the individual nurses have limited opportunity to get to know the client, have limited power over what happens to the client, and feel frustrated professionally and very isolated personally, too.

13. *Coping versus Helplessness.* Coping requires the nurse to assess, support, maintain, and augment the client's abilities to achieve an optimum level of functioning in one's ongoing existential state.

Coping, according to the dictionary,[11] means to encounter problems and difficulties in such a manner that one is "on even terms with" or "is successful"; it is willingness to fight a battle. A person daily encounters problems and difficulties that require continuous striving, choosing, and doing. Coping permeates all areas of human life. The nurse is particularly concerned in determining the client's modes of coping as a living and subjective being. The goal of the nurse is to assist the client in achieving not only survival, but also the fullest expression of being human, even in dying.

Helplessness is the dehumanizing opposite of coping for both client and nurse. The client is helpless when without accurate and complete information on which to develop a plan of action. Without individualized guidance and support of the nurse and others, the client tends to feel overwhelmed and may not grasp the total situation and its implications. Panic tends to develop, along with anger and even revenge (I'll sue for this!) for the dehumanizing treatment. Distrust and rejection of all health-care professionals becomes common as clients turn to self-help groups who understand or to "quick-cure" commercial shams. The nurse feels helpless because of the responsibility for, yet inability to control, the nursing-care plan of even one client. Any decision about a client's care that one nurse makes will probably not be respected and followed by nurses on succeeding shifts in the typical hospital setting. Communication between the nurse and the client's physician tends to be very limited, so that the nurse is often unable to coordinate the nursing-care plan with the medical plan of care.

14. *Power versus Powerlessness.* Power requires the nurse to be accountable for personal and professional choices in one's own life and nursing practice, and to recognize the client's fundamental power and freedom as well as accountability for choice, particularly in regard to health-related issues.

Power requires accountability for one's conduct and obligations and for one's choices of right and wrong. It implicitly assumes responsibility for initiating change and being a cause of some event. One is responsible for one's own communicative behavior. In responsible interpersonal relationships, one evaluates feedback from others, becomes congruent with inner feelings, and changes if one chooses to do so. Responsible interpersonal relationships are at the core of humanistic nursing. Communicative acts on the part of the nurse are embodied in the nursing process and are significant factors in the individual client's plan of nursing care. The nurse needs to respect the client's power to choose and to be responsible for one's own choices. Equally, the nurse also needs to respect the client's feelings of dread, anxiety, and anguish which, inevitably for existentialism, follow choice.

Powerlessness is the dehumanizing opposite of power for both the client and nurse. The client is rendered powerless by nurses and others who ignore, do not consult, or even talk about him or her in the client's presence as if absent. The nurse who is moved from unit to unit to meet emergency staffing needs or who is manipulated (coerced) into working double shifts by the supervisor is as powerless as a tin soldier in a child's toy battalion.

INTERACTION (OR INTERDEPENDENCY) OF CONCEPTS OF COMMUNICATION IN HUMANISTIC NURSING

Concepts of communication in humanistic nursing are interdependent and reciprocal. To the degree one communicates with others in a humanizing way, one will tend to promote humanistic nursing. Some of these interdependencies are as follows:

1. To the degree one receives humanizing communication from others, one will tend to feel recognized and accepted as a human being.
2. To the degree a nurse uses humanizing elements to communicate, the nurse will receive humanizing communication from peers, colleagues, and superiors.

3. In a given environment, if a critical life situation develops for a client, to the degree the nurse uses humanizing communication while applying the nursing process, the health of the client will tend to move in a positive direction.

Trust, self-disclosure, and feedback represent the heart of humanistic communication, that is, communing. These three elements tend to covary: increase trust, and self-disclosure tends to increase, as well as feedback. Decrease any one of these three elements, and the others tend to decrease also. Thus, the following further interdependencies can be cited:

4. To the degree that trust, self-disclosure, and feedback occur, humanizing communication or communing also occurs.
5. In the event one tends to experience dehumanizing communication, for example, monologue rather than dialogue, categoric rather than individualistic, and so forth, then one tends to reciprocate.

With knowledge of both humanizing and dehumanizing communication, it can be assumed that nurses will tend to choose humanizing communication. The nurse can communicate by design in a humanizing way with more predictable results. Thus, a final interdependency of concepts can be cited:

6. To the degree that one is aware of one's own communication choices, one is able to develop communication skills and habits that tend to have predictable results in establishing and maintaining relationships.

Not all situations call for humanizing communication. A nurse may very wisely choose dehumanizing communication in talking to some individuals. For example, a young woman as a nurse may use dehumanizing communication to discourage a potential sexual harasser. If one chooses to discontinue a relationship, then dehumanizing communication attitudes and patterns will probably hasten the process. Nevertheless, in those relationships particularly relevant to providing care to clients, humanizing of communication seems to us to generally be preferable.

HUMANISTIC NURSING—PAST

With some variations, numerous nursing scholars and leaders tend to support the idea of humanistic nursing. Pilette[13] describes the nurse as a "humanistic artist" in an existential philosophic context, and she identifies the "nurse-client relationship as the cornerstone of the art of humanistic nursing." She further states:

> Art, our most basic birthright, can be traced to the Biblical character Phoebe and her charitable manner of ministering to the Romans. . . . In this humanistic era, it is fitting that nursing has reclaimed and updated its birthright. . . . The art of nursing has its deepest roots in the human care transaction and is confirmed in the dialogical process or 'I-Thou' relationship.[14]

This book has focused particularly on communication behaviors that seem to be most relevant to the current practice of nursing, that is, trust, self-disclosure, feedback, assertiveness, confrontation, and conflict resolution. LaMonica[15] specifically identifies positive attitudes as determinants of behaviors congruent with humanistic nursing. Also in this book, sets of humanizing and dehumanizing factors in humanistic communication in nursing have been identified and emphasized. LaMonica,[16] Flynn,[17] Blattner,[18] and Watson[19] describe and discuss nursing as being inherently humanistic. King and Gerwig draw on humanistic education and psychology to develop a perspective on humanistic nursing education. They state the following:

> Somewhere amidst all that equipment, behind all that SOAP charting, among all those nursing care plans, there is a human being—the patient. Have we become so involved in keeping up with the fast-paced technology and science of nursing and the hospital organizational routines, that we have lost sight of the art, the caring humanistic side of nursing?[20]

Many nursing authors describe the nurse and nursing as being inherently humanistic. King and Gerwig[21] state that nursing educators have the responsibility of establishing models of humanistic education and learning so that ultimately this philosophy will permeate nursing practice. Lambertson[22] identified principles of professional education for nursing in colleges and universities, which, according to King and Gerwig,[23] have led to the current humanistic educational goals as we know them today.

HUMANISTIC NURSING—FUTURE

If nursing is indeed inherently humanistic, then interpersonal communication, the very process of humanizing, needs to be highly developed as a major concept in the discipline of nursing. A humanistic definition of the human being, unique to nursing and not borrowed from other disciplines, needs to be a consideration in each plan of nursing care. Giuffra[24] stresses this need, and Travelbee[25] has moved in this direction. Roy[26] focuses on adaptation, Orem[27] on self-care, King[28] on goal-oriented care,

Newman[29] on movement, and Yura and Welsh[30] on nursing process. In each of these theories, the interpersonal communication occurring between the nurse and client is of paramount importance in order for the phenomenon of nursing to be operationalized. General reviews of the nursing literature tend to show that the most basic skill in assessment of clients' needs and use of the nursing process, whether in the context of primary nursing or the more traditional delivery systems, is interpersonal communication. Research has shown that nurses tend to limit the communication of the client by ignoring cues and important disclosures.[31] Faulkner[32] suggests that nurses not only need instruction in communication skills, particularly to become aware of the client's feelings, but also to assist in dealing with the results of such communing so that neither is harmed by the experience.

The humanistic definition of human being can be used in several ways in nursing practice and education. In developing nursing care, the characteristics of a human being (living, communicating, negativing, etc.) can be used as an organizing principle for the entire care plan, or, more easily, used as an additional check list to evaluate the comprehensiveness of care in meeting each need or solving each problem identified. The problem-oriented charting and the SOAPs can continue and may be improved. In nursing education, a theoretical framework based on needs, adaptation, or levels of care need not change, and the biophysical-psychosocial organization of nursing content need not be set aside. The humanistic description of human being is seen as a refinement of all of these perspectives of the client and as being compatible with holistic nursing. It represents one step further toward the establishment of humanistic, primary nursing care as a dominant force in the nursing discipline as discussed and advocated by Fagin.[33]

So what *is* humanistic nursing? How does one know when it has happened? Humanistic nursing is both a philosophic framework and a subjective interpersonal communication experience for the nurse and the client. As a philosophic framework, it is a strongly developed value system that focuses on a concern for human beings, quality of life, and enhancement of the process of being and becoming. As a subjective interpersonal communication experience, it can be identified as that nice, warm feeling arising from the innermost regions of one's body, perhaps accompanied by a long sigh of relief and relaxation. It usually occurs in a distressing situation and during special intimate communication with another person. One just knows it when it happens and it feels so right.

Many people choose the profession of nursing because they value human beings and seek this special subjective interpersonal communication experience with others. Both philosophically and subjectively, humanistic nursing has been nursing's history. It is being reclaimed as nursing's present. It *is* nursing's future.

REFERENCES

1. ALVIN TOFFLER: "Nursing Encounters of a Future Time," keynote speech presented at the National League for Nursing Convention, Atlanta, Ga., April 30, 1979.
2. HOWARD LEVENTHAL: "The Consequences of Depersonalization During Illness and Treatment: An Information-Processing Model," in JAN HOWARD AND AMSEIM STRAUSS, EDS: *Humanizing Health Care* (New York: John Wiley & Sons, 1975), pp. 119–162.
3. BONNIE WEAVER DULDT AND KIM GIFFIN: *Theoretical Perspectives of Nursing* (Boston: Little Brown & Company, expected publication date is 1984, in press). The entire theory by Duldt is presented in this publication.
4. *Ibid.*, p. 123.
5. *Ibid.*, pp. 5–41.
6. CARL R. ROGERS AND CHARLES B. TRUAX: "The Therapeutic Conditions Antecedent to Change: A Theoretical View," in GERALD EGAN: *Encounter Groups: Basic Readings* (Belmont, Calif.: Brooks/Cole Publishing Company, 1971), pp. 264–276.
7. KIM GIFFIN AND BOBBY R. PATTON: *Personal Communication in Human Relations* (Columbus, Ohio: Charles E. Merrill Publishing Company, 1974), p. 124.
8. GEORGE H. MEAD: *Mind, Self and Society* (Chicago: University of Chicago Press, 1934).
9. BOBBY R. PATTON AND KIM GIFFIN: *Interpersonal Communication in Action* (New York: Harper & Row, 1977), pp. 347–348.
10. E. T. HALL: *The Hidden Dimension* (Garden City, N. Y.: Doubleday, 1969), pp. 113–129.
11. HENRY BOSLEY WOLF, ED: *Webster's New Collegiate Dictionary* (Springfield, Mass.: G. & C. Merriam Company, 1979).
12. BONNIE WEAVER DULDT AND KIM GIFFIN: *Theoretical Perspectives of Nursing* (Boston: Little Brown & Company, in press).
13. PATRICIA CHEHY PILETTE: "The Nurse as a Humanistic Artist," in ARLYNE B. SAPERSTEIN AND MARGARET A. FRAZIER: *Introduction to Nursing Practice* (Philadelphia: F. A. Davis Company, 1980).
14. *Ibid.*, pp. 233–234.
15. ELAIN L. LAMONICA: *The Nursing Process: A Humanistic Approach* (Menlo Park, Calif.: Addison-Wesley Publishing Company, 1979).
16. *Ibid.*
17. PATRICIA ANNE RANDOLPH FLYNN: *Holistic Health: The Art and Science of Care* (Bowie, Md.: Robert J. Brady Co., 1980); PATRICIA ANNE RANDOLPH FLYNN: *The Healing Continuum: Journeys in the Philosophy of Holistic Health* (Bowie, Md.: Robert J. Brady Co., 1980).
18. BARBARA BLATTNER: *Holistic Nursing* (Englewood Cliffs, N. J.: Prentice-Hall Inc., 1981).
19. JEAN WATSON: "The Philosophy and Science of Caring: Carative Factors in Nursing," in PATRICIA ANNE RANDOLPH FLYNN, ED.: *The Healing Continuum: Journeys in the Philosophy of Holistic Health* (Bowie, Md.: Robert J. Brady Co., 1980), pp. 109–112.

20. VIRGINIA G. KING AND NORMA A. GERWIG: *Humanizing Nursing Education: A Confluent Approach Through Group Process* (Wakefield, Mass.: Nursing Resources, 1981), p. 19.
21. *Ibid.,* pp. 32–33.
22. E. LAMBERTSON: *Education for Nursing Leadership* (Philadelphia: J. B. Lippincott, 1958).
23. KING AND GERWIG: *Humanizing Nursing Education,* pp. 25–28.
24. M. J. GIUFFRA: "Humanistic Nursing in a Technological Society," *Journal of New York State Nurses' Association,* 11 (March, 1980): 17–22.
25. JOYCE TRAVELBEE: "Interpersonal Aspects of Nursing Concept: The Human Being," in PATRICIA ANNE RANDOLPH FLYNN, ED.: *The Healing Continuum: Journeys in the Philosophy of Holistic Health* (Bowie, Md.: Robert J. Brady Co., 1980), pp. 71–92.
26. SISTER CALLISTA ROY: *Introduction to a Nursing Adaptation Model* (New York: Prentice-Hall, 1976).
27. DOROTHEA E. OREM: *Nursing Concepts of Practice* (St. Louis: McGraw-Hill Co., 1971).
28. IMOGENE M. KING: *A Theory for Nursing* (New York, Wiley, 1981).
29. MARGARET NEWMAN: *Theory Development in Nursing* (Philadelphia: F. A. Davis Company, 1979).
30. H. YURA AND M. B. WALSH: *The Nursing Process: Assessing, Planning, Implementing and Evaluation,* 2nd ed. (New York: Appleton-Century-Crofts, 1973).
31. A. FAULKNER: "Aye, There's the Rub—Communication Skills," *Nursing Times,* 77 (Feb. 19, 1981): 332–336; J. HAYWOOD: *Information!, A Prescription Against Pain* (London: Royal College of Nursing, 1975); M. JOHNSON: "Communication of Patient's Feelings in Hospital," in A. E. BENNETT, ED.: *Communication Between Doctors and Patients* (New York: Oxford University Press, 1976).
32. A. FAULKNER: *Ibid.*
33. C. M. FAGIN: "Primary Care as an Academic Discipline," *Nursing Outlook,* 26 (December, 1978): 750–753.

INDEX

A "t" following a page number indicates a table. A page number in *italics* indicates a figure.

ABSTRACTNESS, word, 85–86
Abuse, verbal, 238–241
"Abused nurse syndrome," 239–241
Acceptance, judgment versus, 266
Accommodating relationship, 140
Accurate empathy, 143–144
Advances, unwanted sexual. *See* Sexual harassment
Affect, 125
Affection, 47, 126–127, 194
Affiliation, 45
Age, interview problems caused by, 250–251
Alienation, 45, 224–225
  anger and, 230
    dealing with, 230–233
  communication behaviors related to, 225–226
  communication denial and, 226–228
  "double bind" and, 228–230
Analysis
  Interaction Process, 198–199, *204*
  problem, *153*, 153–155, *155*
Anger, 45
  alienation and, 230
  dealing with, 230–233
Antagonism, 45

Anxiety, defensiveness and, 217
Appearance, physical, 37–39
Appraisal, interviews for, 246
Assessment
  of communication competencies, 196–197
  of interactions, 197–209, *198*, *204*, 205t, 206t, 207t, 208t
  of interpersonal needs, 193–196, *195*
  of leadership behavior, 209–213
Assumptions of humanistic nursing, 260–262
Attack, personal, defensiveness and, 218
Attempt to control, defensiveness and, 219
Attending, anger and, 230–231
Attention, audience, public speaking and, 175–177
Attitude, racial, 90–91
Attraction, 45
Audience, attention of, public speaking and, 175–177
Authenticity, role playing versus, 267

BALES' system of categories, 197–209, *198*, *204*, 205t, 206t, 207t, 208t

Barriers
communication, dehumanization and, 4
overcoming of, 156–157
Battered wife syndrome, 239–241
Behavior(s)
communication, alienation and, 225–226
control, 47
defensive, 218–221
dominant, relationships and, 125–126
generation of defensiveness by, 218–221
leadership, 209–213
nonverbal communication, 107–108
face and eyes in, 111–112
personal appearance as, 108–109
postures, gestures, and body language as, 112–115
touching as, 115–116
vocal tones as, 109–111
submissive, relationships and, 125–126
Body language, 99–100, 112–115
Bracket markers, 133
Business and management concepts in health-care systems, 1

CARELESSNESS, caring versus, 267–268
Caring, carelessness versus, 267–268
Categories, individuals versus, 263
Chairs, as environmental factors, 54–57
Challenging relationship, 139–140
Child, speech and, 82
Choice, directive versus, 264
Choosing, 8
Client
definition of, 7
interview of, 249–252
Closed-mindedness, 42–43
Closing, interviewing and, 249
Collaboration, conflict and, 161–162
Collection, data, problem solving and, 156
Colors, connotations of, racial attitudes and, 90–91
Communicating, 7–8
Communication
definition of, 9
group, 149
conflict management and, 159–162
decision making and, 149–159
meetings and, 162, 163
problem solving and, 149–159, 153
psychiatric teams and, 162–165

therapeutic groups and, 162–165
interpersonal, 10–11
assessing interactions in, 197–209, 198, 204, 205t, 206t, 207t, 208t
communication competencies and, 196–197
concepts of, in humanistic nursing, 262–271
interaction of, 271–272
dialogue in, 13–15
existentialism and meaning and, 12–13
facts and feelings and, 13
interpersonal needs and, 193–196, 195
leadership behavior and, 209–213
process of, 11–12
interview and, 245–246
client, 249–252
humanizing versus dehumanizing in, 257
nurse, 252–257
sequence of, 247–249
nonverbal, 99–100
behaviors and, 107–108
face and eyes in, 111–112
personal appearance as, 108–109
postures, gestures, and body language as, 112–115
touching as, 115–116
vocal tones as, 109–111
feedback and, 116
verbal/nonverbal interface and, 100–103
semiology and, 103
pragmatics and, 103–104
semantics and, 105–106
syntactics and, 104
in public
audience attention and, 175–177
body of speech and, 179–185
conclusion of speech and, 185–187
developing a speech and, 171–174
establishment of credentials for, 177–178
organization of ideas and, 175
presentation of speech and, 187–189
self-perception and, 167–171
special problems of
alienation as, 224–233
behaviors that generate defensiveness, 218–221
distrust and defensiveness as, 217–218

gaps between groups as, 221–224
sex role and, 233–234
sexual harassment and, 234–238
verbal abuse and, 238–241
verbal
language characteristics and, 82
abstractness as, 85–86
creation of "social reality" as, 90–92
incompleteness as, 87–88
reflection of personality and culture
as, 88–90
word meanings, 83–85, *84*
understanding of, 92
feedback and, 95–96
listening and, 94–95
speaking and, 92–94
Communication barriers, dehumanization and, 4
Communication competencies, 196–197
Communication denial, alienation and,
226–228
Communication skills, 196–197
Communing, interviewing and, 248
Competencies, communication, 196–197
Competition, 43–45
Compromise, conflict and, 161
Concepts, business and management, in
health care, 1
Concern, lack of, 1–2
defensiveness and, 219
Conclusion of speeches, 185–187
Conflict management, 159–162, 196–197
Conformity, 61–65
Confronting relationships, 140
Congruence among perceived data, 34–36
Connotative meaning, 83–85
Contracting, interviewing and, 247–248
Control, 194
attempt to, defensiveness and, 219
relationships and, 125–126
Control behavior, 47
Cooperativeness, 43–45
Coping, helplessness versus, 270
Cost/reward ratio of relationships, 143
Counseling, interviews for, 246
Credentials for public speaking, 177–178
Critical life situation, definition of, 9
Criticism, defensiveness and, 219
Culture(s), 68–75
gaps between, as communication prob-
lem, 223–224
interview problems caused by, 250
language as reflection of, 88–90

D-A-S-H paradigm, 126–128, *127*
Data collection, problem-solving and, 156
Decision, 158
Decision making, group, 149–159
Defensiveness, 217–218
Definitions, word, 83–85, *84*
Degradation, equality versus, 264–265
Dehumanization, 2, 3–5
Dehumanizing, interviews and, 257
Denial
communication, alienation and, 226–
228
conflict and, 161
Denotative meaning, 83, 85
Describing, anger and, 231–232
Despair, dehumanization and, 4
Development, group, 150–152
Diagram, force-field, 154, *155*
Dialogue
communication and, 13–15
monologue versus, 262–263
Differences, cultural, 68–75
Directive, choice versus, 264
Discipline
interviews for, 246
of nursing, 5–6
Disregard, positive regard versus,
265–266
Distance
intimate, 56
personal, 56
public, 56
social, 56
Distortion of message, defensiveness
and, 218
Distrust, 217–218
Dogmatism, defensiveness and, 219
Dominance, 126–127
conflict and, 161
Dominant behavior, relationships and,
125–126
Dominant-submissive relationships
degree of rigidity in, 137–138
punctuation of interaction in, 136–137
rules in, 128–135
significance of rules in, 135–136
"Double bind," alienation and, 228–230
Dreaming, 8

EDUCATING relationship, 140
Egocentric speech, 82
Emblems, nonverbal, 114–115

Emotional distress, dehumanization and, 4
Emotional tone, 125
Empathy
  accurate, 143–144
  tolerance versus, 266–267
Entertainment, as purpose of public speaking, 172
Environment
  culture as, 68–75
  definition of, 9
  organizational influence, 66–68
  physical settings, 51–52
    chairs and tables as, 54–57
    rooms and places as, 52–54
    time as, 57–59
  social factors, 59
    group membership as, 60–66
    presence of others, 59–60
Equality, degradation versus, 264–265
Equity theory, 185–186
Evaluation of problem solution, 159
Exchange, information, 196–197
Existentialism, 12–13
Exit interview, 256–257
Expendable, irreplaceable versus, 268–269
Expert witness, 254–255
Eyes, nonverbal communication behaviors and, 111–112

FACE, nonverbal communication behaviors and, 111–112
Facts, communication and, 13
Fear, 45
  defensiveness and, 217
Feedback, 116
  understanding and, 95–96
Feelings, communication and, 13
Femininity, 40
FIRO, 194–195
Focusing, interviewing and, 247
Force-field diagram, 154, 155
Forming, group development and, 150

GAMES, relationship, 140–142
Genuineness, 144–145
Gestures, 112–115
Goal commitments, 61, 65
Group communication, 149
  conflict management and, 159–162
  decision making and, 149–159
  meetings and, 162, 163
  problem solving and, 149–159, 153

psychiatric teams and, 162–165
  therapeutic groups and, 162–165
Group development, 150–152
Group membership, as environmental factor, 60–66
Group objective, 155–156
Groups
  gaps between, as communication problem, 221–224
  reference, 221–222
  therapeutic, 162–165

HARASSMENT, sexual, 234–238
Hate, 45
Health, definition of, 9
Health-care providers. See also Nurses; Nursing
  lack of concern by, 1–2
Health-care systems, business and management concepts in, 1
Helplessness, coping versus, 270
History, humanism in, 3
Holism, 263–264
Hopelessness, dehumanization and, 4
Hostility, 45, 126
  verbal abuse and, 239–240
Human being(s)
  communicators as, 15–16
  definition of, 7–9
Humanism, 2–5
Humanistic nursing communication theory, 259–260
  assumptions of, 260–262
  concepts of communication in, 262–271
    interaction of (relationship statements), 271–272
  future of, 273–274
  past of, 272–273
Humanizing, interviews and, 257

ICON, 105–106
Iconic gestures, 113–115
Ideas, organization of, public speaking and, 175
Identification of areas of mutual concern, 152–153, 153
Identifying, anger and, 232–233
Impressions of others, formation of, 34–38
Inclusion, 47, 194
Incompleteness of language, 87–88
Independence, 45–46
Index, 105–106

Indexical gestures, 114
Individuals, categories versus, 263
Inferences about others, accuracy of, 29–31
Influence of organizations, 66–68
Information
  exchange of, 196–197
  as purpose of public speaking, 172
Instructing, 196–197
Integration, conflict and, 161–162
Interaction
  assessment of, 197–209, *198, 204,* 205t, 206t, 207t, 208t
  punctuation of, 136–137
Interaction Process Analysis, 198–199, *204*
Interface, verbal/nonverbal, 100–103
Interpersonal behavior reflex, 137
Interpersonal communication. *See also* Communication
  assessing interactions in, 197–209, *198, 204,* 205t, 206t, 207t, 208t
  communication competencies and, 196–197
  concepts of, in humanistic nursing, 262–271
  interpersonal needs and, 193–196, *195*
  leadership behavior and, 209–213
Interpersonal involvement, 123–125
Interpersonal needs, 193–196, *195*
Interpersonal perception. *See* Perceptions, interpersonal
Interpersonal Perception Scale, *195,* 195–196
Interview, 245–246
  of client, 249–252
  exit, 256–257
  humanizing versus dehumanizing, 257
  of nurse, 252–257
  sequence of, 247–249
Intimacy, isolation versus, 269–270
Intimate distance, 56
Introducing, interviewing and, 247
Inventing, 8
Involvement, interpersonal, 123–125
IPA system, 198–199, *204*
Irreplaceable, expendable versus, 268–269
Isolation
  dehumanization and, 4
  intimacy versus, 269–270

JOB pressures, interview problems caused by, 250–251
Judgment
  acceptance versus, 266

defensiveness and, 219

LACK of concern
  defensiveness and, 219
  by health-care providers, 1–2
Language characteristics, 82
  abstractness as, 85–86
  creation of "social reality" as, 90–92
  reflection of personality and culture, 88–90
  word meanings as, 83–85, *84*
Language, interview problems caused by, 250
Leadership behavior, 209–213
Leadership Style Questionnaire, 211–212
  scoring sheet for, 213
Leadership Style Scoring Sheet, 213
Listening, 196–197
  understanding and, 94–95
Living, 7
Love, 45

MANAGEMENT
  concepts of, in health-care systems, 1
  conflict, 159–162, 196–197
Manipulative styles of relationships, 139–140
Markers, bracket, 133
Masculinity, 40
Meaning, 12–13
  connotative, 83–85
  denotative, 83, 85
  word, 83–85, *84*
Meetings, planning and conducting, 162, *163*
Messages
  distortion of, defensiveness and, 218
  nonverbal, 99–100
    behaviors and, 107–108
      face and eyes in, 111–112
      personal appearance as, 108–109
      postures, gestures, and body language as, 112–115
      touching as, 115–116
      vocal tones as, 109–111
    feedback and, 116
    verbal/nonverbal interface and, 100–103
    semiology and, 103
      pragmatics and, 103–104
      semantics and, 105–106
      syntactics and, 104
  verbal
    language characteristics and, 82

Messages—*continued*
    abstractness as, 85–86
    creation of "social reality" as, 90–92
    incompleteness as, 87–88
    reflection of personality and culture
      as, 88–90
    word meanings as, 83–85, *84*
    understanding of, 92
      feedback and, 95–96
      listening and, 94–95
      speaking and, 92–94
Monologue, dialogue versus, 262–263
Mourning, group development and,
    151–152

NEED(S)
    to control, defensiveness and, 219
    interpersonal, 46–47, 193–196, *195*
Negativing, 8
Negotiation, conflict and, 161
Nonpossessive warmth, 144
Nonverbal messages, 99–100
    behaviors and, 107–108
      face and eyes in, 111–112
      personal appearance as, 108–109
      postures, gestures, and body lan-
        guage as, 112–115
      touching as, 115–116
      vocal tones as, 109–111
    feedback and, 116
    verbal/nonverbal interface and, 100–103
    semiology and, 103
      pragmatics and, 103–104
      semantics and, 105–106
      syntactics and, 104
Norming, group development and, 151
Nurse
    client interview by, 249–252
    definition of, 7, *84*
    interview of, 252–257
    lack of private office for, 53
Nursing
    definition of, 6–7
    discipline of, 5–6
    humanistic, 16–18
    humanistic communication theory of,
      259–260
      assumptions of, 260–262
      concepts of communication in,
        262–271
        interaction of (relationship state-
          ments), 271–272
      future of, 273–274
      past of, 272–273

humanistic theory of, 6–10
Nursing process, definition of, 9
Nurturing relationship, 139

OBJECTIVE, group, 155–156
Open-mindedness, 42–43
Ordering, 8
Organization
    of ideas, in public speaking, 175
    influence of, 66–68
Orientations toward people, 42
    cooperative-uncooperative, 43–45
    meeting interpersonal needs, 46–47
    moving toward, away, or against, 45–46
    open-closed, 42–43

PARADIGM, D-A-S-H, 126–128, *127*
Part, whole versus, 263–264
People, orientations toward, 42
    cooperative-uncooperative, 43–45
    meeting interpersonal needs through,
      46–47
    moving toward, away, or against, 45–46
    open-closed, 42–43
Perception, interpersonal, 21–22
    accuracy of inferences and, 29–31
    estimated relationship potential and,
      38–39
    forming impressions through, 35–38
    process of, 22–24
    reciprocal perspectives and, 40–41
    sensory bases of, 24–25
      sight as, 25–26
      sound as, 26–27
      touch as, 27–29
    stereotyping and, 31–34
Perception, selective, 34–36
Performing, group development and, 151
Person perception
    accuracy of inferences and, 29–31
    forming impressions through, 35–38
    process of, 22–24
    sensory bases of, 24–25
      sight as, 25–26
      sound as, 26–27
      touch as, 27–29
    stereotyping and, 31–34
Personal attack, defensiveness and, 218
Personal attitudes, 61–62
Personal distance, 56
Personality, language as reflection of,
    88–90
Perspectives, reciprocal, 40–41
Persuasion

interviews for, 246
as purpose of public speaking, 172
Philosophy, humanism in, 2
Physical appearance, 37–39
Physical settings, 51–52
  chairs and tables as, 54–57
  rooms and places as, 52–54
  time as, 57–59
Places, as environmental factors, 52–54
Plan, implementation of, in problem solving, 158–159
Planlessness, dehumanization and, 4
Positive regard, disregard versus, 265–266
Postures, 112–115
Potential for relationship, 38–39
Power, 61–62
  conflict and, 161
  powerlessness versus, 271
  relationships and, 126
Powerlessness, power versus, 271
Pragmatics, 103–104
Prejudice, 90–91
  language as creator of, 90–91
Presence of others, as environmental factor, 59–60
Pressure, job, interview problems caused by, 250–251
Problem(s)
  analysis of, 153, 153–155, 155
  of communication
    alienation as, 224–233
    behaviors that generate defensiveness, 218–221
    distrust and defensiveness as, 217–218
    gaps between groups as, 221–224
    sex role and, 233–234
      sexual harassment and, 234–238
      verbal abuse and, 238–241
Problem solving, group, 149–159, 153
Process, communication, 11–12
Psychiatric teams, 162–165
Psychology, humanism in, 2–3
Public distance, 56
Public speaking
  audience attention and, 175–177
  body of speech and, 179–185
  conclusion of speech and, 185–187
  developing a speech and, 171–174
  establishing credentials in, 177–178
  organization of ideas and, 175
  presentation of speech and, 187–189
  self-perception and, 167–171

Punctuation of interaction, 136–137

QUESTIONNAIRE, Leadership Style, 211–212
  scoring sheet for, 213

RACIAL attitudes, 90–91
Rambling, interview problems caused by, 250
Ratio, cost/reward, of relationships, 143
Reciprocal perspectives, 40–41
Recording, interviewing and, 248
Reference groups, 221–222
Reflex, interpersonal behavior, 137
Regard, positive, disregard versus, 265–266
Rejection, sexual harassment and, 235–237
Relationship potential, estimated, 38–39
Relationships, 121–123
  accommodating, 140
  bad habits in
    games as, 140–142
    manipulative styles as, 139–140
  challenging, 139–140
  confronting, 140
  control and, 125–126
  cost/reward ratio of, 143
  D-A-S-H paradigm and, 126–128, 127
  dominant-submissive
    degree of rigidity in, 137–138
    punctuation of interaction in, 136–137
    rules in, 128–135
    significance of rules in, 135–136
  educating, 140
  emotional tone of, 125
  improvement of, 143–145
  interpersonal involvement and, 123–125
  nurturing, 139
  supporting, 139
Religion, humanism and, 3
Rerun signals, 130
Research, preparing a speech and, 173–174
Retaliation, sexual harassment and, 235–237
Rigidity, degree of, in dominant-submissive relationships, 137–138
Role(s)
  group, 65
  sex
    communication and, 233–234
    sexual harassment and, 234–238
    verbal abuse and, 238–241

Role playing, authenticity versus, 267
Rooms, as environmental factors, 52–54
Rules
  in dominant-submissive relationships,
    128–135
  significance of, 135–136

SCALE, Interpersonal Perception, 195,
    195–196
Scoring sheet, leadership style, 213
Selection, interviews for, 246
Selective perception, 34–36
Self-perception, public speaking and,
    167–171
Self-reflecting, 9
Self-sufficiency, 45–46
Semantics, 105–106
Semiology, 103
  pragmatics and, 103–104
  semantics and, 105–106
  syntactics and, 104
Separation, dehumanization and, 4
Sex role
  communication and, 233–234
  sexual harassment and, 234–238
  verbal abuse and, 238–241
Sex, touching and, 115–116
Sexism, language as creator of, 91–92
Sexual advances, unwanted. See Sexual
    harassment
Sexual harassment, 234–238
Sight, person perception and, 25–26
Signaling, 114–115
Signals, rerun, 130
Signs
  icon, 105–106
  indexical, 105–106
  science of, 103
    pragmatics and, 103–104
    semantics and, 105–106
    syntactics and, 104
  symbolic, 105–106
Size, group, 65–66
Skills, communication, 196–197
Small group communication, 196–197
"Smoothing over," conflict and, 161
Social distance, 56
Social factors, 59
  group membership as, 60–66
  presence of others as, 59–60
"Social reality," created by language,
    90–92
Social speech, 82
Solutions, problem, 157–158

Sound, person perception and, 26–27
Speaking
  public
    audience attention and, 175–177
    body of speech and, 179–185
    conclusion of speech and, 185–187
    developing a speech and, 171–174
    establishing credentials in, 177–178
    organization of ideas and, 175
    presentation of speech and, 187–189
    self-perception and, 167–171
    understanding and, 92–94
Speech
  body of, 179–185
  conclusion of, 185–187
  development of, in public speaking,
    171–174
  egocentric, in children, 82
  presentation of, 187–189
  social, in children, 82
Stereotypes, voice and, 110
Stereotyping, 31–34
Storming, group development and,
    150–151
Styles of relationships, manipulative,
    139–140
Subcultures, gaps between, as communi-
    cation problem, 223–224
Submission, 126–127
Submissive behavior, relationships and,
    125–126
Superiority, defensiveness and, 219
Supporting relationship, 139
Suppression, conflict and, 161
Suspicion, 45
Symbol, 105–106
Syndrome
  "abused nurse," 239–241
  battered wife, 239–241
Syntactics, 104
System, IPA, 198–199, 204

TABLES, as environmental factors, 54–57
Task commitments, 61, 65
Teams, psychiatric, 162–165
Testimony, court, 254–255
Theory, equity, 185–186
Theory, humanistic nursing communica-
    tion, 259–274
Therapeutic groups, 162–165
Time, as environmental factor, 57–59
Tolerance, empathy versus, 266–267
Tone(s)
  emotional, 125

vocal, 109–111
Touch, person perception and, 27–29
Touching
  as nonverbal communication behavior,
    115–116
  sex and, 115–116
Trust, 45
  interpersonal, 121

UNCERTAINTY, dehumanization and, 4
Uncooperativeness, 43–45
Understanding one another, 92
  feedback and, 95–96
  listening and, 94–95
  speaking and, 92–94
Unwanted sexual advances, 235–237

VERBAL abuse, 238–241
Verbal messages
  language characteristics and, 82
    abstractness as, 85–86
    creation of "social reality" as, 90–92

incompleteness as, 87–88
reflection of personality and culture
    as, 88–90
word meanings as, 83–85, *84*
understanding of, 92
  feedback and, 95–96
  listening and, 94–95
  speaking and, 92–94
Verbal/nonverbal interface, 100–103
Vocal tones, 109–111

WARMTH, nonpossessive, 144
Whole, part versus, 263–264
Withdrawal, 45
  conflict and, 161
Witness, expert, 254–255
Word meanings, 83–85, *84*
Words
  connotative meaning of, 83–85
  degree of abstractness of, 85–86
  denotative meaning of, 83, 85